Alison Stewart

Palliative Medicine Handbook

Third Edition

Ian N. Back MA(Cantab) MB BChir MRCGP DA
Consultant in Palliative Medicine
Holme Tower Marie Curie Centre, Penarth, Wales
Pontypridd & Rhondda NHS Trust, Wales

GW00566909

August 2001

Published by:
BPM Books
P.O. Box 5023
Cardiff
CF5 2XB
U.K.

Printed by Cambrian Printers, Aberystwyth, Ceredigion

© I.N. Back, 2001

First edition 1997
Second edition 1998
Third edition 2001

Note
The author has, as far as it is possible, taken care to ensure that the
information given in this text is accurate and up-to-date. However, readers
are strongly advised to confirm that the information, especially with regard
to drug usage, complies with the latest legislation and standards of practice.
The author does not accept responsibility or legal liability for any errors in
the text, or for the misuse or misapplication of material in this work.

Corrections and further information may be found at:
http://www.pallmed.net

ISBN 0-9542246-0-4

Contents

Preface

This is the third edition of a handbook originally written for trainee doctors working in specialist palliative care units. It is intended to be a pocket reference source, aide-memoir, and formulary, containing notes on prescribing and management guidelines for symptom control.

The main section of notes on prescribing broadly follows the familiar British National Formulary format, being divided by body system and then by symptom. Notes on general management of the symptoms are sometimes included, but the emphasis is on prescribing. It is assumed that accurate diagnosis and careful assessment of the patient precedes any prescribing. Non-pharmacological treatments (e.g. nursing care for pressure sore pain) and other psychosocial issues (e.g. addressing anxiety or depression when treating pain) are an essential part of palliative care. This does not aim to be a comprehensive textbook, and omissions of these aspects of palliative care do not mean that they should be ignored.

Although these notes on prescribing may be relevant to conditions other than cancer which are being managed in a palliative way, they have been put together with treatment of advanced malignancy as the main emphasis; thus, where it is not specifically stated it should be assumed that comments relate to cancer patients.

Many drugs are used in palliative care outside their licensed use at the doctor's discretion. Details of these, together with 'typical' doses and maximum doses are included as an aide-memoir. However, the inclusion of a drug or treatment in this handbook does not dissolve the doctor of their personal responsibility in providing treatment that they are confident with, and can justify, and that is tailored to the individual patient's circumstances. The extensive references aim to help the prescriber to know the evidence supporting its use.

Non-specialists (GPs and junior hospital doctors) quite commonly find themselves obtaining advice on symptom control from specialist palliative care nurses. This is a difficult area from the point of view of responsibility for the prescribing. The classification of unlicensed drug use *(p.xiii)* is intended to help the non-specialist prescriber in particular, to differentiate between the routine e.g. using metoclopramide for hiccups, and cases where more specialist prescribing knowledge should be sought.

Further information on most of the topics can be found in three standard textbooks on palliative care that are strongly recommended:

Twycross R, Wilcock A, Thorp S. *Palliative Care Formulary*, 1998;[1] also available on-line.[2]

Doyle D, Hanks GWC, MacDonald N, eds. *Oxford textbook of palliative medicine*. 2nd ed, 1997.[3]

Twycross R. *Symptom management in advanced cancer*. 3rd ed, 2001.[4]

The text is also extensively referenced to journal articles. Where possible, references have been included to journals likely to be held by palliative care centres e.g. *Palliative Medicine, Journal of Pain and Symptom Management,* and *European Journal of Palliative Care*.

Acknowledgements

I am grateful to the following (and many other colleagues) who have contributed to the development of this book: Anthony Byrne, Sue Closs, Alison Duncan, Ilora Finlay, Jane Fleming, Andrew Fowell, Pola Grzybowska, Melanie Jefferson, Rhian Owen, Vanessa Skingle, Helen Taylor.

Abbreviations & Symbols

AF - atrial fibrillation
AIDS - auto immune deficiency syndrome
amp. - ampoule
b.d. - twice daily
BP - blood pressure
Caps. - capsules
CCF - congestive cardiac failure
CNS - central nervous system
COPD - chronic obstructive airways disease
COX-1/COX-2 - cyclo-oxygenase 1/2
CSCI - continuous subcutaneous infusion
CT - computerised tomography
CVA - cerebrovascular accident
Disp. - dispersible (tablets)
DVT - deep vein thrombosis
EAPC - European Association of Palliative Medicine
ECG - electrocardiogram
EPSE - Extrapyramidal side-effects
FBC - full blood count
FFP - fresh frozen plasma
g - gram
GERD - gastro-oesophageal reflux disease
GI - gastrointestinal
h - hour
HRT - hormone replacement therapy
ICP - intracranial pressure
IM - intramuscular
Inj. - injection
INR - international normalised ratio
IV - intravenous
IVI - intravenous infusion
IVP - intravenous pyelography
JVP - jugular venous pressure
L - litre
LFT - liver function tests
LVF - left ventricular failure
MAOI - monoamine oxidase inhibitor
µg - microgram
mL - millilitre
mmol - millimole
MND - motor neurone disease (AML)
MRI - magnetic resonance imaging
MS - multiple sclerosis
neb. - nebuliser
NG - nasogastric
nocte - at night
NSAID - non-steroidal anti-inflammatory drug

o.d. - daily
OTFC - oral transmucosal fentanyl citrate
PE - pulmonary embolism
PEG - percutaneous endoscopic gastrostomy
PO - by mouth
PPI - proton pump inhibitor
PR - rectal
PRN - as required
PV - per vagina
q.d.s. - four times a day
RBL - renal-bone-liver includes U&E LFT and serum calcium
RT - radiotherapy
SC - subcutaneous
sol. - soluble
SR - slow (or modified) release
SSRI - selective serotonin reuptake inhibitor
stat. - immediately
Supps. - suppositories
Susp. - suspension
SVC - superior vena cava
SVCO - superior vena caval obstruction
Tabs. - tablets
t.d.s. - three times a day
TENS - transcutaneous electrical nerve stimulator
TIA - transient ischaemic attack
TSD - typical starting dose
u - units
U&E - urea & electrolytes
UTI - urinary tract infection
VTE - venous thromboembolism

⇨ - Refers to other relevant sections of the handbook
⬚ - References to further reading
‡ - Drug preparation needing special arrangements for prescribing
☑ - Suggested first choice of drug within group e.g. PPI or NSAID
☼ - Off-label prescribing (see below)
⃠ - Non-Formulary drug or preparation
   (Non-Formulary refers to the Bro Taf Formulary, currently under
   development in South Wales - *http://www.bro-taf-ha.wales.nhs.uk* -
   follow links to District Medical Committee → Drug & Therapeutics
   Committee → Hospital Formulary)

£ - Costs, where given, are for 28 days at the Typical Starting Dose quoted,
based on BNF Vol. 41 March 2001.

☼ Off-label prescribing, and suggested guidance on prescribing

	Unrestricted	Specialist	Consultant
Licensed	(not marked)	oo	ooo
Licence partially / unclear	⊙	⊙⊙	⊙⊙⊙
Not licensed	●	●●	●●●

Off-label drug use

Off-label prescribing is a term used to include:

- Unlicensed drugs - manufactured by a licensed manufacturer, but may be awaiting a UK licence, withdrawn from the market etc. Usually available on a 'named patient basis'. Also indicated in the text as †
- 'Specials' - prepared by a manufacturer with a Specials Manufacturing Licence. Also indicated as †
- Prescribing a licensed drug outside its product licence, whether by altering its formulation, indication, dose or route.

Off-label prescribing is the responsibility of the individual prescribing physician. The practice is common in palliative care.[5,6]

Off-label use is indicated with the symbol ● whilst use that is partially covered by license or is questionable is indicated with the symbol ◉. Examples of a 'partly licensed' drug use would be carbamazepine for neuropathic pain, where the licence only covers trigeminal neuralgia.

Off-label drug use is not marked in this book when use is outside the product licence only by way of using the sc route as an alternative to im or iv use.
For further details on the subcutaneous route for injections ⇨ *p.178*.
For combinations of drugs mixed for subcutaneous infusion ⇨ *p.173*.

Guidance on prescribing

Guidance on prescribing has been indicated throughout the book. Although this is mainly for off-label drug prescribing, it occasionally relates to licensed use also. The categories are suggestions only, taking note of whether a drug is mentioned in the BNF, standard textbooks in palliative medicine, or national guidelines; also the level of supporting evidence (from case reports to systematic reviews), potential adverse reactions, and cost implications.

- **Unrestricted** (1 symbol) - unlicensed ● or partly licensed ◉ drug use, but which is considered already to be part of general prescribing practice, or which can safely be so; drugs which the generalist doctor should be familiar with; no special precautions needed; e.g. amitriptyline for neuropathic pain, metoclopramide for hiccups. As the drug is being prescribed off-label, consider warning the patient that the drug information that is provided from pharmacy with the drug, may be misleading or inappropriate in the circumstances you have prescribed it. No additional steps need be taken to obtain consent when prescribing.
- **Specialist** (2 symbols) - unlicensed ●●, partly licensed ◉◉, or licensed ◎◎ drug use, where additional knowledge should inform prescribing; drugs which the generalist doctor may not be familiar with, or where special precautions may be relevant to the unlicensed indication; e.g. stanozolol for pruritus in cholestatic jaundice. If prescribing off-label, consider discussing with the patient the use of a drug outside its product licence, and whether it is appropriate to obtain specific consent.
- **Consultant-level** (3 symbols) - unlicensed ●●●, partly licensed ◉◉◉, or licensed ◎◎◎ drug use, where advanced specialist knowledge (at a level one would expect in a consultant in palliative medicine) should inform prescribing; evidence for its use may be very weak; significant risks, side-effects, interactions or cost implications may exist; e.g. methadone for neuropathic pain, erythropoietin for anaemia. If prescribing off-label, consider discussing with the patient the use of a drug outside its product licence, and whether it is appropriate to obtain specific consent.

NOTES ON PRESCRIBING

GASTROINTESTINAL

Dyspepsia

Gastro-oesophageal reflux / Oesophagitis
Assessment
- Exclude or treat oesophageal candida. *(p.44)*
- Consider oesophageal spasm. *(p.49)*
- Review drugs which cause oesophagitis - potassium, NSAIDs, antimuscarinics.
- Consider pain of cardiac origin.

Treatment
1) Raise head of bed to reduce acid reflux.
2) Consider paracentesis for tense ascites.
3) Metoclopramide 10mg t.d.s. if signs of gastric stasis or distension.
4) Antacid e.g. *Gaviscon* 10mL q.d.s. for mild symptoms.
5) Proton pump inhibitor PPI e.g. lansoprazole 30mg daily for moderate or severe symptoms; start with treatment dose then step-down after a few weeks.[7]

Prophylactic use of a PPI is indicated for a stent or Celestin/Atkinson tube that bypasses the gastro-oesophageal junction.

NSAID- and steroid-related dyspepsia
Treatment of dyspepsia
1) Consider stopping or reducing dose of NSAID/steroids.
2) PPI e.g. lansoprazole 30mg o.d. for severe symptoms or proven pathology, start with treatment dose then reduce dose after four weeks; milder symptoms start with maintenance dose and increase later if needed.[7]
3) If symptoms persist on treatment dose of PPI, consider changing to a selective COX-2 inhibitor.

Indications for prophylaxis
- prescribing NSAID with recent history of dyspepsia or ulcer
- prescribing steroids with recent history of dyspepsia or ulcer
- co-prescribing NSAID with steroids, anticoagulants, or aspirin
- prescribing NSAID in elderly patient > 70 years (less clear - use judgement)

Prophylaxis
- PPI at maintenance dose[7] e.g. lansoprazole 15mg daily

(NSAID with misoprostol is as effective. Requires fewer tablets per day. Risk of diarrhoea, which may be less of a concern in some palliative care patients.)

ThinkList

- metoclopramide ⊛ for non-ulcer dyspepsia in cancer[8,9]
- very high risk patients - in palliative care it is sometimes appropriate for a patient to continue on an NSAID despite symptoms or very high risk of GI toxicity; misoprostol and PPIs afford protection by different mechanisms and may work synergistically - no trials have been done
- oral lidocaine ●●● - 30mL antacid and 15mL 2% viscous lidocaine for oesophagitis[10]

SEE ALSO
⇨ *NSAIDs & COX inhibitors (p.61), Haematemesis (p.39)*
📖 NICE Guidelines[7]

Drugs for Dyspepsia
PROTON PUMP INHIBITORS (PPIs)
There is little difference between the PPIs available.[7] Pantoprazole may have least drug-drug interactions, but this may not be clinically significant.[11,12] A single daily dose is appropriate for the **PPIs**, rather than divided doses. Lansoprazole and omeprazole can be taken before or after food with equal efficacy.[13,14]
Despite the variations in dose recommendations in the product literature, omeprazole, lansoprazole and pantoprazole display similar dose-response relationships with similar potency at the same milligram doses. Daily doses of 15-20mg **PPI** are appropriate for maintenance therapy, prophylaxis, or less severe **GERD**; doses of 30-40mg daily are appropriate for treatment.[15,16] Too little information is available yet to include rabeprazole, which may be more potent.

LANSOPRAZOLE ☑
Caps. 15mg, 30mg; Susp. 30mg sachets
TSD: Prophylaxis & maintenance - 15mg daily PO (£12.98), treatment - 30mg daily (£23.75; Susp. £34.14)

OMEPRAZOLE
Caps. 10mg, 20mg, 40mg; Disp. tabs. *(MUPS)* 10mg, 20mg, 40mg
TSD: Prophylaxis & maintenance - 20mg daily PO (£28.56), treatment - 40mg daily (£57.12)
Inj. 40mg amp ☑
Increases phenytoin blood levels (risk of toxicity), blood diazepam levels (increase sedation), and enhances anticoagulation effect of warfarin

PANTOPRAZOLE ◎
Tabs. 20mg, 40mg; Inj. 40mg amp
TSD: Prophylaxis & maintenance - 20mg daily PO (£12.88), treatment - 40mg daily (£23.65)

RABEPRAZOLE ◎
Tabs. 10mg, 20mg
TSD: Prophylaxis & maintenance - 10mg daily PO (£12.43), treatment - 20mg daily (£22.75)

ANTACIDS
Aluminium-containing antacids cause constipation; magnesium-containing antacids are laxative. Dimeticone in *Asilone* is a defoamer, useful for gastric distension/hiccups. Oxethazaine in *Mucaine* has local anaesthetic properties; said to be helpful for oesophagitis, but evidence is poor.[17] It is also used gargled, for a sore mouth e.g. mucositis.

GAVISCON ☑
Tabs. (Na. alginate 250mg, Na. bicarbonate 134mg, Ca. carbonate 80mg) Peppermint or lemon flavour
Liquid (Alginic acid, Al. hydroxide, Mg. Trisilicate, Na. bicarbonate) Peppermint or aniseed flavour
TSD: 2 tabs. q.d.s. PO (£8.40); 10mL q.d.s. PO (£6.05)

ASILONE ◎
Susp. (Al. hydroxide 420mg, dimeticone 135mg, Mg. oxide/5mL)
TSD: 10mL q.d.s. PO (£4.37)

MUCAINE
Susp. (Al. Hydroxide, Mg. Hydroxide, Oxethazaine)
TSD: 10mL q.d.s. PO (£4.26)

PROSTAGLANDIN ANALOGUES

Misoprostol is effective at preventing **NSAID**-induced ulcers, but is less well tolerated than **PPIs**, and diarrhoea is a common side-effect; in some palliative care patients this may be an advantage. Misoprostol is available in combination with diclofenac ⇨ *NSAIDs (p.61)*

MISOPROSTOL

Tabs. 200µg

TSD: Prophylaxis & maintenance - 200µg b.d. (£10.40), treatment - 400µg b.d. PO (£20.80)

H2 ANTAGONISTS

H2 antagonists are less effective at acid suppression than **PPIs**, and are less effective clinically at healing ulcers. Ranitidine has significantly fewer drug interactions and adverse affects than cimetidine.

RANITIDINE

Tabs. 150mg, 300mg; Tabs. sol. 150mg, 300mg; Syrup 75mg/5mL

TSD: Prophylaxis & maintenance - 150mg nocte PO (£8.06), treatment - 300mg daily (£15.82)

Additional Information

Corticosteroids alone have not been proven to cause an increased risk of gastric ulcer, but when prescribed together with an **NSAID**, significantly increase the risk of **NSAID**-induced ulcer.[18]

Risk of **NSAID**-induced ulceration is increased by: history of peptic ulcer disease, advanced age, high doses, co-administration of aspirin or corticosteroids. With the possible exception of age, patients with any of these risk factors should receive prophylaxis with a **PPI** when prescribed an **NSAID**.[19]

Risk factors which increase the incidence of peptic ulceration in patients prescribed corticosteroids include: total dose of corticosteroid, previous history of peptic ulceration, advanced malignant disease and concurrent prescribing of **NSAIDs**. It is suggested that prophylaxis should be considered for those patients with two or more risk factors.[20]

SSRIs may increase the risk of **GI** bleeding, especially in patients taking **NSAIDs**.[21-25]

Nausea & Vomiting

Management of Nausea & Vomiting

1) Identify any causes of nausea and vomiting that can best be treated specifically e.g.
   - constipation - remember to do a rectal examination
   - gastritis - epigastric discomfort & tenderness
   - raised intracranial pressure - neurological signs
   - oropharyngeal candida - typical white plaques seen
   - hypercalcaemia - dehydration, confusion
   - drug induced - recent introduction of morphine?
   - intestinal obstruction *(p.25)*

2) Choose an antiemetic based on the most likely cause of nausea and vomiting (see below):
   - drug or metabolic → haloperidol
   - gastric stasis → metoclopramide
   - GI tract involvement or cerebral tumour → cyclizine

3) If first choice drug unsuccessful or only partially successful after 24h, increase dose or use different antiemetic(s)
   - nausea & vomiting in cancer is often multifactorial
   - if confident of diagnosis of a single cause, consider increasing the dose of antiemetic (especially metoclopramide), or changing to a second-line specific antiemetic (e.g. ondansetron for drug-induced nausea)
   - if not confident of cause, empirically try one of the other first-line antiemetics (metoclopramide, haloperidol, cyclizine)
   - combinations of antiemetics with different actions (e.g. at different receptor sites) are often needed and can act additively
   - if using more than one antiemetic, one from each class of antiemetics should be used
   - cyclizine and haloperidol is a logical combination that is often effective
   - levomepromazine (methotrimeprazine) acts at several receptor sites, and alone may replace a previously unsuccessful combination
   - levomepromazine may be useful as a non-specific second-line antiemetic for nausea & vomiting of any or unknown aetiology[26-29]
   - cyclizine may antagonise the prokinetic effects of metoclopramide, and they should not usually be mixed

General points

- Always give antiemetics regularly - not PRN.
- If vomiting is preventing drug absorption, use an alternative route e.g. CSCI.
- Dexamethasone 4mg daily often contributes an antiemetic effect of unknown mechanism.
- Check blood urea and electrolytes, liver function tests and calcium:
  - renal failure - consider lowering the dose of opioids
  - hypercalcaemia - can be easily treated with intravenous bisphosphonates
- Monitor carefully if giving prokinetic drugs (e.g. metoclopramide) in intestinal obstruction in case they increase vomiting.
- Always reassess the patient regularly as the cause of nausea and vomiting can change with time.

Antiemetic Ladder

	2nd line narrow spectrum	e.g. ondansetron
	OR combination	e.g. cyclizine + haloperidol
	OR broad spectrum	e.g. levomepromazine
	Step 2	

Selected narrow spectrum antiemetic
- metoclopramide
- cyclizine
- haloperidol

Step 1

± administer by CSCI
± dexamethasone
- for intestinal obstruction -
± prokinetic drugs (cisapride) or antiperistaltic drugs (*Buscopan*)
± antisecretory drugs (*Buscopan* or octreotide)

First-line antiemetics	Second-line
Metoclopramide	Levomepromazine
Haloperidol	Dexamethasone
Cyclizine	Hyoscine hydrobromide
	5-HT₃ antagonists
	Corticosteroids

Specific Causes of Nausea & Vomiting

First and second-line antiemetics are given where theory or experience suggests they have a specific place for this type of vomiting. Levomepromazine is often used as a second-line antiemetic in any of these situations.

Drugs, metabolic, toxins

Causes	Drugs - opioids, anticonvulsants, chemotherapy. Metabolic - hypercalcaemia, renal failure, liver failure. Tumour toxins
Clinical notes	Nausea and retching more prominent than vomiting. Nausea usually persistent and not relieved by vomiting. Renal failure causes opioids to accumulate; both can cause nausea and vomiting.
Antiemetic	Haloperidol Metoclopramide 5-HT₃ antagonist e.g. ondansetron
Other considerations	Corticosteroids Review opioid use in renal failure. Check serum Ca⁺⁺, LFT, U&E Hypercalcaemia may be treated easily and effectively.

Opioid-induced nausea & vomiting

Opioids can cause nausea and vomiting through a number of different possible mechanisms: stimulation of chemoreceptor trigger zone (as above), increased vestibular sensitivity, gastric stasis, or impaired intestinal motility and constipation.

Haloperidol is usually recommended as first-line for opioid-induced nausea and vomiting, however metoclopramide (for gastric stasis), cyclizine or hyoscine hydrobromide[30] may all be effective in certain patients. 5-HT₃ antagonists have also been shown to be useful,[31-34] but are expensive for long term use.

Gastric motility disorders

Causes	Hepatomegaly Ascites Upper abdominal tumour Linitis plastica Upper GI surgery Carcinoma of pancreas Antimuscarinic drugs
Clinical notes	Post-prandial bloating, epigastric fullness, discomfort. Flatulence, hiccough or heartburn. Post-prandial vomiting of undigested food. Pancreatic tumours can cause a functional as well as a pathological gastric outlet obstruction.
Antiemetic	Metoclopramide 40-80mg/24h Add haloperidol 2.5-5mg/24h
Other considerations	Physical obstruction may be present (↪ p.25). Give by CSCI - stasis may reduce absorption. Antiflatulent (Asilone) or antacid. Ascites - paracentesis/diuretics. Hepatomegaly - steroids. Dietary advice. Erythromycin[35-48] acts as a pro-motility agent: 250mg t.d.s. as suspension[49] PO or 250-500mg/day IV

Gastritis

Causes	NSAIDs (may be exacerbated by steroids); Antibiotics
Clinical notes	Epigastric discomfort; Often post-prandial vomiting; Usually resistant to antiemetics
Antiemetic	Metoclopramide may help, but aim to treat gastritis specifically
Other considerations	PPI e.g. Lansoprazole (↪ Dyspepsia p.16) Antacid Stop the offending drug

Vomiting centre directly stimulated

Causes	Raised intracranial pressure from cerebral tumour. Direct involvement of vomiting centre or VIIIth nerve. Cranial radiotherapy
Clinical notes	Neurological signs e.g. Papilloedema. Often associated with headaches or drowsiness. Vertigo may be present.
Antiemetic	Cyclizine Hyoscine hydrobromide
Other considerations	Corticosteroids Radiotherapy

Pharyngeal stimulation

Causes	Sputum Candida infection
Clinical notes	Vagal stimulation results from thick sputum in the throat
Antiemetic	Cyclizine Hyoscine hydrobromide
Other considerations	Saline nebulisers or antibiotics. Treat candida

Intestinal Obstruction

Causes	Tumour
	Adhesions
	Faecal impaction (pseudo-obstruction)
Clinical notes	Pattern of vomiting from several times daily to once every few days.
	Vomiting often relieves nausea.
	Large volume vomits.
	Faeculent vomiting.
	Colic may be present.
	History of bowels not open.
Antiemetic & Other considerations	⇨ p.25

Psychological and Emotional

Causes	Pain
	Fear and anger
	Anxiety & depression
Clinical notes	Distress often exacerbates symptoms; vomiting is rarely purely psychogenic.
Antiemetic	Levomepromazine (methotrimeprazine)
Other considerations	Counselling & reassurance
	Ensure good pain control
	Diazepam/midazolam
	Antidepressant

PRESCRIBING STATUS

- ☼ Levomepromazine ⊛
- ☼ Corticosteroids ●
- ☼ 5-HT₃ antagonists ⊛⊛
- ☼ Erythromycin ●●

ThinkList

- acupuncture & acupressure at P6 - good evidence of efficacy in chemotherapy, pregnancy and post-operatively, and motion sickness;[50-53] effective in morphine-induced emesis in ferrets;[54] only one small study in terminally ill (6 patients) was ineffective[55,56]
- gastroenterostomy with jejunal feeding for gastric stasis in pancreatic cancer[57]
- olanzapine and other atypical antipsychotics ●●● have pharmacological actions that would suggest they may be useful antiemetics; olanzapine[58,59] has a similar profile to levomepromazine, whilst risperidone has potent dopamine D_2 and 5-HT₂ activity[2,58,59]
- cannabinoids ●●● are antiemetic, but probably little to offer over current antiemetics[60-63] - (⇨ p.180)
- nifedipine ●● for motion sickness[64]

SEE ALSO

⇨ *Intestinal obstruction (p.25)*
📖 Reviews[65-67] & Guidelines[68,69]

Antiemetic Drugs

ANTIHISTAMINES

The central *vomiting centre* is rich in histamine and acetylcholine receptors. Most antihistamine drugs are also antimuscarinics.

Cyclizine is a commonly used antihistamine antiemetic. Acting at the vomiting centre, it is useful for vomiting of many causes (although antipsychotics have a more specific action at the CTZ). Dose: 25-50mg t.d.s. orally or 100-200mg/24h CSCI. Side effects: antimuscarinic effects like dry mouth and drowsiness often abate after a few days.

CYCLIZINE ☑

Tabs. 50mg; Inj. 50mg/1mL
TSD: 50mg t.d.s. PO; 150mg/24h CSCI

ANTIMUSCARINICS

Hyoscine hydrobromide is a potent anti-muscarinic. It is especially useful if there is intestinal obstruction or colic as it reduces peristalsis. Side effects of dry mouth, drowsiness or confusion may be more severe than with cyclizine. It is available as buccal tablets *(Kwells)*, transdermal patch[70,71] *(Scopoderm TTS)*, and can be used by CSCI. 200-800μg/24h CSCI.

HYOSCINE HYDROBROMIDE (SCOPOLAMINE HYDROBROMIDE)

Tabs. 300μg; Patch *(Scopoderm TTS)* 1mg/72h; Inj. 400μg/1mL, 600μg/1mL
TSD: 300μg q.d.s. PO; 1 patch every 3 days; 400μg/24h CSCI

ANTIPSYCHOTICS

Drugs and metabolic disturbances cause vomiting by stimulating the chemoreceptor trigger zone (CTZ). Antipsychotics (as potent dopamine antagonists) block this pathway and are very effective against drug or metabolic induced nausea and vomiting (e.g. opioids and renal failure).

Haloperidol is a good standard drug. Dose: 1.5mg nocte orally (0.5-1.5mg b.d.) or 2.5-5mg/24h CSCI.

Side effects: sedation and extrapyramidal effects are rare at these low doses. Prochlorperazine[72] is relatively more sedative but is available in buccal *(Buccastem)* and suppository form.

Levomepromazine (methotrimeprazine) is sedative, but low doses can be effective as antiemetic. Some patients show a narrow therapeutic window. It may be considered a 'broad-spectrum' antiemetic, as it also has antimuscarinic, antihistamine and 5-HT$_2$ antagonist effects, and an anxiolytic effect. Dose ranges: 6mg - 25mg nocte or b.d. orally or 6.25-25mg/24h CSCI.

Phenothiazines and haloperidol used concomitantly with amiodarone increase the risk of ventricular arrhythmias and the advice is to avoid use. The low doses of haloperidol (antiemetic) used in palliative care probably carry a low risk.

HALOPERIDOL ☑

Tabs. 1.5mg, 5mg; Caps. 0.5mg; Liquid 2mg/mL; Inj. 5mg/1mL
TSD: 1.5mg nocte PO; 2.5mg/24h CSCI

Indometacin given with haloperidol can cause severe drowsiness.

LEVOMEPROMAZINE (METHOTRIMEPRAZINE)

Tabs. 6mg[‡◯] 25mg; Susp. 25mg/5mL[‡◯]; Inj. 25mg/1mL *(Nozinan)*
TSD: 12.5mg nocte or b.d. PO; 12.5mg/24h CSCI

6mg tablets are available on named patient basis from Link Pharmaceuticals *(Levinan)*

Suspension available from Rhone-Poulenc Rorer (Canada); contact Idis World Medicines Ltd, Kingston-upon-Thames, Surrey[29]

Oral bioavailability of levomepromazine is approx. 40%.[1] Use half the daily oral dose by CSCI.

Avoid concurrent use with MAOIs (p.211)

PROCHLORPERAZINE

Buccal tabs. 3mg *(Buccastem)*; Supps. 5mg, 25mg *(Stemetil)*
TSD: 1 tab. t.d.s. PO; 5mg t.d.s. or 25mg PRN PR

PROKINETIC DRUGS / DRUGS ALTERING GASTRIC MOTILITY

Metoclopramide acts peripherally on the gut restoring normal gastric emptying. It also acts at the CTZ and thus helps drug-induced nausea. Dose: 10mg t.d.s. - 20mg q.d.s. PO; 30-80mg/24h CSCI. Side effects: extra-pyramidal effects are rare, but most common in young female patients.

Domperidone is very similar to metoclopramide but is less likely to cause extrapyramidal effects, and is available as suppositories.

METOCLOPRAMIDE ☑

   Tabs. 10mg; Syrup 5mg/5mL; Tabs. SR 15mg *(Gastrobid)*◊   Inj. 10mg/2mL
   TSD: 10mg q.d.s. PO; 15mg SR b.d. PO; 40mg/24h CSCI

DOMPERIDONE

   Tabs. 10mg; Susp. 5mg/5mL; Supps. 30mg *(Motilium)*
   TSD: 10mg t.d.s. PO; 30mg t.d.s. PR

5-HT$_3$ ANTAGONISTS

5-HT$_3$ receptors are found in the chemoreceptor trigger zone. They are very effective against acute-phase chemotherapy- and radiotherapy-induced[73] nausea with little to choose between ondansetron and granisetron,[74] but their place in other situations (e.g. intestinal obstruction) is as yet uncertain.

Ondansetron has been shown to be ineffective in motion sickness,[75] but effective at treating morphine-induced nausea & vomiting.[31-34] 5-HT$_3$ antagonists may work synergistically with haloperidol in some cases.[76,77]

Tropisetron[78] is a mixed 5-HT$_3$ and 5-HT$_4$ antagonist,[79] but the clinical implications of this are uncertain, and clinically appears to be very similar to the others.[80]

Ondansetron[81] is well absorbed by sublingual, SC, and rectal routes.[82]

5-HT$_3$ antagonists are licensed for chemotherapy-induced and post-operative emesis.

ONDANSETRON ☑

   Tabs. 4mg, 8mg; Syrup 4mg/5mL; Melts 4mg◊ 8mg◊ ; Supps. 16mg
   TSD: 8mg b.d. PO (£433.22)
   Inj. 4mg/2mL, 8mg/4mL◊
   TSD: 16mg/24h CSCI (£721.84)

GRANISETRON ◊

   Tabs. 1mg, 2mg; Inj. 1mg/1mL, 3mg/3mL
   TSD: 1mg b.d. PO or 2mg o.d. (£512.00)

TROPISETRON ◊

   Caps. 5mg; Inj. 2mg/2mL, 5mg/5mL
   TSD: 5mg o.d. PO (£301.62) or 5mg/24h CSCI (£340.48)

OTHER DRUGS

Corticosteroids *(p.126)* often have a non-specific benefit in reducing nausea and vomiting.

Additional Information

A Cochrane review is in preparation on acupuncture and chemotherapy-induced nausea and vomiting.

Newer atypical antipsychotics may be expected to show antiemetic effects. Olanzapine has a similar pharmacological profile to levomepromazine[83] and there is weak anecdotal evidence that it may be an effective antiemetic;[58,59] risperidone has potent 5-HT$_2$ antagonist effects as well as being antidopaminergic[84] but there is no published evidence to date of any antiemetic effect.

Gastric pacing is a novel treatment described for gastroparesis.[85,86]

Intestinal obstruction

Intestinal obstruction is not uncommonly partial or subacute in palliative care, often precipitated by constipation. Careful use of stimulant laxatives, and rectal measures may resolve the obstruction. Severe constipation with faecal impaction may mimic obstruction.

Clinical notes
- pattern of vomiting from several times daily to once every few days
- vomiting often relieves nausea
- large volume vomits
- faeculent vomiting
- colic may be present
- history of bowels not open

Drug management
The optimum treatment for intestinal obstruction is surgery, however this is often inappropriate in advanced cancer.

1) Relieve nausea and reduce vomiting as much as possible:
    - metoclopramide - may increase colic or vomiting in complete obstruction, but may resolve partial upper GI tract obstruction;[87] metoclopramide 80-160mg/24h CSCI should be tried initially, provided colic is not present
    - cyclizine 150mg + haloperidol 2.5mg/24h CSCI
    - if nausea persists replace with levomepromazine (methotrimeprazine) 12.5-25mg/24h CSCI
    - haloperidol 2.5-5mg/24h can be added to levomepromazine for persistent nausea
2) Ensure constant pain is adequately relieved with diamorphine as required.
3) Stop any stimulant laxatives.
4) Prescribe docusate 200mg t.d.s. (capsules, not liquid) if obstruction may be partial.
5) Dexamethasone 8mg daily SC (or CSCI) 5-day initial trial (stop if obstruction does not resolve) should be started for:
    - high-level GI obstruction e.g. gastric outlet
    - lymphoma (tumour response to steroid)
6) Dexamethasone 8mg daily SC (or CSCI) 5-day initial trial may also be tried for large intestinal obstruction that continues unresolved, and no contraindications to steroids exist.
7) Colic may be helped by hyoscine butylbromide *(Buscopan)* 20mg SC stat and 80-160mg/24 CSCI:
    - if unsuccessful, glycopyrronium 400µg/24h CSCI if sedation important to avoid,[88] or
    - hyoscine hydrobromide 800µg/24h CSCI: also antiemetic, so can replace cyclizine
8) If vomiting remains frequent, start octreotide 250µg/24h CSCI to reduce volume and frequency of vomits to once or twice daily;[89-93]
    - increase dose every 1-2 days as below

PRESCRIBING STATUS
- Corticosteroids •
- Hyoscine butylbromide *(Buscopan)* - to ↓ volume of vomiting ••
- Octreotide ••

Think List

- nasogastric tube to reduce vomiting - should usually only be considered a temporary procedure
- stenting gastric outlet, duodenum or proximal small bowel for physical obstruction[94-103]
- percutaneous venting gastrostomy[104,105]
- stenting colonic or rectal obstruction[106-113]
- palliative chemotherapy[114]

SEE ALSO

⇨ *Nausea and vomiting (p.19), Colic (p.27)*

📖 EAPC Guidelines[115] & Reviews[116-120]

Drugs used in intestinal obstruction

OCTREOTIDE
Inj. 50µg/1mL, 100µg/1mL, 500µg/1mL, 1mg/5mL
  TSD: 250µg/24h CSCI (£386.96). Max. 1000µg/24h
Increase dose by 250µg increments every 1-2 days if no response, to 750µg/24h. If still no response, then discontinue. Tolerance may develop; consider increasing dose if response seems to reduce over a week or two. Long acting depot injections of somatostatin analogues are available, but 2 weeks are needed to achieve plasma levels[121]

HYOSCINE BUTYLBROMIDE (SCOPOLAMINE BUTYLBROMIDE)
Inj. 20mg/1mL *(Buscopan)*
  TSD: 80mg/24h CSCI (£22.40)

GLYCOPYRRONIUM BROMIDE (GLYCOPYRROLATE)
Inj. 200µg/1mL, 600µg/3mL
  TSD: 400µg/24h CSCI (£33.60)

HYOSCINE HYDROBROMIDE (SCOPOLAMINE HYDROBROMIDE)
Inj. 400µg/1mL, 600µg/1mL
  TSD: 800µg/24h CSCI (£151.76)

Additional Information

Corticosteroids

Corticosteroids have been used to try and resolve intestinal obstruction. Despite large trials, results are inconclusive, although the trend is towards helping resolution, and with little evidence of adverse effects.[122-124]

Anti-secretory drugs

Hyoscine butylbromide has been reported to reduce GI tract secretions in intestinal obstruction as well as helping colic,[125] and is cheaper than octreotide. However, studies suggest octreotide is more effective.[89,90] Both drugs have been used together.[126]

Bezoars

Bezoars[127-130] are large conglomerates or concretions of various substances in the stomach, small intestine, or rarely oesophagus, which can present with obstruction. Pharmacobezoars are bezoars comprised of medications. Contributory factors include: casein-containing enteral feeding formulas, decreased oesophageal pH, presence of a prosthetic device (NG tube, stent), functional oesophageal spasm, regurgitation of stomach contents, gastric paresis, antacids, altered motility or anatomy of the gastrointestinal tract, dehydration, concomitant use of antimuscarinics and opioids. Sucralfate has been associated with bezoar formation, as well as: aluminium hydroxide gel, enteric-coated aspirin, guar gum, colestyramine and nifedipine XL.

Intestinal colic

Management
- Stop stimulant laxatives.
- Immediate treatment:
    - hyoscine butylbromide *(Buscopan)* 20mg stat. sc☑ or
    - glycopyrronium 0.1-0.2mg stat. sc
- Continuing treatment:
    - glycopyrronium 0.2-0.6mg/24h csci☑ or
    - hyoscine butylbromide *(Buscopan)* 40-160mg/24h csci, or
    - propantheline 15mg t.d.s. po
- Mebeverine or peppermint have direct muscle relaxant effect on smooth muscle of bowel - generally milder effects than the antimuscarinics.

PRESCRIBING STATUS
☼ Glycopyrronium ●

ThinkList
- many other drugs have antimuscarinic action, which may add to, or overlap with, the effect of these drugs:
    - antimuscarinics e.g. hyoscine hydrobromide
    - tricyclic antidepressants (e.g. amitriptyline)
    - phenothiazine antipsychotics
- *Entonox* (nitrous oxide) - NB cautions *(p.86)*

SEE ALSO
⇨ *Intestinal obstruction (p.25)*

Drugs used for Intestinal colic
Hyoscine butylbromide *(Buscopan)* po is poorly and variably absorbed and is not recommended.

GLYCOPYRRONIUM BROMIDE (GLYCOPYRROLATE)
Inj. 200µg/1mL, 600µg/3mL
TSD: 400µg/24h csci for colic

HYOSCINE BUTYLBROMIDE (SCOPOLAMINE BUTYLBROMIDE)
Inj. 20mg/1mL; Tabs. 10mg *(Buscopan)*
TSD: 80mg/24h csci; 10mg q.d.s. po

PROPANTHELINE
Tabs. 15mg
TSD: 15mg t.d.s. po

MEBEVERINE
Tabs. 135mg *(Colofac)*
TSD: 1 tabs. t.d.s. po

PEPPERMINT WATER
Solution
TSD: 10mL t.d.s. po

Additional Information
Glycopyrronium (Glycopyrrolate)
Glycopyrronium is an antimuscarinic drug with actions similar to hyoscine hydrobromide:
- onset of action is approximately 30 minutes
- effects last approximately 6-8h after a single injection
- unlike hyoscine hydrobromide, it does not cross the blood-brain barrier, and is thus devoid of the central effects of hyoscine i.e. sedation,

paradoxical agitation, and anti-emetic activity
- can be given by SC injection or CSCI
- it has been mixed in syringe drivers with diamorphine, haloperidol, cyclizine, levomepromazine (methotrimeprazine), and midazolam; mixing with dexamethasone should be avoided[131]
- approximately twice as potent as hyoscine in single doses i.e. 1 ampoule of glycopyrronium (200μg) is roughly equivalent to 1 ampoule of hyoscine hydrobromide (400μg)

Biliary Colic

Management
- Consider cholangitis and treat as appropriate, especially if obstructed.
- Immediate treatment:
  - NSAID e.g. diclofenac 75mg stat.☑ or
  - hyoscine butylbromide *(Buscopan)* 20mg stat. SC, or
  - glycopyrronium 0.1-0.2mg stat. SC
- Continuing treatment:
  - glycopyrronium 0.2-0.6mg/24h CSCI☑ or
  - hyoscine butylbromide *(Buscopan)* 40-160mg/24h CSCI, or

PRESCRIBING STATUS
☼ Glycopyrronium •

ThinkList
- many opioids cause spasm of biliary tract smooth muscle; if biliary colic is present, consider changing to fentanyl. *(p.76)*
- glyceryl trinitrate •• [132]
- stenting biliary duct for symptomatic relief
- *Entonox* (nitrous oxide)

Drugs used for Biliary colic
Hyoscine butylbromide *(Buscopan)* PO is poorly and variably absorbed and is not recommended.
GLYCOPYRRONIUM BROMIDE (GLYCOPYRROLATE)
    Inj. 200μg/1mL, 600μg/3mL
    TSD: 400μg/24h CSCI for colic
HYOSCINE BUTYLBROMIDE (SCOPOLAMINE BUTYLBROMIDE)
    Inj. 20mg/1mL; Tabs. 10mg *(Buscopan)*
    TSD: 80mg/24h CSCI; 10mg q.d.s. PO
PROPANTHELINE
    Tabs. 15mg
    TSD: 15mg t.d.s. PO
DICLOFENAC
    Inj. 75mg/3mL
    TSD: 75mg SC stat.

Constipation

Causes of constipation
- immobility - general weakness, paraplegia, lymphoedema
- dehydration - reduced fluid intake, vomiting etc.
- drug induced - e.g. opioid analgesics, antacids, phenothiazines
- environment - poor access to facilities - lack of privacy on a ward
- altered dietary intake - anorexia, dysphagia, low fibre, high milk content
- depression
- generally reduced muscle tone - elderly
- abdominal wall muscle paresis - spinal cord compression
- primary or secondary bowel disease - haemorrhoids, secondary to RT
- hypercalcaemia

Complications of constipation
- pain - colic or constant abdominal discomfort
- intestinal obstruction
- urinary retention or frequency
- overflow diarrhoea
- faecal incontinence
- confusion or restlessness if severe

Management
1) Anticipate this common problem.
2) Enquire about bowel function regularly.
3) Start prophylactic laxatives when starting opioid drugs.
4) Use oral laxatives in preference to rectal measures.
5) Use a combination of a stimulant laxative with a softener/osmotic laxative.
   - polyethylene glycol *(Movicol)* used alone is a useful alternative for some patients[133,134]
6) Titrate components to achieve optimum stool frequency and consistency.
7) Ideally the patient should be taught to understand this use of the laxatives.
8) Remember also to:
   - increase fluid intake
   - increase fruit in diet
   - encourage mobility
   - get patient to toilet if possible - avoid bed pans
   - provide privacy
   - raised toilet seat for comfort

Faecal Impaction
If the patient has become very constipated with faecal impaction try:
1) bisacodyl suppositories (must be in contact with rectal mucosa)
2) phosphate enema
3) arachis oil retention enema to soften
4) manual removal (with midazolam, diamorphine, or caudal anaesthesia)

An alternative is *Movicol* taken for 3 days (see below).[135,136] The patient must be able to take the 1 litre of fluid required to be effective.

If the rectum is empty but the patient remains impacted higher up, try a high arachis oil or phosphate enema.

Once successful it is imperative to start oral measures to prevent recurrence of the problem.

Neurogenic constipation

Patients with spinal cord compression or sacral nerve damage who have lost neurological control and sensation to the rectum may present a particular problem. In some of these patients oral laxatives may only produce a softer stool and thence faecal incontinence, but not stimulate defecation. These patients may best be managed by allowing the faeces to become quite hard, and then using a suppository (e.g. *Carbalax*) or enema (or removing faeces manually) every 2-3 days.

Choice of laxative

- A number of laxatives combinations may be equally effective.
- Patient preference may dictate choice.
- Mixed preparations of softener/stimulant (e.g. co-danthramer) keep medications to a minimum.
- Separate softener and stimulant allows titration of components to give optimum stool frequency and consistency.
- Senna has a greater tendency to cause than colic than dantron-containing combination laxatives.[137]

In the absence of specific indications/contraindications the following are recommended:

- magnesium hydroxide and senna syrup mixed
- co-danthramer (suspension or capsules)

Partial intestinal obstruction

- docusate 200mg b.d. (as capsules)

ThinkList

- naloxone PO ••• has been used to treat opioid-induced constipation;[138-143] titration regimen used: day 1 - 3mg t.d.s., day 2 - 6mg t.d.s., day 3 - 9mg t.d.s.[143]

SEE ALSO
Reviews[116,144-148]

Drugs for Constipation

OSMOTIC LAXATIVES

LACTULOSE
Solution (3.35 g/5mL); Powder 10g/sachet
TSD: 10mL PO
May cause unacceptable wind in some patients. Others cannot tolerate the sweet taste of solution. Powder is tasteless and can be sprinkled on food.

MAGNESIUM HYDROXIDE
Mixture
TSD: 10mL PO

ISO-OSMOTIC LAXATIVES

Osmotic laxatives draw fluid into the large intestine by osmotic pressure gradient. A new class of 'iso-osmotic' laxative contains balanced electrolytes and retains water during GI transit. This may be helpful in patients with poor hydration status.

POLYETHYLENE GLYCOL 3350 / MACROGOL *(MOVICOL)* **(LIME OR LEMON)**
Oral powder sachets (polyethylene glycols '3350' 13g)
TSD: 1 sachet b.d. each in 125mL water (£24.36)
Faecal impaction can be treated with 8 sachets in 1 litre water drunk within 6h, for 3 days[135,136]

COMBINATION LAXATIVES WITH DANTRON (DANTHRON)
Co-danthramer and co-danthrusate are licensed only for use in patients with 'terminal illness'

All drugs containing dantron may cause perianal discoloration or a sore rash.[149-151] Patients should be warned that these drugs all will cause urine to turn red (mimicking haematuria).

CO-DANTHRAMER ☑
Caps. (Dantron 25mg + Poloxamer 200mg)
Susp. Dantron 25mg + Poloxamer 200mg /5mL
  TSD: Caps. 2 nocte, Susp. 10mL nocte - b.d. (£12.00 caps.)

STRONG CO-DANTHRAMER
Caps. (Dantron 37.5mg + Poloxamer 500mg)
Susp. Dantron 75mg + Poloxamer 1 gm /5mL

CO-DANTHRUSATE ⊘
Caps. (Dantron 50mg + Docusate 60mg)
Susp. Dantron 50mg + Docusate 60mg /5mL
  TSD: Caps. 1 nocte

Approximate equivalent doses:
- co-danthramer capsules - 3
- strong co-danthramer capsule - 1
- co-danthramer suspension - 15mL
- strong co-danthramer suspension - 2.5mL
- co-danthrusate capsules - 2
- co-danthrusate suspension - 10mL

STIMULANT LAXATIVES
BISACODYL
Tabs. 5mg
SENNA
Tabs. 7.5mg; Syrup 7.5mg/5mL
  TSD: 7.5mg PO
SODIUM PICOSULFATE
Elixir 5mg/5mL
  TSD: 10mL PO

Sodium picosulfate is a useful, potent stimulant laxative; indicated only when other stimulant laxatives failed.

FAECAL SOFTENERS
DOCUSATE SODIUM
Caps. 100mg
  TSD: 200mg b.d. PO

Docusate is available as a liquid, but this tastes disgusting and should not be used. Acts more as a surface wetting agent than a stimulant.

SUPPOSITORIES & ENEMAS
ARACHIS OIL
Enema 130mL
  Contains peanut oil - do not use in patients with nut allergy
BISACODYL
Supps. 5mg, 10mg
CARBALAX ⊘
Supps. (Sodium acid phosphate 1.69g in effervescent base)
GLYCERINE
Supps. 1g, 2g, 4g
MICRALAX
Enema (Sodium citrate - rectal)
PHOSPHATE (FORMULA B)
Enema 128mL

Diarrhoea

Management

Treat or exclude any specific causes:

Subacute small bowel obstruction	⇨ p.25
Laxatives (including self-administered magnesium-containing antacids)[152]	Discontinue and review
Faecal impaction (with anal leakage or incontinence)	Rectal disimpaction/manual evacuation/Movicol (⇨ p.29)
Antibiotic-associated diarrhoea / pseudomembranous colitis (recent broad-spectrum antibiotics)	Check stool for *Clostridium difficile* (metronidazole 400mg t.d.s. for 7-14 days)
Radiotherapy-induced	**NSAID** Ondansetron[153]
NSAID	Try stopping or changing **NSAID**
Misoprostol	Use a **PPI** or other alternative
Pre-existing disease e.g. Crohn's or ulcerative colitis	Corticosteroids or sulphasalazine
Ileal resection (causing bile salt diarrhoea	Colestyramine
Steatorrhoea / fat malabsorption	Pancreatic enzymes ± **PPI** (reduces gastric acid destruction of enzymes)
Carcinoid syndrome	Octreotide 5-HT$_3$ antagonists or clonidine[154]

Infection

A stool culture is always worth sending if no obvious cause is determined. Candida infection has been described causing secretory-type diarrhoea,[155] and can be treated with oral nystatin. Live yoghurt may be an alternative, or used to prevent recurrence, but no evidence supports its use.

Symptomatic management of diarrhoea

Patients on strong opioid analgesics already:

1) Consider converting morphine from SR tablets to normal release preparations to improve absorption, or use diamorphine by CSCI.
2) Titrate dose of strong opioid up to control diarrhoea, as limited by side effects:
   - if the maximum tolerated dose of morphine is low, consider adding codeine 60mg q.d.s. which has a greater antidiarrhoeal effect at equianalgesic doses
3) If ineffective, add loperamide 2mg q.d.s.
   - increase dose up to 4mg q.d.s.

For patients not taking strong opioids already:

1) Loperamide 2mg after each loose stool:
   - if not controlling diarrhoea rapidly, change to 2mg q.d.s.
   - increase dose up to 4mg q.d.s.
2) Substitute codeine 30-60mg q.d.s. PO if ineffective.
3) Use combination of loperamide + codeine.
4) Change to loperamide + morphine:
   - use normal release preparations of morphine, not SR tablets
   - titrate dose upwards as for analgesia, limited by side effects

Further options

- If severe diarrhoea is preventing absorption of oral drugs, use diamorphine starting at 10mg/24h by CSCI, or dihydrocodeine 100-200mg/24h by CSCI if not tolerated.

- Bacterial overgrowth or imbalance of the normal gut flora may cause diarrhoea despite negative stool cultures for pathogens, especially after ileo-colic resection or surgical formation of blind-loops of gut; a course of metronidazole 400mg t.d.s. PO may be tried empirically.

- Glucose is pro-absorptive in the bowel; giving a glucose/electrolyte drink e.g. *Lucozade Sport* or *Dioralyte* may help diarrhoea, as well as replacing important losses.

- Octreotide may reduce high output diarrhoea following ileostomy or colectomy, and has been used in carcinoid syndrome, graft-versus-host disease, and other cancer- and AIDS- related diarrhoeas.[156-162] It is expensive and should be tried after other options.

HIV patients / AIDS

Patients with AIDS frequently have problems with diarrhoea. It is usually infective, but the diagnosis, isolation of pathogens, and treatment can be very complex. A specialist in AIDS should be involved.

PRESCRIBING STATUS
☼ Morphine and Dihydrocodeine ®
☼ Octreotide ●●

ThinkList

- boiled rice, or the water in which it was boiled, is an old remedy for diarrhoea; there is evidence that it is effective[163-165]
- 5-HT$_3$ antagonists ●●● e.g. ondansetron have been used for radiotherapy-induced diarrhoea[153] and carcinoid syndrome[154]
- clonidine ●●● has been used for 'diabetic diarrhoea' due to autonomic neuropathy, and for high output diarrhoea following bowel transplant[166]

SEE ALSO
📖 Reviews[160,162,167,168]

Drugs used for Diarrhoea

LOPERAMIDE
Caps. 2mg; Syrup 1mg/5mL *(Imodium)*
  TSD: 1 caps. q.d.s. PO. Max. 16mg daily.
CODEINE
Tabs. 15mg, 30mg, 60mg; Syrup 25mg/5mL
  TSD: 30mg q.d.s. PO
DIHYDROCODEINE TARTRATE
Inj. 50mg/1mL
  TSD: 100mg/24h by CSCI
OCTREOTIDE
Inj. 50μg/1mL, 100μg/1mL, 500μg/1mL, 1mg/5mL
  TSD: 250μg/24h CSCI (£386.96). Max. 1000μg/24h
Increase dose by 250μg increments every 1-2 days if no response, to 750μg/24h. If still no response, then discontinue. Tolerance may develop; consider increasing dose if response seems to reduce over a week or two. Long acting depot injections of somatostatin analogues are available, but 2 weeks are needed to achieve plasma levels[121]

Additional Information
Loperamide

Loperamide is absorbed when taken orally, but undergoes extensive first-pass hepatic metabolism; it does not penetrate the CNS. At equal doses, loperamide gives longer protection against diarrhoea than diphenoxylate, codeine or morphine. Single doses of up to 60mg do not produce opiate-like effects.

Loperamide binds to opioid receptors, but also exerts its antidiarrhoeal effects by inhibiting calcium channels and calmodulin, and acts mainly on the colon.[169] Loperamide may therefore work synergistically with other opioid drugs.

Equivalent doses

Loperamide 2mg is equivalent in effect to codeine 30mg, morphine 15-30mg, or methadone 15-25mg;[169,170] as it is longer acting than codeine or morphine, loperamide 2mg b.d. may be more equivalent to codeine 30-60mg q.d.s.[171]

Compared with loperamide or codeine, diphenoxylate/atropine is less effective at producing a solid stool and causes more side-effects.[170,172]

Fistulae (entero-cutaneous)

- Octreotide reduces secretions in the small bowel and reduces intestinal motility. It is useful in drying up high-output fistulae.[173,174]
- For large bowel fistulae, consider deliberately constipating the patient, using anti-diarrhoeal drugs *(p.32)*.

PRESCRIBING STATUS
Octreotide ••

ThinkList

- *Cavilon*[175] for skin care
- stent for colo-vaginal fistula[176]
- an intra-vaginal prosthesis has been described to treat an entero-vaginal fistula, incorporated into a urinary catheter[177]
- Histoacryl glue has been used to seal a (tracheo-oesophageal) fistula[178]
- self-polymerising silicone rubber bung[179]
- malignant gastro-colic fistula treated by endoscopic human fibrin sealant injection[180]

SEE ALSO
Review[181]

Drugs used for Fistulae
OCTREOTIDE

Inj. 50µg/1mL, 100µg/1mL, 500µg/1mL, 1mg/5mL
TSD: 250µg/24h **CSCI** *(£386.96). Max. 1000µg/24h*
Increase dose by 250µg increments every 1-2 days if no response, to 750µg/24h. If still no response, then discontinue. Tolerance may develop; consider increasing dose if response seems to reduce over a week or two. Long acting depot injections of somatostatin analogues are available, but 2 weeks are needed to achieve plasma levels[121]

Anorexia & Cachexia

Anorexia

Anorexia is commonly part of a cancer-induced anorexia-cachexia syndrome. Always exclude or treat other causes of poor appetite:

- nausea
- painful mouth
- oral infection
- oesophagitis/oesophageal spasm (odynophagia)
- dysphagia from obstructed oesophagus

Management

Corticosteroids can increase appetite and enjoyment of food in many patients.[182-185] Progestagens are probably as effective as corticosteroids, but are very much more expensive.

1) Symptoms of gastric stasis, such as early satiety, should be sought carefully even if nausea is not prominent, and a trial with metoclopramide considered.[8,186]
2) Dexamethasone 4mg o.d. ⇨ *(p.126)*

Cachexia

Corticosteroids do not cause non-fluid weight gain; progestagens can increase weight, but the effect is quite slow.

PRESCRIBING STATUS

☼ Corticosteroids •

☼ Progestagens (medroxyprogesterone & megestrol acetate) ••

ThinkList

- cannabinoids (dronabinol, nabilone) ••• [187-190] *(p.180)*
- thalidomide ••• [191-193]
- EPA (eicosapentaenoic acid) is being investigated for cachexia *(p.180)*

SEE ALSO

⇨ *Corticosteroids (p.126), Progestagens (p. 129), Hydrazine (p.182)*
📖 Reviews[189,194-201]

Drugs used for anorexia

DEXAMETHASONE ☑

Tabs. 0.5mg, 2mg; Inj. 4mg/1mL, 8mg/2mL, 120mg/5mL
Susp. 2mg/5mL‡ (available from Rosemount)
Dexamethasone is up to twice as potent given **SC** as by the oral route
TSD: 4mg o.d. for anorexia (£4.84)

BETAMETHASONE

Tabs. sol. 0.5mg *(Betnesol)*; Inj. 4mg/1mL
TSD: 4mg o.d. for anorexia (£8.13)
Soluble tablets are useful alternative if cannot manage tablets. Equipotent to dexamethasone. 8mg will dissolve in <=10mL water.

PREDNISOLONE

Tabs. 1mg, 2.5mg, 5mg, 25mg; Tabs. sol. 5mg
TSD: 30mg o.d. for anorexia (£4.02)

MEGESTROL ACETATE

Tabs. 40mg, 160mg *(Megace)*
TSD: 800mg daily (£136.73)

Hiccups (Singultus)

Many drugs and other methods have been reported to successfully stop hiccups, but none are consistently reliable.

Causes

- Via vagus nerve
  - gastric distension
  - gastritis/gastro-oesophageal reflux[202,203]
  - hepatic tumours[204]
  - ascites / intestinal distension / obstruction
- Via phrenic nerve
  - diaphragmatic tumour involvement[205]
  - mediastinal tumour
- CNS
  - intracranial tumours, especially brainstem lesions[206-209]
  - meningeal infiltration by Ca.
- Systemic
  - renal failure
  - corticosteroids[210,211]
  - Addison's disease[212]
  - hyponatraemia[213]

Treatment

1) Pharyngeal stimulation / palatal massage[214] - get the patient to rub the back of their palate with their index finger - as far back as possible without causing gagging - is often effective, at least temporarily.
2) Treat gastritis if present with antacid and/or PPI.
3) Corticosteroids can cause hiccups - consider stopping if recently started.
4) Antiflatulent e.g. *Asilone* (dimeticone) may help if gastric distension present.
5) Metoclopramide - especially likely to help if hiccups associated with gastric distension.[215,216]
6) Paracentesis may help for abdominal distension (and subsequent gastric stasis).
7) Chlorpromazine is often effective - but only on doses that are sedative. A useful fall-back for persistent hiccups, when a dose of 25-50mg nocte will at least allow sleep.[216,217]
8) Baclofen 5mg t.d.s.[218-225]
9) Nifedipine 10mg SR b.d.[218,226-229]
10) Dexamethasone 4-8mg o.d. can help hiccups[230] especially if associated with cerebral or hepatic tumours.
11) Other measures worth considering:
    - nebulised saline[231]
    - haloperidol[232]
    - midazolam[233]
12) Several anticonvulsants have been reported to help: sodium valproate,[234] carbamazepine,[235] phenytoin,[236,237] phenobarbital

PRESCRIBING STATUS

⚖ Asilone, Metoclopramide, Baclofen, Nifedipine, Dexamethasone •
⚖ Midazolam •
⚖ Anticonvulsants ••

Think List

- numerous other drugs have been reported: amitriptyline,[*] ketamine (0.5mg/kg),[***] orphenadrine,[***] amantadine,[***] cisapride (now unavailable, but newer 5-HT4 agonists are being developed), methylphenidate,[***] glucagon,[***] and nikethamide [***] [238-252]
- acupuncture[253-257]
- venting gastrostomy for gastric distension
- digital rectal massage[258,259]!
- implanted phrenic nerve stimulator[260,261]

SEE ALSO

📖 Reviews[262-265] & Comments[266,267]

Drugs used for Hiccups

ASILONE ©
  Susp. (Al. hydroxide 420mg, dimeticone 135mg, Mg oxide)
    TSD: 10mL q.d.s. PO
METOCLOPRAMIDE
  Tabs. 10mg; Tabs. **SR** 15mg *(Gastrobid)*; Syrup 5mg/5mL; Inj. 10mg/2mL
    TSD: 10mg q.d.s. PO; 15mg SR b.d. PO; 40mg/24h CSCI
CHLORPROMAZINE
  Tabs. 10mg, 25mg, 50mg; Elixir 25mg/5mL; Supps. 100mg; Inj. 50mg/2mL
    TSD: 25mg o.d. - t.d.s. PO; 100mg PR
NIFEDIPINE
  Tabs. **SR** (12h) 10mg, 20mg *(Adalat Retard)*
    TSD 10mg SR (Adalat Retard) b.d. PO
  Tabs. **SR** (24h) 20mg, 30mg, 60mg *(Adalat LA)*
  Caps. 5mg, 10mg
  Hypotension and headaches are main side effects. Short-acting preparations
  can cause large falls in blood pressure and are best avoided. Different
  modified-release versions may have different clinical effect; prescribe by
  brand name. Long-acting preparations (especially *Adalat LA* for 24h dosing)
  are best avoided in hepatic impairment.
  Increases phenytoin blood levels (risk of toxicity).
BACLOFEN
  Tabs. 10mg; Liquid 5mg/5mL
    TSD: 5mg t.d.s. PO

Ascites

Symptoms caused by tense ascites

- abdominal distension, discomfort and pain
- dyspnoea
- nausea & vomiting due to 'squashed stomach syndrome'
- dyspnoea
- oesophageal reflux

Treatment options

- chemotherapy - intraperitoneal or systemic
- paracentesis
- diuretics
- peritoneovenous shunt

Management

1) Chemotherapy can be considered if the prognosis warrants, but for most patients, therapy aimed at symptomatic control is appropriate.
2) Paracentesis is the treatment of choice for rapid symptom control.
3) Repeated paracentesis as needed is appropriate for most patients with a poor prognosis e.g. < 4-6 weeks e.g. gross hepatomegaly or jaundice.
4) Commence diuretics if prognosis > 4 weeks, paracentesis not accepted or unsuccessful. Leg oedema is an additional indication for using diuretics. See diuretic regime below.
5) If diuretics unsuccessful, or for persistently recurring ascites, consider a peritoneovenous shunt - can be effective, but shunt obstruction, sepsis and other complications are frequent.[268-270]

Diuretic regime

Spironolactone is the drug of choice for ascites, as increased plasma rennin activity and sodium retention occur in malignant ascites. Doses between 100-400mg o.d. are used. However it takes about 7 days to improve symptoms, and up to 28 days for full effect.[271-274] The addition of furosemide will help achieve a more rapid response until spironolactone works,[274] or may help in cases resistant to spironolactone alone.

1) Start spironolactone 100mg o.d.
2) Add furosemide 40mg o.d. if rapid initial result desired, as long as the patient is not dehydrated/hypovolaemic:
   – aim to withdraw furosemide after a week or so
3) Increase spironolactone by 100mg increments once or twice weekly to maximum 200mg b.d.
4) If ascites is resistant to 400mg spironolactone, add furosemide 40mg o.d. increased if necessary to 80mg o.d.
5) If little or no response to furosemide, change to bumetanide 2mg o.d. or furosemide 100mg/24h by CSCI.[275] (⇨ p.154)

Monitoring

Patients on diuretics should be monitored closely for dehydration (indicated by U&E's, thirst, postural hypotension or confusion). Girth measurements can be used once to twice weekly to monitor the effect of diuretics.

ThinkList

- permanent indwelling peritoneal cannula[276,277] - high incidence of complications
- intraperitoneal triamcinolone hexacetonide 10mg/kg ●●● may lengthen interval between paracentesis (9 to 17 days), but risk of infection (bacterial peritonitis or localised herpes zoster)[278]
- octreotide ●●● [279]
- Corynebacterium parvum 7mg ●●● [280-282]

SEE ALSO
⇨ *Diuretics (p.154), Paracentesis (p.203)*
📖 Reviews[273,283-286]

Diuretics
SPIRONOLACTONE
Tabs. 25mg, 50mg, 100mg; Susp. 10mg/5mL, 25mg/5mL, 50mg/5mL‡
TSD: 100mg mane PO

FUROSEMIDE (FRUSEMIDE)
Tabs. 20mg, 40mg, 500mg; Liquid 1mg/mL, 40mg/5mL‡ 50mg/5mL‡
TSD: 40mg PO
Inj. 20mg/2mL, 50mg/5mL, 250mg/25mL
TSD: 100mg/24h CSCI
CO-AMILOFRUSE 5/40
Tabs. *(Frumil)*
TSD: 1 tab. mane PO
BUMETANIDE
Bumetanide 1mg is approximately equivalent to 40mg furosemide
Tabs. 1mg, 5mg; Liquid 1mg/5mL; Inj. 1mg/2mL, 2mg/4mL
TSD: 1mg mane PO

Gastrointestinal bleeding

Gastric bleeding & melaena

Assessment

Consider the commonest causes:
- tumour bleeding
- clotting disorders ⟹ *Bleeding & haemorrhage (p.147)*
- peptic ulcer ± NSAIDs

SSRIs may increase the risk of GI bleeding, especially in patients taking NSAIDs.[21-25]

Treatment

1) Review or stop NSAIDs, aspirin, corticosteroids, SSRIs.
2) Consider radiotherapy referral.
3) Consider and treat other systemic causes of bleeding *(p.147)*:
   - blood tests for clotting screen and platelets
4) Tranexamic acid 1-2g t.d.s. PO (or by slow IV until able to take PO):[287-294]
   - stop if no effect after 1 week[295]
   - continue for 1 week after bleeding has stopped, then discontinue
   - continue long term (500mg t.d.s.) only if bleeding recurs and responds to second course of treatment
5) Commence PPI in treatment dose e.g. lansoprazole 30mg o.d. when able to take orally. *(p.16)*
6) Small bleeds can herald a larger massive haemorrhage; consider siting an IV cannula to administer emergency drugs. *(p.184)*

PRESCRIBING STATUS
☼ Tranexamic acid ®

ThinkList

- intravenous high-dose PPI ••• e.g. omeprazole 80mg IV stat. then 8mg/hr IV infusion (see below)
- arterial embolisation[296-301]
- oral sucralfate •• [291,302,303]
- octreotide ••• - an accepted medical management for bleeding from oesophageal or colonic varices.[304-306] circumstantial evidence indicates that the actions of octreotide are mainly mediated by a splanchnic vasoconstrictive effect, possibly with gastric acid suppression and enhancement of platelet aggregation;[307] uncertain whether it has a role in gastrointestinal bleeding of other aetiology[308-310]
- etamsylate ® ⟹ *Haemostatic drugs (p.150)*

Rectal bleeding

Assessment

Consider the commonest causes:

- tumour bleeding
- clotting disorders ⇨ *Bleeding & haemorrhage (p.147)*
- pelvic infection
- haemorrhoids

NSAIDs can cause lower gastrointestinal bleeding as well as the better-documented upper GI bleeding.[311,312]

Treatment

1) Review or stop NSAIDs.
2) Treat any evidence or signs suggestive of pelvic infection.
3) Consider radiotherapy referral.
4) Consider and treat other systemic causes of bleeding. *(p.147)*
   - blood tests for clotting screen and platelets
5) Tranexamic acid 1g t.d.s. PO (or by slow IV until able to take PO):
   - stop if no effect after 1 week[295]
   - continue for 1 week after bleeding has stopped, then discontinue
   - continue long term (500mg t.d.s.) only if bleeding recurs and responds to second course of treatment
6) Small bleeds can herald a larger massive haemorrhage. Consider siting an IV cannula to administer emergency drugs. *(p.184)*

PRESCRIBING STATUS

☼ Tranexamic acid ®

ThinkList

- arterial embolisation[296-299,313]
- etamsylate ® ⇨ *Haemostatic drugs (p.150)*
- oral sucralfate for post-radiation proctitis ●● [314]
- *Maalox* for hemorrhagic radiation-proctitis:●●● 50-100 ml of original or 1/2 diluted *Maalox* instilled into rectum and catheter clamped for 30 min. to 1 hr. after sufficient irrigation with 500 ml of 100 times diluted iodine; bleeding should cease within 2 to 8 days after initiation of *Maalox* therapy[315]
- tranexamic acid rectal instillation ●●● for rectal bleeding[316]
- rectal sucralfate ●●● for bleeding from post-radiation procto-sigmoiditis; 20 ml of 10% rectal sucralfate suspension enemas twice daily[317]
- alum solution for rectal carcinoma;●●● used soaked into a ribbon gauze, and inserted under general anaesthetic[318]

Major gastrointestinal or rectal bleeding

If patient's condition is not stable, with history of major haemorrhage or ongoing bleeding:

- Consider if the patient should be transferred to an acute medical/endoscopy unit.
- Site an IV cannula to anticipate need for emergency drugs. *(p.184)*
- Treat anxiety or distress as needed:
  - midazolam 2-5mg initially by slow IV titration (diluted 10mg in 10mL with saline)
  - if no IV access, midazolam 5-10mg SC (or IM if shocked/vasoconstricted)

SEE ALSO
⇨ *Bleeding & haemorrhage (p.147)*, *Dyspepsia(p.16)*
📖 Reviews[309] & Comments[319]

Drugs used for Haematemesis & Melaena

For other preparations of PPIs ⇨ (p.16).
TRANEXAMIC ACID (CYKLOKAPRON)
   Tabs. 500mg; Syrup 500mg/5mL; Inj 500mg/5mL
   TSD 1g t.d.s. PO or by slow IV injection
   Avoid if risk of ureteric obstruction e.g. renal haemorrhage. Discontinue if
      disturbance in colour vision develops.
OMEPRAZOLE
   Inj. 40mg amp ☑
   TSD: see notes below
SUCRALFATE (ALUMINIUM HYDROXIDE AND SULPHATED SUCROSE COMPLEX)
   Tabs. Disp. 1g; Susp. 1g/5mL (aniseed or caramel flavour)
   TSD: 1g q.d.s. PO
   CSM advises caution in seriously ill patients, patients on enteral feeding, or
      with delayed gastric emptying, due to bezoar formation *(p.25)*

Additional Information
PPIs
Acid suppression in early studies did not help in the management of acute GI
bleeding. It has more recently been shown that intensive therapy aimed at
achieving complete acid suppression does substantially reduce the risk of
recurrent bleeding after initial endoscopic treatment. Pharmacokinetic studies
with PPIs have shown that a bolus of 80mg pantoprazole or omeprazole
followed by immediate continuous infusion of 8mg/hour will result in an
intragastric pH of 7 within 20 minutes.[320] This has been continued for 72h in
studies.[321,322] Reports of blindness following intravenous PPIs[323] have later
been disputed.[324]

Haemorrhoids & Anal fissure

Pain from anal fissures can be treated medically using glyceryl trinitrate.[325-327]

SOOTHING HAEMORRHOIDAL PREPARATIONS
ANUSOL
   Rectal ointment, Rectal cream., Supps.

ANAL FISSURE
GLYCERYL TRINITRATE
   Ointment 0.2%‡

HAEMORRHOIDAL PREPARATIONS WITH CORTICOSTEROID
ANUSOL HC
   Rectal ointment, Supps.
XYLOPROCT
   Rectal ointment, Supps. (contains lidocaine)

Tenesmus & Tenesmoid pain

Tenesmus is the painful sensation of rectal fullness, usually caused by local rectal tumour. There may be associated spasm of smooth muscle, or neuropathic pain from lumbosacral plexus infiltration causing stabbing or more continuous pain. May be difficult to distinguish from pudendal neuralgia.[328]

Management

1) Prevent and treat constipation.
2) Opioid analgesics - often resistant.[329]
3) NSAID e.g. diclofenac 50mg t.d.s.
4) Radiotherapy
5) Nifedipine SR 10-20mg b.d.[330]
6) Co-analgesics as for neuropathic pain *(p.51)*
    – amitriptyline
    – anticonvulsants
    – corticosteroids
7) Lumbar sympathectomy: > 80% success rate.[331]

PRESCRIBING STATUS
☼ Nifedipine ●●

ThinkList

- benzodiazepines ● e.g. diazepam 2-5mg b.d. - t.d.s.
- chlorpromazine ● e.g. 25mg nocte
- rectal enema of lidocaine 2% gel PRN ●● [332]
- methadone ●●● [333]
- spinal infusion of local anaesthetic ± opioids
- laser treatment of rectal tumour[334,335]
- rectal instillation of morphine gel ●● [336]
- cryoanalgesia or neurolytic saddle block[337]

SEE ALSO
⇨ *Neuropathic pain (p.51)*
▢ Reviews[332,337]

Drugs used for Tenesmus

NIFEDIPINE

Tabs. SR (12h) 10mg, 20mg *(Adalat Retard)*
   TSD 10mg SR (Adalat Retard) b.d. PO
Tabs. SR 20mg, 30mg, 60mg *(Adalat LA)*
Caps. 5mg, 10mg

Hypotension and headaches are main side effects. Short-acting preparations can cause large falls in blood pressure and are best avoided. Different modified-release versions may have different clinical effect; prescribe by brand name. Long-acting preparations (especially *Adalat LA* for 24h dosing) are best avoided in hepatic impairment.
Increases phenytoin blood levels (risk of toxicity).

Painful mouth & Stomatitis

Management
Diagnose and treat underlying causes of painful mouth where possible:
- bacterial infection *(p.117)*
- oral candida *(p.44)*
- herpes simplex *(p.121)*
- aphthous ulceration (see below)
- tumour
- post-radiotherapy or chemotherapy mucositis
- iron deficiency (angular stomatitis and 'beef-red' glossitis)
- vitamin C deficiency - gingivitis and bleeding *(p.147)*

Symptomatic treatment
- Good oral hygiene ± chlorhexidine mouthwash *(Corsodyl)*.
- Systemic analgesia:
  - NSAID e.g. diclofenac
  - soluble aspirin may be used as mouthwash ± gargled in addition to systemic NSAID or as an alternative
  - opioids are often ineffective
- Analgesic or anaesthetic mouthwash:
  - *Difflam* oral rinse - mild analgesic, or
  - *Mucaine* as mouthwash (topical anaesthetic effect)
- For localised painful ulcers:
  - *Bonjela* oral gel is a mild analgesic, or
  - *Orabase* is a protective ointment that adheres well to the mucosa

Aphthous ulceration
- Topical corticosteroid - *Corlan* lozenges or *Adcortyl in Orabase*.
- Tetracycline mouthwash (see below).

PRESCRIBING STATUS
☼ Mucaine or Tetracycline mouthwash •

ThinkList
- opioids systemically are often ineffective - oral morphine may be tried as a mouthwash • (use *Sevredol* which is alcohol-free and will sting less)
- viscous lidocaine gel •• may be used for severe pain - can cause hypersensitisation, and a risk of aspiration due to pharyngeal anaesthesia
- sucralfate as mouthwash •• - significantly reduces throat pain and analgesic requirement after tonsillectomy[338]
- cocaine mouthwash •• (2%) is used for mucositis in some centres
- thalidomide ••• for aphthous ulcers (in AIDS)[192,193,339,340]

SEE ALSO
📖 Reviews[341-343]

Drugs used for Oral Pain
ORABASE
  Oral paste
    Apply PRN
ADCORTYL IN ORABASE
  Oral paste (Triamcinolone 0.1%)
    Apply b.d.

BONJELA (CHOLINE SALICYLATE ORAL GEL)
  Oral gel (Choline salicylate 8.7%)
    Apply q.d.s.
CHLORHEXIDINE *(CORSODYL)*
  Mouthwash 0.2%
    15mL q.d.s.
BENZYDAMINE HYDROCHLORIDE *(DIFFLAM)*
  Oral rinse
    15mL q.d.s.
    Dilute 1:1 with water if stings
HYDROCORTISONE *(CORLAN)*
  Pellets (hydrocortisone 2.5mg)
    1 q.d.s. PO held against ulcerated area
TETRACYCLINE (MOUTHWASH)
  Caps. 250mg
    TSD: 250mg q.d.s.
    For aphthous ulcers: dissolve contents of 1 cap. in small amount of water;
      hold in mouth for 2-3 minutes, q.d.s. for 3 days. Preferably not swallowed.
    Predisposes to oral candida. Tetracycline can stain teeth.

Additional Information

Cochrane Library review in preparation on interventions for treating oral mucositis and associated pain for patients receiving chemotherapy or radiotherapy.

Oral Candida

Oral candida is present in 80% of patients with metastatic disease, but it is not necessarily symptomatic.
Candidiasis may present with:
• dry mouth
• loss of taste
• smooth reddened tongue
• soreness
• dysphagia (NB oesophageal candidiasis)
• isolated 'salt grain' lesions on the inner aspects of the cheeks or gum
    margins
• severely furred dirty tongue with a central fissure
• angular cheilitis

Treatment

• Confirmation by routine bacteriology swabs is unnecessary.
• Regular oral hygiene is always important.
• Dentures must also be treated (soak in Milton's).
• Mild cases - nystatin 2-5mL q.d.s.
• More severe cases:
    – fluconazole 150mg stat.[344] if causative factors resolved e.g. following a
        course of antibiotics, else give -
    – fluconazole 50mg daily for 1 week
• Recurrent candidiasis - fluconazole 50mg daily.
• Resistant candidiasis - itraconazole.

Notes

Topical preparations (nystatin, miconazole and amphotericin) will give poor results if not used regularly and with appropriate advice.

SEE ALSO

⇨ *Fungal infections (p.120)*

📖 Reviews[345-347] & Guidelines[348]

Drugs for Candidiasis

Fluconazole and miconazole increases phenytoin blood levels (risk of toxicity). Fluconazole, miconazole, itraconazole, and ketoconazole all enhance warfarin anticoagulation. Fluconazole and miconazole increase sulphonylureas e.g. gliclazide, glibenclamide (risk of hypoglycaemia) Fluconazole increases celecoxib levels[349] – halve celecoxib dose Itraconazole, ketoconazole and possibly fluconazole increase sedation with midazolam

FLUCONAZOLE ☑

Tabs. 50mg; Susp. 50mg/5mL
TSD: 50mg o.d. PO

ITRACONAZOLE

Caps. 100mg; Liquid 10mg/mL
TSD: 100mg o.d. PO

KETOCONAZOLE

Tabs. 200mg; Susp. 100mg/5mL
TSD: 200mg o.d. PO

TOPICAL ORAL ANTIFUNGAL TREATMENTS

NYSTATIN ☑

Susp. 100,000u/mL; Pastilles 100,000u
TSD: 2-5mL q.d.s. PO; 1 pastille q.d.s. PO

MICONAZOLE

Oral gel 25mg/mL
Apply q.d.s. PO

AMPHOTERICIN

Lozenges 10mg *(Fungilin)*
TSD: 1 tabs. q.d.s. PO

Additional Information

Cochrane Library review is in preparation on interventions for treating oral candidiasis for patients receiving chemotherapy or radiotherapy.

A number of different species of Candida may be implicated. Fluconazole resistance is not uncommon. It may be overcome in some cases by using a higher dose of fluconazole; alternatively an alternative imidazole is needed e.g. itraconazole.[350,351]

Dry mouth (Xerostomia)

Causes
- opioids[352]
- antimuscarinic drugs
- candida
- dehydration
- renal failure
- radiotherapy
- mouth-breathing (dyspnoea)

Management
- Treat underlying cause if possible.
- Good oral hygiene is important to avoid infection.
- General measures include:
    - adequate availability of drinks
    - sucking ice cubes
    - chewing gum
- Saliva substitute according to patient acceptability:
    - *Saliva Orthana* (NB pork-mucin based)
    - *Salivix* pastilles
    - *OralBalance* gel
- Pilocarpine - licensed for radiation-induced xerostomia or Sjogren's syndrome, but may be effective for other indications including for opioid-induced xerostomia.[353,354]

PRESCRIBING STATUS
- ☼ Pilocarpine •• (for dry mouth - other than radiotherapy-induced)

ThinkList
- pilocarpine 4% eye drops ••• PO 2-3 drops (4-6mg) t.d.s. (2mg/1 drop)
    - add to raspberry syrup (cost £5/month vs. £52/month for *Salagen*)
- acupuncture[355,356]

SEE ALSO
- 📖 Reviews[342,357,358] & Clinical trials[359-362]

Drugs used for dry mouth
SALIVA ORTHANA
  Oral spray 50mL, Refill 450mL; Lozenges
  NB Pork mucin based saliva substitute.
GLANDOSANE$^{\ominus}$
  Aerosol spray: neutral, lemon or peppermint flavour
ORALBALANCE$^{\ominus}$
  Gel, 50g
SALIVIX
  Pastilles
PILOCARPINE
  Tabs. 5mg *(Salagen)*
  TSD: 5mg t.d.s. PO (£51.43). Can increase to 10mg t.d.s.
  Contraindicated in asthma or COPD. Side effects include sweating, nausea and colic.

Sialorrhoea/Drooling

Sialorrhoea is the production of an excessive amount of saliva (uncommon, but consider GERD[363] or oesophageal tumours[364]), whereas drooling describes difficulty or inability to swallow normal amounts of saliva. Drooling may be caused by neuromuscular problems with swallowing, including:

- motor neurone disease / AML
- tumours of head and neck
- brain tumours
- Parkinson's disease
- drug-induced parkinsonism
- severe debility

Management

Antimuscarinic drugs will reduce saliva production. Most patients will not be able to swallow tablets or capsules, or large volumes; a number will have PEG feeding.

Drugs that do not cross the blood-brain barrier minimise the risk of sedation and other central side-effects; however they are usually poorly and unpredictably absorbed when given orally.

Given by injection	
Glycopyrronium 0.1-0.4mg/24h CSCI	Ideal drug, but requires regular or continuous injection. Most reliable way of establishing effective symptom control rapidly.
Glycopyrronium 25-100µg b.d. SC increased as needed	
Hyoscine hydrobromide transdermal patch[365-367]	Central side effects can occur, especially in the elderly.

Given orally/PEG/sublingual	
Glycopyrronium PO 0.6-2mg up to t.d.s.[368,369]	Solution for injection can be used but may need 3-10mL. Powder for oral solution requires pharmacy to prepare, is not routinely available, and is expensive. Titration to effective dose may take longer.
Atropine eye drops 1% 2 drops PO/sublingual q.d.s.[370]	Cheapest; least published experience. Central side effects may occur, but less than hyoscine hydrobromide.

Other drugs with antimuscarinic effects will reduce saliva production e.g. amitriptyline PO 25mg nocte or propantheline 15mg t.d.s. but use is often limited by side effects.

Choice will depend on local availability and patient's circumstances. Suggested regimen for in-patient:

- Glycopyrronium 0.1mg/24h CSCI, with 25-50µg SC PRN, titrating infusion to effective dose, to establish efficacy and gain symptom control rapidly.
- For longer-term maintenance, change to atropine eye drops 1% 2 drops q.d.s. adjusting dose as needed:
  - glycopyrronium can also be prescribed to ensure no loss of control, in a dose of one-third of the effective CSCI 24h-dose given SC t.d.s. PRN

PRESCRIBING STATUS

✿ Hyoscine hydrobromide, Glycopyrronium CSCI/SC, Atropine eye drops •

✿ Amitriptyline or propantheline •

✿ Glycopyrronium PO ••

ThinkList

- beta blockers •• (propranolol or metoprolol) have been used in persistent thick tenacious secretions in AML[371]
- nebulised hyoscine •• has also been used[372,373]

SEE ALSO

📖 Review[374]

Drugs used for sialorrhoea

GLYCOPYRRONIUM BROMIDE (GLYCOPYRROLATE)

Inj. 200µg/1mL, 600µg/3mL ᴼ

Tabs‡ 1mg ᴼ 2mg ᴼ

TSD: 100µg/24h CSCI; 0.6-1mg t.d.s. PO

Tablets are available on named-patient basis from IDIS through pharmacies (020-8410-0700); oral solution can be made from powder, available from Antigen. Injection solution can be used via PEG tube, using filter needle to draw up. Oral solution of 1mg in 10ml can be made up in purified water, this is given an expiry of seven days and refrigerated.[370] The oral dose needed of glycopyrronium is approximately 35 times the parenteral dose.[375]

HYOSCINE HYDROBROMIDE (SCOPOLAMINE HYDROBROMIDE)

Tabs. 300µg; Patch *(Scopoderm TTS)* 1mg/72h; Inj. 400µg/1mL, 600µg/1mL

TSD: 300µg q.d.s. PO; 1 patch every 3 days (£20.07); 400µg/24h CSCI

ATROPINE SULPHATE

Eye drops 1% 10mL, 1% single-use 0.5mL

TSD: 2 drops PO/sublingual q.d.s.

PAIN

Pain Control

- Treat constant pain with regular analgesia.
- Different types of pain respond to different analgesics.
- Psycho-social factors like anxiety or depression, which may reduce tolerance to pain or be exacerbated by pain, must also be assessed and treated[376,377]

A step-by-step guide to pain control

1) Mild pain of many causes will respond to paracetamol.
2) Identify if the type of pain can best be treated by a specific treatment:
   - pain from bone metastases → radiotherapy
   - smooth muscle colic → antimuscarinic
   - infection such as cellulitis → antibiotic
   - pathological fracture → radiotherapy or surgical fixation
   - raised intracranial pressure → corticosteroids
3) For moderate pain, consider an NSAID e.g. diclofenac 50mg t.d.s. if an inflammatory process is thought to be involved and there are no contraindications to an NSAID:
   - bone metastases
   - musculo-skeletal pain
4) Else, try a weak opioid ± paracetamol e.g. codeine, co-proxamol or co-codamol (strong).
5) For more severe pain start a strong opioid and titrate dose (⇨ p.65)
   - morphine PO or diamorphine CSCI are usual first-line strong opioids[378]
   - selected patients may be started on fentanyl (⇨ p.71 & p.76)
6) If this does not relieve the pain or the opioid dose has been escalated to the maximum tolerable side effects - consider:
   - adding an NSAID if not already tried
   - morphine-resistant pain (⇨ p.68)
   - underlying depression or fear lowering the patient's tolerance to pain
   - if disseminated bone pain, consider hypercalcaemia which lowers pain threshold
   - a new pain may have developed
   - vomiting preventing drug absorption
   - poor compliance of medication

Common types of pain

Visceral pain

Tumour infiltration of the viscera causes a constant dull pain, poorly localised, that usually responds very well to opioids.

Liver pain may also be due to stretching of the liver capsule. Dexamethasone 4-6mg o.d. often helps the pain.

Raised intracranial pressure pain is due to stretching of the meninges and may respond well to dexamethasone.

Pancreatic malignancy may produce pain unrelieved by opioids, due to retroperitoneal nerve involvement. A coeliac plexus block has a high success rate.[379-381]

Bone pain
Often described like 'toothache', bone pain is usually well localised, and local tenderness may be elicited. ⇨ *Bone pain (p.58)*

Musculo-skeletal pains
Commonly occur due to general debility. NSAIDs are often successful but a strong opioid may be needed as well.

Soft tissue involvement
(e.g. chest wall involvement in breast or lung cancer)
Dexamethasone may be more effective than a NSAID[382] (usually in combination with an opioid). Consider radiotherapy referral.

Infection
Pain from cellulitis or deep pelvic infection is best treated with an antibiotic if appropriate. NSAIDs may also be helpful.

Smooth muscle colic
Opioids often ineffective. ⇨ *Intestinal and Biliary colic (p.27 & 28)*, and *Bladder spasms (p.137)*

Nerve pain (Neuropathic pain)
Often but not always associated with sensory changes.
Many are at least partially responsive to opioids, which should be titrated first. ⇨ *Neuropathic pain (p.51)*

Odynophagia (painful dysphagia)
Causes include painful mouth *(p.43)*, radiotherapy-induced oesophagitis, candidiasis *(p.44,120)*, acid reflux *(p.16)* and oesophageal spasm. Pain from oesophageal spasm may respond to nifedipine *(p.37)* or glyceryl trinitrate.[383]

Ischaemic pain
When surgery is inappropriate for ischaemic pain from a gangrenous foot, pain relief can be difficult. Spinal analgesia with an opioid and local anaesthetic is probably the treatment of choice. It may not always be possible. Alternatives to consider include liberal use of local anaesthetic (e.g. Emla cream) smothered over the affected part, or a local anaesthetic subcutaneous infusion *(p.84)*. Ketamine and methadone (as described under *Neuropathic pain p.51*) may be helpful.

Episodic pain
Pain that varies significantly with time may be:
- 'end-of-dose' pain requiring a review of analgesic dose or regimen
- pleuritic pain (NSAID, corticosteroid, antibiotic, intercostal nerve block, interpleural anaesthetic infusion)
- pain on movement from bone disease *(p.58)* or nerve compression *(p.51)*
  – pain on movement may respond better to NSAIDs than opioids[384]
- skin hypersensitisation - neuropathic *(p.51)* or inflammatory
- pain related to dressing changes or procedures
  – *Entonox* (nitrous oxide) may be helpful for predictable pain e.g. dressing changes or procedures

PRESCRIBING STATUS
☼ Corticosteroids, Nifedipine or GTN for oesophageal spasm •

ThinkList

- regional anaesthesia techniques, including:
  - intercostal nerve block for chest wall & rib pain
  - continuous brachial plexus blockade[385]
  - interpleural bupivacaine[386-388]
- octreotide••• has been reported helping pancreatic cancer pain[389]
- embolisation of painful bone metastases[390]
- thorascopic sympathectomy for pancreatic pan, as an alternative approach to coeliac plexus block[391]
- complementary methods of pain control[56] including TENS[392] and acupuncture[393]

SEE ALSO

⇨ *Dyspepsia (p.16), Painful mouth & stomatitis (p.43), Tenesmus (p.41)*
⇨ *Skeletal muscle spasm (p.112) and Leg cramps (p.113)*
⇨ *Malignant ulcers & pressure sores (p.161)*
📖 SIGN Guidelines (recommended)[377]
📖 Guidelines[394-396] & Reviews[397] - nerve blocks[398]

Neuropathic pain

Up to 40% of cancer-related pain may have a neuropathic mechanism involved.[399] Neuropathic pain may be difficult to control. A wide variety of treatments may be needed:

1st line	2nd line
Opioids **NSAIDs** **TENS** Radiotherapy Corticosteroids Antidepressants (tricyclic) Anticonvulsants	Ketamine Spinal (epidural & intrathecal) Methadone Lidocaine infusion Mexiletine Flecainide Neurolytic procedures e.g. coeliac plexus block, cordotomy Capsaicin

1st line management

- Some patients with mild to moderate neuropathic pain may respond to paracetamol and weak opioid analgesics.
- Consider radiotherapy for all cancer-related neuropathic pain.
- TENS (or acupuncture) may help neuropathic pain, and can be used as an adjunct at any stage.
- Consider a coeliac plexus block for pancreatic pain (80% success rate).
1) Strong opioid analgesic titrated to maximal tolerated dose.
2) Dexamethasone 8mg o.d. - trial for 3-5 days.
3) NSAID - trial for 3-5 days.
4) Amitriptyline 25mg nocte - trial for 5 days.
5) Gabapentin day 1 - 300mg, day 2 - 300mg b.d., day 3 - 300mg t.d.s.
    – wait 2-3 days then titrate further to maximum 1800-2400mg/day if some response

Notes

- If pain is very severe and/or prognosis short, consider moving on to 2nd line treatment which can act rapidly e.g. ketamine or spinal analgesia, after step 2 (opioids and corticosteroid).
- If chronic non-malignant neuropathic pain with no active tissue damage occurring e.g. thoracotomy scar pain:
  - there is little evidence that corticosteroids or NSAIDs[400] help
  - antidepressants and anticonvulsants may be used first-line
  - opioids are increasingly being used, but usually after other options
- Stop each drug after a trial period if there is no clear response so that the patient does not end up on unnecessary medication; the exception to this is that many people add the anticonvulsant to the antidepressant even in the absence of a response to antidepressant alone, in the belief that there is synergy between the two.
- For most cancer patients, it is appropriate to use each drug for a fixed trial period and move on to another option fairly rapidly to avoid wasting time and losing confidence.
- Longer trial periods (e.g. increasing doses of antidepressants or trying alternative opioids or anticonvulsants) are appropriate for patients with longer prognosis or milder pain.

Opioid analgesics

Opioids are effective in both cancer-related and non-malignant neuropathic pain.[401-404] Opioids other than morphine/diamorphine have been shown to be effective including tramadol,[405,406] fentanyl,[407,408] and oxycodone.[409]

Opioids are used first-line in cancer-related neuropathic pain as:

- many patients will have a different, co-existing nociceptive pain
- there may be a nociceptive element of the pain when tumour is causing nerve damage
- opioids alone may control a third of neuropathic pain, and partially control a further third [410]

If the pain seems to be resistant to first-line opioid:

- an alternative opioid analgesic may be tried for better tolerance (p.71)
- psychostimulants can be given to counteract sedative side-effects
- ⇨ Morphine-resistant pain (p.68)
- move on to the next step

Methadone can be considered different from the other opioids with respect to neuropathic pain; it can either be tried as an alternative to a first-line opioid, or introduced later, when other options have failed (p.81).

Corticosteroids

Corticosteroids (usually dexamethasone) may help cancer-related neuropathic pain, either by reducing inflammatory sensitisation of the nerves, or by reducing pressure on nerves caused by oedema. A high initial dose is used to achieve rapid results (dexamethasone 8mg/day will work in 1-3 days); the dose should then be rapidly reduced to the minimum that maintains benefit. Although long-term corticosteroids may be best avoided, they can sometimes buy useful time whilst allowing other methods (e.g. radiotherapy or antidepressants) time to work.

NSAIDs

NSAIDs are sometimes effective in cancer-related neuropathic pain, either because there is mixed nociceptive pain or because they reduce inflammatory sensitisation of the nerves.[411,412]

Antidepressants

Amitriptyline has been used most commonly, but many tricyclic antidepressants have been shown to have similar efficacy.[413] The doses needed for neuropathic pain may be lower, and speed of onset faster (1-7 days) than for depression.[413-415]

SSRIs have been used successfully, but are probably less effective than tricyclic antidepressants, and in some studies no better than placebo.[404,413]

Newer antidepressants are being used, including venlafaxine,[416] but their role is as yet unclear. Mirtazapine is a noradrenergic and specific serotonergic antidepressant (NaSSA);[417,418] there are a few reports of its use in neuropathic pain.[419,420]

Note that amitriptyline can increase the bioavailability of morphine[421,422] leading to opioid side-effects.

- Start with amitriptyline 25mg nocte.
- If no response by day 5, either increase dose or move on to try an anticonvulsant:
  - some patients do not see benefit until after 4-6 weeks of treatment, and/or doses of up to 100-150mg/day
  - severity of pain and the patient's prognosis will dictate how long to persevere with antidepressants
  - many patients do not tolerate amitriptyline especially in higher doses,[423] therefore consider changing to dosulepin (dothiepin) or lofepramine if increasing dose
- Use lofepramine for frail, elderly, or those already with antimuscarinic side effects from other drugs:
  - start at 70mg nocte
  - may increase to 70mg b.d. on day 5-7

Anticonvulsants

Anticonvulsants have for a long time been considered better than tricyclic antidepressants for lancinating or paroxysmal pain, but evidence from studies does not support this.[424]

There is little to choose overall between antidepressants and anticonvulsants for neuropathic pain in terms of efficacy or adverse-effects.[404,425]

A number of different anticonvulsants have been successfully used, including: gabapentin, carbamazepine, sodium valproate, phenytoin, and clonazepam. There is little data to compare anticonvulsants in terms of efficacy[424], although in one trial comparing the efficacy of different anticonvulsants for lancinating pain, the results suggested Clonazepam > Phenytoin > Valproate > Carbamazepine.[426]

Carbamazepine has been used most extensively, but is often tolerated poorly by elderly, frail or ill patients, and has numerous drug interactions. Valproate has therefore been recommended by many in palliative care, but there is little data on its efficacy.[427] Clonazepam has been used in cancer-related pain[428] and has an advantage of being usable by CSCI. Lamotrigine has had mixed results[429-431] Topiramate is under investigation for neuropathic pain; it acts on AMPA receptors.[432-435]

Gabapentin[436] is the only drug licensed for all types of neuropathic pain. Trials have shown it effective in non-malignant and cancer-related pain.[437-444] It appears to be well tolerated in palliative care patients. Doses up to 2400mg/day have been used successfully (with a few studies up to 3600mg/day).[437,438,441]

Unlike the antidepressants, anticonvulsants are pharmacologically diverse in their actions, and there is good theoretical reason to try alternative anticonvulsants if one is ineffective.

All anticonvulsants are used in their typical 'anticonvulsant' doses'.

- Start with gabapentin: day 1 - 300mg nocte, day 2 - 300mg b.d., day 3 - 300mg t.d.s.
- If no response by day 5, either increase dose in 300mg increments every few days (maximum 1800-2400mg/day), use an alternative anticonvulsant, or move on to another method:
  - some patients do not see full benefit from anticonvulsants until after 4-6 weeks of treatment
  - severity of pain and the patient's prognosis will dictate how long to persevere with gabapentin, or with anticonvulsants in general

2nd line management

- ketamine *(p.83)*
- methadone *(p.81)*
- spinal injection or catheter
  - caudal injection of steroid and local anaesthetic[445]
- local anaesthetic by sc infusion *(p.84)*
- flecainide or mexiletine (see below)
- neurolytic blocks
  - coeliac plexus block for pancreatic pain[379-381]
  - cordotomy for unilateral pain, especially from mesothelioma[446,447]
- return to untried options from 1st line management e.g. alternative anticonvulsants

Numerous other methods have been used to help neuropathic pain, but there is no comparative data from which to recommend optimal management. Factors such as patient characteristics and preferences, and availability of local resources (e.g. anaesthetists) will guide decisions.

	Notes
Ketamine	Drug not routinely available in community. Easier to initiate as in-patient. Can be used orally or by CSCI.
Methadone	Complicated to manage dose titration, especially in the community. Risks of accumulation and overdose. Easier and safer to initiate as in-patient. Parenteral route not used routinely (irritant sc).
Spinal injection or catheter & neurolytic blocks	In-patient. Rapid onset of effect. Dependent on local availability of necessary skills. Single injection sometimes gives lasting effect. Indwelling catheter carries risk of complications, and complicated to arrange continuing care in community.
Local anaesthetic by sc infusion	Easier and safer to initiate as in-patient, as requires close monitoring for side effects. Requires CSCI, unless converted to flecainide or mexiletine
Flecainide or mexiletine	Risks of cardiac arrhythmias need careful assessment versus potential benefits. Mexiletine poorly tolerated - flecainide better? Can be initiated as outpatient. Delayed onset of effect

Local anaesthetics, flecainide & mexiletine

Infusions of lidocaine (lignocaine) have been shown to be effective in
neuropathic pain, and have been used long-term over many weeks. *(p.84)*
As a continuous infusion is not always acceptable, oral drugs with similar
sodium-channel blocking properties have been used (flecainide and
mexiletine).

A positive response to lidocaine infusion may predict a response to
mexiletine,[448] and possibly therefore flecainide.

Mexiletine

Mexiletine reduces neuropathic pain in doses between 250-625mg/day, but
the reduction in pain may not be clinically very great. Minor side effects mean
that it is not very well tolerated. Serious cardiac arrhythmias have not been
reported in patients receiving mexiletine for painful diabetic neuropathy;
however, transient tachycardia and palpitations have been reported. There are
significant differences in the metabolism of mexiletine between people who
have different cytochrome P450 CYP2D6 isoenzymes.[415,449,450]

One study identified that stabbing or burning pain, heat sensations, or
formication may benefit most by mexiletine therapy.[451]

- Start with mexiletine 100-200mg/day.
- Increase dose slowly.
- Contraindicated with 2nd and 3rd degree heart block or any cardiac
  arrhythmias.
- Avoid using concurrently with drugs that affect cardiac conduction e.g.
  tricyclic antidepressants.
- An ECG before and during dose titration should ideally be performed.

Flecainide

Flecainide has been used as an alternative in cancer patients, and may be
better tolerated, but there is little evidence supporting its use.[452,453] It has been
used rectally.[454]

- Start with flecainide 100mg b.d.
- Flecainide has a long half-life; if effective, try to reduce the dose after 5-7
  days to 50mg b.d.
- Use reduced doses in renal failure (accumulation of the drug).
- Contraindicated with 2nd and 3rd degree heart block or any cardiac
  arrhythmias.
- Avoid using concurrently with drugs that affect cardiac conduction e.g.
  tricyclic antidepressants.
- An ECG before use should ideally be performed.

PRESCRIBING STATUS

- ☼ Amitriptyline and other tricyclic antidepressants ●
- ☼ Sodium valproate ●
- ☼ Carbamazepine and phenytoin ●
- ☼ Corticosteroids ●
- ☼ SSRIs, Ketamine ●●
- ☼ Methadone ○○○
- ☼ Flecainide, Mexiletine, Lidocaine CSCI, Clonidine ●●●

Think List

- hypomagnesaemia should be corrected (see additional notes below)
- *Opsite* has been applied to the skin of painful diabetic peripheral neuropathy with success;[455] *Opsite* spray has also been used
- baclofen •• [456-460] - may specifically help paroxysmal pain; up to 60mg daily used
- levomepromazine •• (methotrimeprazine) appears to have intrinsic analgesic activity;[461] the sedative/anxiolytic effect may also benefit distressed patients
- amantadine ••• 200mg/24h IV, then 100mg o.d. for 2 weeks – duration of relief 6 months[462-464]
- doxepin cream (topical) ••• [465]
- clonidine ••• - used extensively in spinal infusions (cf); given systemically its tolerance is limited by hypotension and sedation - 25µg t.d.s. increasing to 100 µg t.d.s.;[466-468] transdermal patch 0.3mg/day[469] has been effective, in one study selectively helping those with sympathetically maintained pain[470]; IV infusion helped post-operative pain but caused more sedation than epidural use[471]; other studies show no benefit[472]
- capsaicin cream ••• has proved useful in neuropathic pain,[473] especially post herpetic neuralgia; the application of the cream can itself cause stinging, this can be relieved by the use of *Emla* cream applied prior to the capsaicin
- dextromethorphan ••• has been reported to successfully relieve neuropathic pain in doses up to 400mg/day;[404] other studies using up to 90mg/day have shown no benefit[474,475]
- cannabinoids ••• are no more effective than codeine for most pain, but may have a place in neuropathic pain, or pain associated with muscle spasm[476,477] ⇨ *(p.180)*

SEE ALSO
⇨ *Alternative strong opioids (p.71), Methadone (p.81), Ketamine (p.83)*
⇨ *Local anaesthetic infusions (p.84), Corticosteroids (p.126)*
📖 Reviews[404,415,435,478-485] & Systematic reviews[413,424,425,486]

Drugs used for Neuropathic Pain
ANTIDEPRESSANT DRUGS
Tricyclic antidepressants used concomitantly with amiodarone increase the risk of ventricular arrhythmias and should be avoided. The low doses of TCA's used for neuropathic pain probably carry a low risk.

AMITRIPTYLINE ☑
    Tabs. 10mg, 25mg, 50mg; Syrup 25mg/5mL, 50mg/5mL
    TSD: 25mg nocte PO
DOSULEPIN (DOTHIEPIN)
    Caps. 25mg; Tabs. 75mg *(Prothiaden)*
    TSD: 25mg nocte PO
LOFEPRAMINE
    Tabs. 70mg; Susp. 70mg/5mL
    TSD: 70mg nocte PO
DOXEPIN
    Cream 5% 30g
    TSD: Apply t.d.s to q.d.s., maximum 12g daily

ANTICONVULSANT DRUGS

GABAPENTIN ☑

Caps. 100mg, 300mg, 400mg; Tabs. 600mg[○] 800mg[○]

*TSD: Day 1 - 300mg nocte, day 2 - 300mg b.d., day 3 - 300mg t.d.s. **PO**
(£44.52 at 300mg t.d.s.)*

Usual maintenance: 0.9-1.2g/24h. Maximum recommended dose 1.8g/24h, but doses up to 2.4g/24h (and even higher) have been used[437,438,441]

SODIUM VALPROATE

Tabs. 200mg, 500mg; Syrup 200mg/5mL

*TSD: 200mg t.d.s. **PO** or 500mg nocte **PO** (£8.23 at 500mg b.d.)*

Increase 200mg/day at 3-day intervals. Usual maintenance 1-2g/24h. Max. 2.5g/24h in divided doses. Suppositories are available as special orders.

CARBAMAZEPINE

Tabs. 100mg, 200mg, 400mg; Liquid 100mg/5mL; Supps. 125mg, 250mg

*TSD: 100mg b.d. **PO** (£5.90 at 400mg b.d.)*

Increase from initial dose by increments of 200mg every week. Usual maintenance dose 0.8-1.2 g/24h in two divided doses. Max. 1.6-2 g/24h. Equivalent rectal dosage: 125mg **PR** ≅ 100mg **PO**

Carbamazepine levels are increased (risk of toxicity) by dextropropoxyphene[487,488] (co-proxamol), clarithromycin, erythromycin, fluoxetine, fluvoxamine.

CLONAZEPAM

Tabs. 500µg, 2mg
Inj. 1mg/1mL

TSD: 1mg nocte for 4 nights (£3.14 at 2mg b.d.)

Increase gradually to usual maintenance dose 4-8mg/24h. Oral solutions in various strengths are available from several sources.

ANTI-ARRHYTHMIC DRUGS

FLECAINIDE ☑

Tabs. 50,100mg; Liquid 25mg/5mL

*TSD: 100mg b.d. **PO***

Flecainide used concomitantly with amiodarone increase the risk of ventricular arrhythmias and should be avoided. Flecainide blood levels (and risk of toxicity) increased by fluoxetine, tricyclic antidepressants, and quinine.

MEXILETINE[○]

Caps. 50mg, 200mg

*TSD: 100mg b.d. **PO***

OTHER DRUGS FOR NEUROPATHIC PAIN

AMANTADINE

Caps. 100mg; Syrup 50mg/5mL; Inj.‡

*TSD: 100mg o.d. **PO** (£7.68)*

CAPSAICIN

Cream 0.075% 45g *(Axsain)*

TSD: Apply topically 3-4 times daily (£15.04 - 45g)

CLONIDINE[○]

Tabs. 25µg *(Dixarit)*; Tabs. 100µg, 300µg; Caps. **SR** 250µg *(Catapres)*

*TSD: Neuropathic pain 25µg t.d.s. **PO** increasing to 100 µg t.d.s.*

BACLOFEN

Tabs. 10mg; Liquid 5mg/5mL

*TSD: 5mg t.d.s. **PO***

Additional Information

NMDA receptor

The NMDA receptor is thought to be involved in the development of the 'wind-up' phenomenon of neuropathic pain. Ketamine, dextromethorphan, and amantadine are all NMDA antagonists[489,490] which may explain their benefit on neuropathic pain.

The site of action of opioid analgesics is closely related to the NMDA receptor, and anecdotal reports suggest that opioid analgesics may be needed for NMDA receptor antagonists to work.

Magnesium is also required for the normal function of the NMDA receptor. An IV infusion of 0.5g-1g magnesium relieved neuropathic pain in > 50% cancer patients for up to 4h;[491] although this offers no practical therapeutic option, it may demonstrate the importance of correcting hypomagnesaemia.

Efficacy of drugs for neuropathic pain (NNT)[404,425]

	Diabetic neuropathy	Postherpetic neuralgia
Oxycodone		2.5
Tramadol	3.4	
Tricyclic antidepressants	2.4	2.3
SSRIs	6.7	
All antidepressants	3.4	2.1
Carbamazepine	3.3	
Gabapentin	3.7	3.2
All anticonvulsants	2.7	3.2
Mexiletine	10.0	
Baclofen	1.4	
Capsaicin	5.9	5.3

(NNT is the number of patients needed to treat in order to see a response in one patient who would not have responded to placebo.)

Bone pain

1) Radiotherapy is usually effective for pain from bone metastases
2) NSAID e.g. diclofenac 50mg t.d.s.
3) Strong opioids (morphine)
4) Corticosteroids
5) Bisphosphonates

Bisphosphonates & Bone Pain

Bisphosphonates have a role in a long-term strategy to reduce skeletal complications, including pain, from bone metastases.

Bisphosphonates may also have a role in the 'acute' management of metastatic bone pain:

Indications
- pain from bone metastases of any origin, where treatment with conventional analgesics, radiotherapy or surgery is unsuccessful or inappropriate

Treatment
- pamidronate 90mg IV infusion
  - dilute to 500mL 0.9% N saline (minimum 375mL)
  - infuse over 2-4hr (minimum 1½hr, or 4½hr in renal failure)
- alternative - clodronate IV infusion 1500mg

Follow-up

- analgesic effect should be expected within 14 days[492,493]

If pain responds fully:

- re-treatment with same regimen is appropriate if and when pain recurs
- analgesic response should be expected to last 4-8 weeks.

In patients who do not respond to first dose:

- treatment may be repeated after 2 weeks
- lack of response after two treatments makes further treatment inappropriate

If pain responds partially to one or two treatments:

- consider regular pamidronate 90mg IV every 4 weeks

PRESCRIBING STATUS

✵ Bisphosphonates ●●

Think List

- strontium[90] is effective against pain from multiple bony sites, but may take 12 weeks to have full effect; hemi-body irradiation is an alternative for multiple-site pain[494,495]
- local infiltration or intra-lesional injection with depot corticosteroid ± local anaesthetic[496]
- surgical fixation of unstable bone weakness
- spinal injection or infusion
- calcitonin 200u q.d.s. SC (licensed use) or 800u/24h by CSCI;●● [497] CSCI may reduce side effects of nausea & vomiting, and stinging at SC injection sites; discontinue after 48h, repeat as necessary
- injection of acrylic cement percutaneously into unstable fractures of pelvis or vertebrae[498-507]
- alcohol injection (percutaneous CT-guided into bone metastases)[508]
- bone pain in prostate cancer may be helped by Vitamin D ●●● [509]

SEE ALSO

⇨ *Bisphosphonates (p.141)*

📖 Guidelines[492,510] & Reviews[511]

Drugs for Bone Pain

DISODIUM PAMIDRONATE ☑

Inj. 15mg, 30mg ⊘ 90mg (dry powder for reconstitution)
TSD: See relevant sections (90mg £155.80)

SODIUM CLODRONATE

Inj. 300mg/5mL ⊘ 300mg/10mL
TSD: See relevant sections (1500mg £68.90)
Caps. 400mg ⊘ 520mg *(Loron)* ⊘ Tabs. 800mg
TSD: 800mg or 520mg b.d. PO (£162.55)

CALCITONIN (SALMON)

CSCI may reduce side effects of nausea & vomiting, and stinging at SC injection sites[497]

Inj. 100u/1mL ⊘ 400u/2mL
TSD: 200u q.d.s. SC, or 800u/24h CSCI (for 2 days £102.48)

Additional Information

A Cochrane Library review is in preparation on bisphosphonates as analgesics for bone pain.

Although it is a commonly held belief, there is no convincing evidence from studies that NSAIDs are better than opioids for bone pain[512,513]

Calcitonin has been shown to be helpful in pain from osteoporotic vertebral fractures[514] 50-100IU daily for 4 weeks either SC or intra-nasal.

In a number of the studies on bisphosphonates, patients had not previously been treated with radiotherapy, NSAIDs or opioid analgesics, and persistent bone pain was investigated rather than incident pain on movement.[515-517] Any expected benefit from bisphosphonates may be influenced by these factors.

Paracetamol & Weak Opioids

Codeine
5-10% Caucasians are CYP2D6 poor-metabolisers, an hepatic enzyme necessary to convert codeine to morphine. These patients will not obtain equivalent analgesia using codeine-containing analgesics.[518-520] This bioactivation is markedly inhibited by antipsychotics (chlorpromazine, haloperidol, levomepromazine, and thioridazine), metoclopramide, and tricyclic antidepressants (amitriptyline etc.).[521] If hepatic metabolism is decreased in patients taking these drugs, or with liver disease, the analgesic action of codeine may also be compromised.[522]

Co-proxamol
Systematic reviews suggest that co-proxamol is no more effective as an analgesic than paracetamol.[523] However this view has been challenged on the basis that most studies are on single dose administration, and not for cancer-related pain.[524] Dextropropoxyphene has a longer elimination half-life than paracetamol and will therefore accumulate to higher blood levels during repeated dosing.[525] It also has other effects such as NMDA-receptor antagonism[489,526] which may be relevant to some cancer-related pain.

SEE ALSO
📖 Reviews[527] & Systematic review[523,528]

Paracetamol & weak opioids
Compound analgesics containing sub-therapeutic doses of opioids should not be used for pain control in cancer patients.[377]

PARACETAMOL ☑
   Tabs. 500mg; Tabs. sol. 500mg
   TSD: 2 tabs. q.d.s. PO
   Paracetamol may affect warfarin anticoagulation.[529-535]

CO-CODAMOL 30/500 ☑
   Caps. *(Kapake/Tylex)*; Tabs. sol. *(Solpadol)* (Codeine 30mg, Paracetamol 500mg)
   TSD: 2 tabs. q.d.s. PO

CO-CODAMOL (8/500)
   Tabs.; Tabs. disp. (Codeine 8mg + Paracetamol 500mg)
   TSD: 2 tabs. q.d.s. PO

CO-PROXAMOL
   Tabs. (Dextropropoxyphene 32.5mg + Paracetamol 325mg)
   TSD: 2 tabs. q.d.s. PO
   Dextropropoxyphene (in co-proxamol) increases blood levels of carbamazepine up to 6-fold[487,488] ***(risk of toxicity). Also enhances anticoagulation effect of warfarin.***

CODEINE ☑
   Tabs. 15, 30, 60mg; Linctus 15mg/5mL; Syrup 25mg/5mL
   TSD: 30mg q.d.s. PO

NSAIDs

Non-steroidal anti-inflammatory drugs (NSAIDs) are helpful in treating cancer pain[513,536] especially associated with inflammation e.g. bone metastases or soft tissue infiltration by cancer. They may also help in neuropathic pain associated with cancer.[411,412]

Prescribing an NSAID

- Always consider whether an alternative method of analgesia is suitable, especially when risk factors are present.
- Use NSAID with lower risk of GI toxicity e.g. diclofenac 50mg t.d.s.
- Prescribe a gastro-protective drug prophylactically e.g. lansoprazole 15mg o.d. if at least one other risk factor present *(p.16)*:
  - past history of peptic ulcer disease
  - co-administration of corticosteroids, anticoagulants or aspirin
  - advanced age - over 70 years (optional - use judgement)

Gastrointestinal toxicity

Lower	Ibuprofen
	Diclofenac
	Naproxen
Higher	Piroxicam
	Indometacin
	Ketorolac

Specific issues with prescribing NSAIDs

Problem	Solution
Symptoms of dyspepsia, or has recently been treated for ulcer/dyspepsia	Add PPI *(p.16)* If symptoms persist with PPI → increase PPI to treatment dose If symptoms still persist change NSAID to a COX-2 inhibitor
Symptomatic thrombocytopenia, or platelet count < 20	Use a COX-2 inhibitor
Co-administering warfarin	Ibuprofen, diclofenac and naproxen do not normally have a clinically significant interaction with warfarin.[537] INR should nevertheless be monitored carefully, for if GI bleeding does occur it may be severe. Other NSAIDs, including the COX-2 inhibitors, may potentiate the effect of warfarin.
Renal failure or poorly controlled cardiac failure	There is no evidence that any NSAIDs such as sulindac,[538] or the COX-2 inhibitors are safer in impaired renal function.[539-541] All should be avoided if possible, balancing the risks with benefit for the individual.
History of asthma or bronchospasm	CSM data suggests COX-2 inhibitor cross-reactivity to aspirin may be low,[2] but more studies are needed to estimate the safety in asthma/bronchospasm. All NSAIDs should be avoided if possible.

Problem	Solution
Taking low-dose aspirin as prophylaxis for MI or TIAs	Most NSAIDs give a comparable effect on platelets to aspirin.[542] Unlike aspirin, NSAIDs' effect on platelet function is reversible, and waxes and wanes with blood levels of the drug. Therefore they may be less effective at prevention than aspirin (no trials have compared).
	Aspirin should be continued in patients when starting an NSAID, unless prognosis is short and there are other risk factors for GI bleeding, or the burden of medication is too great for the patient.
Unable to swallow medication	Ketorolac may be used by CSCI - see notes below. Naproxen and diclofenac have both been used by CSCI,[543-545] but do not mix well with other drugs, and probably carry a higher chance of site inflammation.
	Suppositories may be used.

In all cases: consider whether use of an NSAID can be avoided.

Ketorolac

Ketorolac is a potent analgesic NSAID with relatively little anti-inflammatory action. It is licensed for post-operative short-term use only. In high doses of 60-90mg/24h there is a high risk of GI toxicity and licensed use is restricted to 48h. In one study with 60-120mg/day, 11% patients had a gastrointestinal bleed, despite being on misoprostol.[546] It has been used by CSCI for cancer pain of various kinds for longer periods when the benefit is seen to outweigh the risk. Lower doses of 30-40mg/day probably have a similar tolerability to other NSAIDs.[411,547-565]

Indications
- severe cancer pain unresponsive to opioids and standard NSAID, especially bone pain:
  - ketorolac 60mg/24h CSCI
  - review after 48h and document clearly if ketorolac is to be continued; add PPI for prophylaxis e.g. lansoprazole 15mg o.d.
  - increase to maximum dose 90mg/24h if partially effective
  - reduce if possible to 30mg/24h
- starting or continuing an NSAID in a patient who cannot take PO medication:
  - ketorolac 30mg/24h CSCI
  - convert to usual NSAID by oral route as soon as possible

Topical NSAIDs

Topical NSAIDs are more effective than placebo for musculo-skeletal pain.[566] They may be useful in selective cases of superficial inflammatory pain in patients who cannot take oral NSAIDs, e.g. chest wall tumour infiltration.

SEE ALSO
⇨ Dyspepsia (p.16), Pain control (p.49)
📖 Reviews[512,567] COX-2[19,568,569] NICE guidelines[570]

NSAID Drug Preparations

Diclofenac and naproxen have similar efficacy and tolerability in treating cancer pain.[571] Ibuprofen is less potent than diclofenac or naproxen, but also carries a lower risk of GI toxicity. Indometacin is more potent anti-inflammatory, but has a higher incidence of both GI toxicity and side effects such as confusion.

Although it has been common practice, there is no evidence to support the view that changing from one class of NSAID to another will achieve any better results, unless changing to a more potent NSAID e.g. indometacin or ketorolac.

See below for COX-2 inhibitors.

DICLOFENAC ☑

Tabs. 25, 50mg; Tabs. disp. 50mg
TSD: 50mg t.d.s. PO (£6.13, disp. £20.60)
Tabs. SR 75mg, (Voltarol 75mg SR) Tabs. SR 100mg (Voltarol Retard)
TSD: 75mg b.d. PR (£17.35) or 100mg o.d. PR (£12.72)
Supps. 50mg, 100mg
TSD: 100mg o.d. PR
Inj. 75mg/3mL
TSD: 75mg SC stat.

DICLOFENAC WITH MISOPROSTOL

Tabs. 50mg/200µg (Arthrotec 50); Tabs. 75mg/200µg (Arthrotec 75)
TSD: Arthrotec 50 1 tab. t.d.s. PO (£18.63)

NAPROXEN

Tabs. 250mg, 500mg; Susp. 125mg/5mL; Supps. 500mg
TSD: 500mg b.d. PO (£8.12, Susp. £17.03); 500mg b.d. PR

IBUPROFEN

Tabs. 200, 400, 600mg; Syrup 100mg/5mL
TSD: 400mg t.d.s. PO

INDOMETACIN (INDOMETHACIN)

Caps. 25mg, 50mg; Susp. 25mg/5mL; Supps. 100mg
TSD: 50mg t.d.s. PO; 100mg nocte PR
Caps. SR 75mg (Flexin Continus)
TSD: 75mg b.d. PO
Indometacin given with haloperidol can cause severe drowsiness.

KETOROLAC

Inj. 10mg/1mL, 30mg/1mL ☑
TSD: 30 or 60mg/24h CSCI
See notes above. Risk of GI bleeding is high when used for >48h.

NSAIDS - SELECTIVE COX-2 INHIBITORS

Clinical studies show a lower rate of GI toxicity with selective COX-2 inhibitors than other NSAIDs, although this effect is lost if aspirin is co-prescribed.[572] However they are not entirely free of GI side-effects, and the same precautions should be taken when prescribing COX-2 inhibitors as for NSAIDs generally, regarding contraindications and side effects. They appear to have no effect on platelet function.[573] There is evidence that COX-1 contributes to inflammation and pain, so selective inhibition of COX-2 will not necessarily produce the same degree of analgesic efficacy that is seen with mixed inhibitors of COX-1 and COX-2.[574] Rofecoxib is the most selective COX-2 inhibitor available, significantly more so than meloxicam and celecoxib: rofecoxib > etodolac > meloxicam > celecoxib.[575]

ROFECOXIB ☑

Licensed for pain and inflammation in osteoarthritis. Max. dose 25mg o.d.
Tabs. 12.5mg, 25mg; Susp 12.5mg/5mL, 25mg/5mL (Vioxx)
TSD: 12.5mg o.d. PO (£21.58 tabs. or susp.)

CELECOXIB ○

Licensed for pain and inflammation in osteoarthritis and rheumatoid arthritis.
Caps. 100mg, 200mg (Celebrex)
TSD: 100mg b.d. PO (£17.12) Max. dose 200mg b.d.
Plasma levels increased by fluconazole[349] – halve celecoxib dose.

TOPICAL NSAIDS

ALGESAL
Gel, (diethylamine salicylate) 50g
TSD: Apply 3 times daily (50g £0.75)

BALMOSA
Gel, (camphor, capsicum oleoresin, menthol, methyl salicylate) 40g
TSD: Apply 3 times daily (40g £0.88)

INTRALGIN
Gel, (benzocaine, salicylamide) 50g
TSD: Apply 3 times daily (50g £0.47)

IBUPROFEN
Gel, ibuprofen 5% 100g, 10% 100g
TSD: Apply 3-4 times daily (5% £5.95, 10% £6.50)

Morphine & Diamorphine

Morphine is the strong opioid of first choice for moderate to severe cancer pain. Alternative opioids may be as effective, and are appropriate for certain patients.[378] *(p.71)*

Starting a patient on morphine

- Start with normal-release morphine 2.5-10mg 4-hourly as liquid or tablets. Starting doses:
  - adult, not pain-controlled on regular weak opioids: 10mg 4-hourly morphine
  - elderly, very cachectic, or not taking regular weak opioids: 5mg 4-hourly morphine
  - very elderly and frail: 2.5mg 4-hourly morphine
- Although 4-hourly morphine gives greatest flexibility for initial dose titration, patients with less severe pain, difficulties with compliance and especially outpatients, can be started on 12-houly slow-release morphine:
  - adult not pain-controlled on regular weak opioids: 30mg 12-hourly morphine SR
  - elderly, very cachectic, or not taking regular weak opioids: 20mg 12-hourly morphine SR
  - very elderly and frail: 10mg 12-hourly morphine SR
- Always prescribe a laxative concurrently (e.g. senna & magnesium hydroxide 10mL of each o.d. - b.d.)
- Consider prescribing a regular anti-emetic for those with a history of nausea/vomiting, e.g. haloperidol 1.5mg nocte: this can usually be stopped after a week if the nausea was purely opioid-induced. If not prescribed prophylactically, warn the patient to report any sickness so that an antiemetic can be prescribed as soon as possible.
- Explain to the patient that they may feel a little drowsiness, but that this will usually wear off after a few days.
- Advise the patient that they should not drive, for at least one week after starting morphine, or after any increase in dose.

Titrating dose of morphine

- Arrange to review the patient regularly and if the pain is severe the dose can be increased twice a day. If less severe, increase every day or two as needed to minimise side effects.
- Increase the dose as needed by increments of 30% - 50% rather than by a fixed amount. The increment percentage tends to decrease a little as the dose increases e.g. 5 - 10 - 15 - 20 - 30 - 40 - 60 - 80 - 100 - 130 - 160 - 200mg. There is no pre-set maximum dose of opioids as long as increasing the dose gives further analgesia. Very few patients will require more than 600mg daily.
- Once the patient is seen to tolerate the morphine, a double dose can be given at bedtime omitting the need for a dose in the middle of the night.
- When pain is reasonably controlled consider converting to slow-release 12-hourly morphine for convenience of b.d. administration.

Converting to 12-hourly morphine

- Divide daily morphine intake by half to give 12-hourly dose (10mg elixir 4-hourly → 30mg morphine SR 12-hourly).
- Ensure the patient has access to normal-release morphine for breakthrough pain. A dose of morphine elixir of 50-100% of the 4-hourly dose equivalent may be taken for breakthrough pain.
- Increase the dose of PRN oral morphine proportionally if the dose of 12-hourly morphine is increased.
- A 'loading dose' of normal-release morphine together with the first dose of 12-hourly morphine is not required, when converting a patient who is on stable doses and is pain-controlled.[576]

Using diamorphine

Diamorphine is more soluble in water than morphine, and is commonly used as the injectable strong opioid in a syringe driver for subcutaneous infusion.
Starting doses: To convert from oral morphine, divide the 24-hourly total dose of oral morphine by 3 e.g.
10mg 4-hourly morphine elixir
≅ 60mg oral morphine total dose in 24h
≅ 20mg diamorphine by CSCI over 24h
Morphine 3mg PO ≡ Diamorphine 1mg by sc injection
Increments in dose should be between 25-50% as for morphine. Additional SC doses for 'breakthrough' pain should be 50-100% of the equivalent 4-hourly dose.

- If vomiting or no longer able to swallow medication, convert to a subcutaneous infusion of diamorphine via a syringe driver by dividing the 24-hourly total dose of oral morphine by three, as for starting dose.

Breakthrough doses

Use 50-100% of the equivalent 4-hourly dose currently being used e.g. for a patient on 270mg morphine SR 12-hourly:
≅ 540mg oral morphine in 24h
≅ 180mg diamorphine parenterally in 24h
≅ 30mg diamorphine SC 4-hourly
≅ 90mg morphine PO 4-hourly
i.e. use breakthrough doses of 15-30mg diamorphine SC 4-hourly, or 45-90mg morphine PO 4-hourly PRN

Intravenous use for pain emergencies

Various different protocols have been described for intravenous titration of opioids for severe pain 'emergencies'.[577-579]

- monitor respiratory rate and conscious level regularly
- draw up diamorphine diluted to 10mL with water
  - diamorphine 5mg if opioid naïve
  - use equivalent 4-hourly dose based on previous opioid use in last 24h (see 'Breakthrough doses' above)
- give diamorphine IV at 1mL/minute (total over 10 minutes)
- stop if pain ≤ 5/10 or toxicity develops
- repeat the above after a further 10-20 minutes if required
- calculate the total dose of diamorphine administered and multiply by 6
- start maintenance infusion with CSCI, or regular oral analgesic with the dose above given over 24h (or morphine equivalent)

SEE ALSO
⇨ *Alternative strong opioids (p.71)*
▢ EAPC Guidelines[378]

Morphine & Diamorphine preparations

Mixtures of morphine containing 10mg/5mL are not concentrated enough to fall under the prescription requirements of the Misuse of Drugs Regulations ('controlled drugs'). However, it is usual practice to manage these preparations as though they were controlled drugs.

Morphine blood levels may be increased by amitriptyline leading to opioid toxicity.[421,422] Rifampicin may reduce the analgesic efficacy of morphine, by an unexplained mechanism.[580] Metoclopramide increases the speed of onset, and sedation from modified-release morphine preparations.[581]

MORPHINE PREPARATIONS - NORMAL RELEASE (4-HOURLY)
MORPHINE (NORMAL RELEASE)
  Mixture 10mg/5mL *(Oramorph/Sevredol)*
  Mixture 20mg/mL *(Oramorph concentrated/Sevredol concentrated)*
  Tabs. 10, 20, 50mg - scored tabs. *(Sevredol)*

MORPHINE (NORMAL RELEASE) UNIT DOSE VIALS ⊘
  Vials. 10, 30, 100mg all in individual 5mL vials *(Oramorph Unit Dose Vials)*

MORPHINE PREPARATIONS - SLOW RELEASE (12-HOURLY)
MST and *Zomorph* can be used interchangeably.[582]
MST CONTINUS (MORPHINE SR)
  Tabs. **SR** 5, 10, 15, 30, 60, 100, 200mg
  Susp. 20, 30, 60, 100, 200mg
  Sachets to prepare suspension
ZOMORPH CAPSULES (MORPHINE SR)
  Caps. **SR** 10, 30, 60, 100, 200mg
  Can be broken and administered via a **NG/PEG** tube, or sprinkled on food.
      Bioequivalent to *MST* [582]

MORPHINE PREPARATIONS - SLOW RELEASE (24-HOURLY)
MXL (MORPHINE SR) ⊘
  Caps. **SR** 30, 60, 90, 120, 150, 200mg
MORCAP SR (MORPHINE SR) ⊘
  Caps. **SR** 20, 50, 100mg
  May not be bioequivalent to MST

MORPHINE PREPARATIONS - RECTAL (4-HOURLY)
MORPHINE SUPPOSITORIES
  Supps. 10mg⊘ 15mg⊘ 20mg, 30mg
  Equianalgesic dose by oral and rectal routes is the same[378]

MORPHINE PREPARATIONS - RECTAL (24-HOURLY)
MORAXEN (MORPHINE SR RECTAL TAMPONS) ⊘
  Rectal tampons 35mg, 50mg, 75mg, 100mg
  Up to 2 tampons can be inserted at one time. Should be removed and replaced
      after 24h, or replaced after defecation immediately. [583,584] Equianalgesic
      dose by oral and rectal routes is the same[378]

DIAMORPHINE
DIAMORPHINE
  Inj. 5mg, 10mg, 30mg, 100mg, 500mg

Morphine-resistant pain

Pain that cannot be adequately controlled by morphine, may present a
number of clinical pictures:

The pain responds to opioids, but side-effects limit the dose of morphine
The patient reports improvement in pain with each dose increment, but side-
effects become unacceptable.
- Ensure dose is carefully titrated ('fine-tuned') to maximise analgesia and
  minimise side-effects.
- ⇨ *Opioid side effects & toxicity (p.69)* for further management.

The pain is unresponsive to increasing doses of morphine
Some pain types (typically some neuropathic pain) may not be controlled by
morphine alone. Typically the patient will report that the last increment of the
morphine dose did not help the pain, or only helped by causing drowsiness.
- Consider a second dose increment if no side effects, to ensure that the
  patient is not merely under-dosed.
- Stop (if no response to starting opioid), or reduce opioid back to previous
  dose.
- Try an alternative analgesic method e.g. co-analgesics.
- For further details ⇨ *Neuropathic pain (p.51), Bone pain (p.58),* and
  Pain control (p.49).
- Methadone may be considered an alternative method for neuropathic,
  ischaemic or inflammatory pain. *(p.81)*

Response to morphine is partial or equivocal and side effects unacceptable
Perhaps most common is a partial or equivocal response to the last dose
increase, together with the development of unacceptable side effects.
Alternatively side effects may occur on starting doses of strong opioids, with
unacceptable side effects and no (or only partial) pain relief. This suggests that
more benefit **may** be derived from persevering with opioids, but may only
ever achieve partial pain control with opioids.
Further management can be justified along either of the above lines (i.e.
persevering with opioids, or changing tack), taking into account:
- previous response to opioids
- likelihood of pain being responsive to opioids
- availability of alternative approaches
- individual patient characteristics

Emotional or spiritual pain (morphine-irrelevant pain)
Anxiety or depression are often associated with pain in cancer, and may be
the cause, or result, of poor pain control. Psycho-spiritual issues should always
be dealt with concurrently.[376]

SEE ALSO
📖 Reviews[585,586]

Opioid side effects & toxicity

Always ensure opioid doses are carefully titrated ('fine-tuned') to maximise analgesia and minimise side effects.[587]
Side effects that start whilst on regular doses of strong opioid may be due to:
- dehydration or renal failure
- other change in disease status e.g. hepatic function, weight loss
- pain relieved by other methods[588]
- co-administration of amitriptyline - increases the bioavailability of morphine[421,422] leading to opioid side-effects

General management
A number of different approaches may be used in general to manage persistent opioid-related side effects:
- treat the side effect
- use an alternative opioid *(p.71)*
- use an alternative analgesic method
- spinal opioids - may cause less systemic or central side-effects
- parenteral rehydration - may help neuropsychiatric toxicity (hallucination, sedation, myoclonus)[589]

Drowsiness & cognitive impairment
Initial mild drowsiness on initiating opioid therapy will often abate over a few days as the patient adjusts; in this case it is often appropriate to wait for the drowsiness to wear off.
For persistent drowsiness, sedation or subtler cognitive impairment:
- parenteral rehydration if appropriate
- alternative opioid
- psychostimulants have been used to combat sedation *(p.103)*.

Hallucinations or Delirium
- parenteral rehydration if appropriate
- alternative opioid
- antipsychotic e.g. haloperidol 3-5mg nocte or by CSCI *(p.105)*

Myoclonus
Consider renal failure - renal failure alone can cause myoclonus, but also causes opioid metabolites to accumulate which increase the risk of opioid toxicity. Myoclonus may be more likely in patients also taking antidepressants, antipsychotics or NSAIDs.[590]
- parenteral rehydration if appropriate
- review other medication which may exacerbate myoclonus
- alternative opioid[591]
- clonazepam 2-8mg/24h[592,593]
- diazepam or midazolam probably less effective than clonazepam but may be appropriate if sedation is also desirable
- gabapentin 600-1200mg/24h divided doses may help opioid-induced myoclonus[594]

Constipation
- constipation can usually be treated acceptably with laxatives
- fentanyl causes less constipation than morphine if change needed *(p.71)*

Paradoxical pain

Hyperalgesia and allodynia have been reported with high-dose morphine.[589,595-597] It is usually associated with myoclonus, and an increase in the morphine dose may lead to worsening of the pain, thus it has been called paradoxical pain.[598,599] It is reported most frequently with morphine, but other opioids including sufentanil (similar to fentanyl) have been implicated.[600] Substitution of an alternative opioid often resolves the symptoms.

Switching to methadone has been reported most effective, but a reduction of dose and addition of an alternative co-analgesic e.g. ketamine or clonazepam may also be tried.

Nausea & vomiting

Initial nausea may wear off after a week and usually responds to:
- haloperidol 1.5mg nocte (➪ *Nausea & Vomiting p.19*)
- metoclopramide may be needed for opioid-induced gastric stasis, and
- cyclizine or 5-HT₃ antagonists may be helpful in other patients
- alternative opioid

Sweating

- alternative opioids
- exclude other causes of sweating
- antimuscarinic drugs
➪ *Sweats (p.166)*

Pruritus (itching)

More common with spinal opioids but can occur with systemic.
- alternative opioids
- if unsuccessful, treat pruritus with 5-HT₃ antagonists or paroxetine *(p.159)*

Respiratory depression/sedation

- Reduction of the dose is usually all that is required immediately. Infusion by a syringe driver should be temporarily stopped to allow plasma levels to decrease, before restarting at a lower dose.
- Naloxone is only indicated if significant respiratory depression is present; opioid withdrawal symptoms and pain can be severe in patients on long-term opioids.[601]
- It is important to titrate the dose carefully, so as not to produce an acute opioid withdrawal.
- Naloxone has a half life of 5-20 minutes. As the half life of most opioids is longer than this, it is important to continue assessment of the patient and give naloxone at further intervals if necessary.

Naloxone

Indications for naloxone

- respiratory rate <8 breaths/min, or
- <10-12 breaths/min, difficult to rouse and clinically cyanosed, or
- <10-12 breaths/min, difficult to rouse and SaO₂ <90% on pulse oximeter

Use of naloxone[1]

- Dilute Naloxone 0.4mg vial in 10mL saline for injection.
- Use an IV cannula or butterfly.
- Administer 0.5mL IV every 2 minutes until respiratory status satisfactory.
- Repeat further doses as needed.

PRESCRIBING STATUS

☼ Clonazepam & other benzodiazepines ●●
☼ Gabapentin ●●

SEE ALSO

⇨ *Alternative opioids (p.71), Opioid resistant pain (p.68)*
📖 Review[589]

Additional Information

Donepezil (acetylcholinesterase inhibitor) shows moderate effect in reducing opioid-induced sedation.[602]

Alternative Strong Opioids

A number of alternative strong opioid analgesics are available which have their place in palliative care:

Morphine & similar drugs	Morphine
	Diamorphine
	Hydromorphone
	Oxycodone
Fentanyl & similar drugs	Fentanyl
	Alfentanil
	Sufentanil
Methadone	Methadone
Intermediate weak-strong opioid	Tramadol
Other opioids occasionally used	Dextromoramide
	Phenazocine
	Buprenorphine
Not recommended	Pethidine

Differences between these drugs are not fully understood, but include patient factors and drug factors. In clinical practice they may be divided into:

Morphine-like opioids

Oxycodone and hydromorphone, like morphine and diamorphine, are available in a wide range of doses in normal (4-hourly) and slow-release oral preparations. They can be used by CSCI, although neither are routinely available in injection form in the UK at present.

Although there may be small intrinsic differences between the side-effect profiles of these drugs (e.g. hydromorphone appears to cause less pruritus than morphine overall), inter-individual variability seems to be a greater factor in determining the clinical picture. Substituting one of these drugs for another may reduce side-effects in up to 75% of selected individuals.[603]

Oxycodone and hydromorphone may cause less toxicity than morphine in patients with renal failure, but neuro-excitatory side-effects are reported.

Fentanyl and its analogues

Fentanyl and its analogues (alfentanil, sufentanil and remifentanil) are *selective* μ–receptor agonists, unlike morphine. They cause less sedation, cognitive impairment and constipation than morphine-like drugs. They are largely inactive orally because of high first-pass hepatic metabolism, but can be used by transdermal patch, oral lozenge (buccal absorption) or CSCI.

Fentanyl does not appear to accumulate and cause toxicity in renal failure.

Methadone

Methadone is an agonist at the μ- and δ-opioid receptors, and also an NMDA receptor antagonist and monoamine reuptake inhibitor. These actions make it a useful treatment for neuropathic and other pain states not fully responsive to morphine. However, it has a long and variable elimination half-life, making it difficult to use safely, and should be reserved for neuropathic, ischaemic or inflammatory pain, or use as third- or fourth-line opioid.

Tramadol

Tramadol may be classed somewhere between the weak and strong opioids. It has additional pharmacological actions to its opioid effects. It is not classed as a 'controlled drug' which has some practical advantages for its prescribing.

Other opioid analgesics

Pethidine has a short duration of action, and when given regularly, active metabolites accumulate and can cause convulsions. Causes more dysphoria than morphine. Best avoided.

Dextromoramide is a short acting opioid that is occasionally used for incident pain that can be predicted e.g. painful dressing changes.

Most other opioid analgesics are too limited in their range of preparations, doses available, or routes of administration to have any routine place in cancer pain.

Indications for starting with an opioid other than morphine

- patient acceptability
- history of subacute/partial intestinal obstruction - to minimise constipation
- patient reluctant to take 'morphine' despite appropriate counselling
- patient reluctant to take oral medication regularly
- renal failure

Indications for changing to alternative opioids

This practice is known as opioid rotation or opioid substitution.
- unacceptable opioid side-effects *(p.68 & 69)*
- renal failure

In daily clinical practice rotation to another opioid should be required in less than 2-3% of cases.[604]

Choice of alternative opioid

	Able to take oral medication	Unable to take oral
Pain well controlled and stable [a]	Fentanyl transdermal patch	Fentanyl transdermal patch
Pain uncontrolled or unstable	Oxycodone [b]	Fentanyl CSCI (or alfentanil) - convert to patch when stable. Oxycodone CSCI suitable if available.

[a] Also for patients starting strong opioid whose pain has increased slowly over time, is mild to moderate, and fairly stable.

[b] Evidence is strongest for hydromorphone as causing less pruritus than morphine.[605,606]

Rationale

- Hydromorphone, oxycodone and fentanyl are useful alternatives to morphine and diamorphine.[378]
- Methadone is difficult to use safely, and should be reserved for neuropathic, ischaemic or inflammatory pain, or use as third- or fourth-line opioid.
- No other strong opioids have the range of doses and preparations needed to be suitable for routine use in cancer pain.
- Hydromorphone and oxycodone are available in a wide range of oral preparations, but parenteral preparations are not routinely available in the UK.
- There is little to choose between oxycodone and hydromorphone, but oxycodone is chosen in preference because:
  - a liquid normal release preparation is available
  - doses are simpler to calculate (e.g. 1.3mg versus 5mg)
  - there is less variation in the reported equianalgesic ratios for oxycodone
  - the manufacturer's recommended conversion of 7.5:1 for morphine to hydromorphone is higher than the more commonly used ratio of 5:1; this makes the tablet doses of 1.3mg even more complicated
- Fentanyl causes less side effects (sedation, cognitive impairment, constipation, myoclonus and pruritus) than any of the morphine family, and has greater patient acceptability.
- Transdermal patch or csci are the only methods of administering fentanyl regularly for chronic pain.
- Rapid dose titration for unstable pain control is more flexible and predictable with oral normal-release oxycodone than with fentanyl, even using fentanyl csci or otfc lozenges.

Renal impairment / Renal failure

Metabolites of morphine accumulate in renal failure and can cause neurotoxic side effects such as myoclonus and confusion.[589,607] Fentanyl is mainly eliminated by hepatic metabolism to inactive metabolites, and case reports support its use in renal failure with less toxicity.

Oxycodone and hydromorphone do have active metabolites that are renally excreted, and their value in renal failure is less clear. However, case reports suggest they may be better than morphine, at least in individual patients switched from morphine.

SEE ALSO
⇨ *Oxycodone (p.74), Hydromorphone (p.75), Fentanyl (p.76)*
⇨ *Alfentanil (p.80), Sufentanil (p.80), Remifentanil (p.80)*
⇨ *Methadone (p.81), Tramadol (p.71)*
📖 Reviews[603,604,608-618]
📖 EAPC Guidelines[378]

Alternative Strong Opioid Drugs

(For other preparations see under individual drug.)
DEXTROMORAMIDE
  Tabs. 5mg, 10mg *(Palfium)*
  TSD: 5mg PRN PO

Tramadol

Tramadol is a synthetic analogue of codeine that binds to μ-opioid receptors and inhibits norepinephrine and serotonin reuptake. It is rapidly and extensively absorbed after oral doses and is metabolized in the liver. Analgesia begins within one hour and starts to peak in two hours. In patients with moderate postoperative pain, parenteral tramadol is roughly equal in efficacy to morphine, but for severe acute pain, tramadol is less effective than morphine. In studies comparing oral tramadol (up to 300 mg/d) with oral morphine for moderate cancer pain, analgesic efficacy was equivalent, but constipation, nausea, neuropsychological symptoms, and pruritus were reported more frequently with morphine.[619,620] Slow release formulations have also been shown to provide effective relief of moderate cancer pain.[621] It is not classed as a 'controlled drug' which has some practical advantages for its prescribing.

SEE ALSO
⇨ *Alternative opioids (p.71)*
📖 Review[622]

Drug preparations
TRAMADOL

Caps. 50mg; Sachets effervescent powder 50mg[○] Sol. tabs. 50mg
Tabs. **SR** (12-hourly) 75mg[○] 100mg, 150mg, 200mg[○]
Caps. **SR** (12-hourly) 50mg, 100mg, 150mg, 200mg[○]
Tabs. **SR** (24-hourly) 150mg[○] 200mg[○] 300mg[○] 400mg[○]
   TSD: 50mg q.d.s. PO or 100mg b.d. PO (12-hourly SR)
Inj. 100mg/2mL

Oxycodone

Oxycodone is a strong opioid analgesic very similar to morphine. It is available in 4-hourly normal release, and 12-hourly slow release preparations, but the injection is not routinely available in the UK.

It is a useful alternative opioid in selected patients who develop side effects with morphine ⇨ *Alternative opioids (p.71)*. Oxycodone has been used successfully and without toxicity in renal failure.[616]

Oxycodone is approximately 1.5-2 times as potent as morphine orally.

Indications
• alternative opioid when morphine causes unacceptable side-effects

Using Oxycodone
• oxycodone should be used in the same way as morphine (remember a laxative)

SEE ALSO
⇨ *Alternative opioids (p.71), Opioid potency ratios (p207)*
📖 Reviews[623]

Drug preparations
OXYCODONE
Caps. 5mg, 10mg, 20mg *(OxyNorm)*
Caps. **SR** (12-hourly) 10mg, 20mg, 40mg, 80mg *(OxyContin)*
Liquid 5mg/5mL, 10mg/1mL
Manufacturers recommend conversion from oral morphine, divide dose by 2
Injection available as a special order ‡

Additional Information
Comparison with morphine
In comparative studies with morphine, there are inconsistent reports of side effect profiles. More vomiting has been reported with morphine, whereas constipation was more common with oxycodone.[624] Other studies have shown no difference.[625]

When selectively switching patients with side effects from morphine to oxycodone, improvements in almost all side effects have been reported: less nausea, hallucinations, drowsiness, sweating and pruritus, but especially confusion/delirium.[623,626,627] These reports do not necessarily reflect an overall difference between the drugs, but may reflect inter-individual variation.[628]

Hepatic metabolism
Oxymorphone, a potent analgesic metabolite of oxycodone, is formed by the hepatic enzyme CYP2D6, which is under polymorphic genetic control.[629] The role of oxymorphone in the analgesic effect of oxycodone is not yet clear.[628] Oxycodone conversion to oxymorphone may be important for analgesic effect in some patients,[630] and genetically 'poor-metabolisers' may not obtain the expected analgesia from oxycodone.[627]
See also codeine *(p.60)*.

Synergy between opioids
In animal models, a combination of sub-analgesic doses of oxycodone and morphine showed synergy producing analgesia.[631]

Hydromorphone

Hydromorphone is a strong opioid analgesic very similar to morphine, although it is a more selective μ-receptor agonist. It is used widely in North America as an alternative for diamorphine which is not available. It is available in 4-hourly normal release, and 12-hourly slow release preparations, but the injection is not routinely available in the UK.
It is a useful alternative opioid in selected patients who develop side effects with morphine ⇨ *Alternative opioids (p.71)*. Hydromorphone has been used successfully and without toxicity in renal failure,[632] but it has also been reported to cause neuro-excitatory effects in some patients.[633]
Hydromorphone is approximately 5-7.5 times as potent as morphine orally.

Indications
▸ Alternative opioid if morphine causes unacceptable side-effects, especially -
▸ Opioid-induced pruritus[605]

Using Hydromorphone
Hydromorphone should be used in the same way as morphine (remember a laxative).
The capsules can be broken open and sprinkled on soft cold foods.

SEE ALSO
⇨ Alternative opioids (p.71), Opioid potency ratios (p207)
📖 Reviews[605]

Drug preparations

HYDROMORPHONE [◎]

Caps. 1.3mg, 2.6mg *(Palladone)*
Caps. SR (12-hourly) 2mg, 4mg, 8mg, 16mg, 24mg *(Palladone SR)*
Manufacturers recommend conversion from oral morphine, divide dose by 7.5
Inj. 10mg/1mL[‡] 20mg/1mL[‡] 50mg/1mL[‡]
Injections available as a special from Martindale

Additional Information

Cough & dyspnoea

Information about the efficacy of alternative opioids for symptoms other than
pain is limited. Hydromorphone has been shown to help cough in doses lower
than analgesia; it also helps dyspnoea.[605]

Conversion ratios with other opioids

Conversion ratios between hydromorphone and other strong opioid analgesics
seem more variable and uncertain than for other opioids, perhaps representing
greater variability in metabolism and bioavailability (10-65%) between
individuals.[605,634] When converting from oral morphine to oral
hydromorphone, the manufacturers recommend a ratio of 7.5:1 (i.e. 1.3mg
hydromorphone ≈ 10mg morphine). The reported average is probably closer
to 5:1.[605,635,636]

Subcutaneous morphine to hydromorphone has given ratios between 3.1:1
and 8.5:1.[605,635,637] Hydromorphone PO to SC is often quoted as 5:1,[605] but
this does not square with a morphine PO to SC ratio of 1:2[638] ⇨ *Opioid
potency ratios (p.207)* for other ratios.

It is suggested that the lowest potency ratio is used for any conversion, with
the expectation of titrating up the dose rapidly if needed.

Side-effects

Hydromorphone and morphine generally have the same side-effects, except
pruritus, nausea and vomiting, sedation and cognitive impairment, which may
be less common with hydromorphone.[605] There may also be individual
variation in side-effect profile between patients ⇨ *Alternative opioids (p.71)*.

Fentanyl

Fentanyl is a selective μ-receptor agonist (morphine acts on μ and κ). It
causes less constipation, sedation, and cognitive impairment than morphine or
hydromorphone[605,627,639-642] (and probably oxycodone). Fentanyl may be
associated with a slightly higher incidence of nausea than morphine.[643]

As it has inactive metabolites and is metabolised mainly in the liver it is less
likely to cause adverse effects in uraemic patients (who accumulate
morphine).[644] The disposition of fentanyl does not appear to be significantly
affected in liver disease.[522]

As it is more selective than morphine, fentanyl will not relieve pain that is
insensitive to morphine, but may help in patients with morphine-responsive
pain who develop intolerable side effects.

Fentanyl is inactive when swallowed and is only available as a transdermal patch, oral lozenge (buccal absorption), or CSCI.[645-647]

CSCI is better than a patch for establishing effective blood levels rapidly, and should be used when speed is important, or when more flexibility is desired. Converting a patient from morphine to fentanyl can lead to a modified withdrawal syndrome of shivering, diarrhoea, bowel cramps, sweating and restlessness, even though pain relief is maintained. These symptoms can be relieved with morphine given PRN for a few days.[648-651]

Fentanyl toxicity from too high doses is subtler than morphine toxicity due to a lack of hallucinations, myoclonus etc. and may present as vagueness, drowsiness or 'not feeling well'.

Indications

- Alternative opioid when morphine causes unacceptable side-effects.
- Starting a strong opioid in a patient with:
  - a history of subacute bowel obstruction - not if obstructed (less constipating than morphine)
  - renal failure (which can lead to myoclonus or confusion with morphine due to metabolite accumulation)
  - biliary colic/obstructed bile duct (see additional notes below)
- First-line strong opioid for reasons of patient acceptability.[643,652]

Transdermal fentanyl patch

- Start with 25μg/h, or convert dose from morphine. (⟿ p.207)
- It takes 12-24h to achieve therapeutic blood levels, and approximately 72h to reach steady-state:
  - CSCI of fentanyl or alfentanil will achieve more rapid blood levels
- If converting from morphine, give last dose of 12-hourly SR morphine when applying patch (or 3 more doses morphine elixir) except when accumulation of opioids in renal failure has occurred.
- If converting from morphine, continue to use morphine PRN for withdrawal symptoms:
  - may just present as restlessness
  - may occur over next 24h (or more)
  - not necessarily pain
- Change patches every 72h.
- Up to 25% patients need patch changing every 48h.[642]
- Use either oral morphine or oral transmucosal fentanyl for breakthrough pain.
- Fever may increase drug absorption due to vasodilation.[653]
- Sweating may decrease drug absorption because it prevents the patch from sticking to the skin.
- After removal of the patch, blood levels decrease by 50% in 18h.
- Mild to moderate skin erythema or pruritus have been reported in <5% of patients.[643,654]

Subcutaneous fentanyl

- Calculate dose as equivalent to transdermal patch[647] e.g. 25μg/h = 600μg/24h; for convenience (and considering the widely variable absorption from a patch[655]) use 500μg/24h CSCI ≈ 25μg/h patch.
- Large volumes are needed for high doses: consider substituting alfentanil (see next section).
- Compatible with most commonly used drugs in palliative care. (p.173)

Oral transmucosal fentanyl citrate (OTFC)

Fentanyl lozenges (on a stick)[655,656] are rapidly absorbed through the buccal mucosa, leading to onset of pain relief within 5-10 minutes. The maximum effect is reached within 20-40 minutes, and a duration of action of 1-3h. Bioavailability is about 50%.[657] One comparative study suggests they may give better results than normal-release oral morphine.[658]

Indication
• Breakthrough pain in patients on regular strong opioid therapy.

Use
The optimal dose is determined by titration, and cannot be predicted by a patient's regular dose of opioid.[659,660]
Approximately 25% of patients fail to obtain relief even at the highest dose, or have unacceptable adverse effects.
• Lozenge should be placed in the mouth and sucked, constantly moving it from one cheek to the other.
• Should not be chewed.
• Water can be used to moisten the mouth beforehand.
• Aim to consume the lozenge within 15minutes.
• Partially consumed lozenges should be dissolved under hot running water, and the handle disposed out of reach of children.

Dose titration
• Initial dose is 200µg, regardless of dose of regular opioid.
• A second lozenge of the same strength can be used if pain is not relieved after 15 minutes.
• No more than two lozenges should be used to treat any individual pain episode.
• Continue with this dose for a further 2-3 episodes of breakthrough pain, allowing the second lozenge when necessary.
• If pain still not controlled, increase to the next higher dose lozenge.
• Continue to titrate in this manner until dose is found that provides adequate analgesia with minimum adverse effects.
• No more than 4 doses per day should be used (regular strong opioid dose should be increased).

ThinkList
• absorption rate from a transdermal patch is *roughly* proportional to the surface area in contact with the skin; various techniques have been used to allow only half of the area to contact with the skin - to approximate to a 12.5µg/hour dose delivery; *Tegaderm* or *Opsite* dressings, with the fentanyl patch placed half on skin/half over the dressing, have been used, but note these dressings are semipermeable; others have folded the patch in half and covered with adhesive tape; neither is recommended by the manufacturers[2]
• initial iv PCA dose titration before conversion to transdermal patch[661]
• some patients develop itching and irritation at the site of transdermal patches - reports suggest spraying the skin with aerosol corticosteroid spray is effective[662] (use beclometasone dipropionate aerosol inhaler 50µg/dose)•
• sublingual fentanyl for breakthrough pain using the injection preparation[663]

SEE ALSO

⇨ *Alternative opioids (p.71), Opioid potency ratios (p207)*
📖 Reviews - transdermal patch[664] & OTFC[665]

Fentanyl preparations

FENTANYL

Patches 25, 50, 75, 100μg/hr *(Durogesic)*
>   TSD: *1 (25μg/hr) patch every 3 days*

Inj. 50μg/1mL[Ⓢ] 100μg/2mL, 500μg/10mL
>   TSD: *500μg/24h CSCI*

Lozenge with applicator 200, 400, 600, 800, 1200, 1600μg *(Actiq)*[Ⓢ]
>   TSD: *200μg lozenge regardless of regular opioid dose (£6.48 per lozenge)*

Additional Information

Inflammatory & neuropathic pain

A few observations suggest that fentanyl (and similar analogues) may be less effective than morphine for inflammatory or neuropathic pain.[645,666] This may be explained by the additional effects of morphine (e.g. at kappa or delta receptors). However, the reduced side effects of fentanyl may allow the dose to be increased, thereby giving better analgesia than morphine.

Dose equivalence

Manufacturer's recommended dose conversion from oral morphine to transdermal fentanyl patch (⇨ *p.207)* is based on a ratio of 150:1 (i.e. 25μgm/h patch ≅ 15mg morphine PO 4-hourly). Other studies suggest this may overestimate the potency of fentanyl, and calculate a ratio of 100:1 (i.e. 25μgm/h patch ≅ 10mg morphine PO 4-hourly)[667] or for CSCI 68:1 (i.e. 25μgm/h by CSCI ≅ 30-40mg morphine/24h CSCI).[645]

Bile duct obstruction

Many opioid μ-receptor agonists, including morphine and diamorphine, have been shown to increase the common bile duct pressure. Fentanyl or sufentanil have no discernable effect on common bile duct diameter, therefore, these μ-receptor agonists seem to be safe in patients in whom spasm of the common bile ducts should be avoided.[668]

Topical use of fentanyl

Fentanyl has been used topically for painful skin ulcers.[669]

Fentanyl versus morphine

μ₁ and μ₂ opioid receptors have been described, with fentanyl binding with greater affinity than morphine to both.[670] However, more recent research shows that there is only one gene encoding for a mu receptor,[671-673] calling into question whether μ₁ and μ₂ exist. A unique binding mode of fentanyl at the μ-receptor may explain the difficulties encountered in defining models of recognition at the μ-receptor and suggest opioid receptors may display multiple binding epitopes.[674]

Alfentanil

Alfentanil is a selective mu-receptor opioid agonist, similar to fentanyl. It is mainly metabolised in the liver to inactive compounds. It has been given by csci in a syringe driver, and appears to mix with most other commonly used drugs in palliative care.[131] It should be diluted with water.

Compared to fentanyl, an equianalgesic dose can be used in a much smaller volume, making csci of large doses possible. It is thus a useful substitute for fentanyl if csci use is desired.

Alfentanil is rapidly eliminated (t½ 90mins)[675] and elimination appears unaffected by renal failure.[676-678] Its onset is more rapid than for fentanyl.[679] Its short-lasting effect means it has been used for incident pain (dressing change).[680]

SEE ALSO
⇨ *Opioid potency ratios (p207)*
▢ Reviews[679,681,682]

Drug preparations
ALFENTANIL
  Inj. 1mg/2mL, 5mg/10mL◯   5mg/1mL
    TSD: 500µg/24h CSCI

Sufentanil

Sufentanil is a synthetic opioid very similar to fentanyl, but with more rapid onset and shorter duration of action.[682] It can be used as an alternative to alfentanil if the fentanyl dose necessitates too large a volume for the portable syringe driver in use. It has also been used sublingually.[683] The clinically derived sufentanil to fentanyl relative potency is approximately 20:1[645]

Remifentanil

Remifentanil is a very short-acting µ-receptor opioid agonist, similar to fentanyl. Remifentanil undergoes metabolism by blood and tissue non-specific esterases, resulting in an extremely rapid clearance that is independent of hepatic or renal function (half-life approximately 3 minutes). The potency of remifentanil is somewhat less than that of fentanyl. Speed of onset of effect is very rapid and is similar to that of alfentanil, approximately 1 to 2 minutes.[684] Its rapid distribution around the body probably leads to a significant risk of apnoea seen when used for painful medical procedures, and its use is not recommended in palliative care.[685]

Methadone

Methadone is a strong opioid analgesic, with several non-opiate actions. It differs from morphine/diamorphine in a number of ways:

- δ-opioid receptor agonist
- NMDA receptor antagonist
- serotonin re-uptake inhibitor[686]
- long and variable elimination half-life
- potential for numerous and complex drug interactions
- inactive metabolites (lower toxicity in renal failure)

The first three of these actions may help account for reports of its effectiveness in managing neuropathic pain.[687]

The pharmacology of methadone is complex and very variable, so it must be used with the utmost care and supervision. The commonest mistake in its use is to underestimate its duration of action, since up to 10 days may be required to reach steady state plasma levels. The greatest tendency to accumulate the drug is in the elderly or those with liver failure.

Drug interactions

Methadone metabolism is increased by a number of other drugs, which can cause opiate withdrawal symptoms when started in a patient on regular methadone. Other interactions which inhibit metabolism can lead to overdose and toxicity:

Decrease methadone levels	Increase methadone levels
Phenytoin	Fluconazole (and probably ketoconazole)
Phenobarbital	
Carbamazepine (not valproate or gabapentin)	SSRIs (venlafaxine little or no effect)
Rifampicin	

Subcutaneous Methadone

Subcutaneous methadone has been used but there is a problem with skin reactions, partly because methadone in solution is acid. If necessary to use, dilute as much as possible; hyaluronidase may also be added. In conversion of oral to subcutaneous or intravenous dosing, use a daily parenteral dose that is half the oral dose.[688]

Use of methadone

Indications

- Pain only partially responsive to morphine e.g. inflammatory, ischaemic or neuropathic pain.
- Alternative opioid when side effects develop with morphine (or other opioid).
- Renal failure
- Morphine tolerance - patients requiring ever increasing doses of opioids with no overall improvement in pain.
- Use with especial caution in the elderly, COPD or asthma.

Guidelines for use

Methadone's efficacy compared to morphine increases with chronic dosing and with higher dose. This is in part due to a long elimination half-life, and in part due to its non-opioid action. The dose ratio of methadone to morphine is inversely proportional to the daily morphine dose. Many studies have shown the difficulty in converting doses from another opioid to methadone or vice versa. At least two guidelines have been published.

Guidelines (A) are most commonly used in the UK, and are recommended for general use, and especially for patients switching opioid because of lack of effect. Guidelines (B) may be helpful for use in patients who have exhibited opioid toxicity.

Guidelines (A) for use of methadone[688]

- Stop all other strong opioids.
- Give fixed doses of methadone PO calculated as one-tenth of the 24h oral morphine dose (or equivalent), to a maximum of methadone 30mg.
- The fixed dose is taken as needed, but not more frequently than every 3h.
- On day 6, add the total dose of methadone given in last 48h, divide by 4, and give at 12-hourly intervals.
- Subsequent dose changes are by percentage increments as for morphine.
- Re-assess carefully as accumulation can occur up to 10 days after.

Guidelines (B) for use of methadone[689]

- Stop all other strong opioids.
- Give methadone at fixed intervals, every 8 hours:

24h oral morphine dose (or equivalent)	8-hourly methadone dose
<90mg	24h morphine dose divided by 12 (3-7.5mg)
90-300mg	24h morphine dose divided by 24 (3.5-12.5mg)
>300mg	24h morphine dose divided by 36 (8.5mg up)

- 10% dose of the **daily** methadone dose may be used for breakthrough pain.
- Re-assess carefully as accumulation can occur up to 10 days after.

PRESCRIBING STATUS
Methadone °°°

SEE ALSO
⇨ *Alternative opioids (p.71)*
📖 Reviews[690-692] & Guidelines[688,689]

Drug preparations
METHADONE
Mixture 10mg/mL‡ ⊘ ☑
Mixture 1mg/mL
Tabs. 5mg; Linctus 2mg/5mL (for cough)
Inj. 10mg/1mL, 20mg/2mL⊘ 50mg/5mL⊘

Additional Information
Side effects
All the typical opioid side effects can be expected, although hallucinations and myoclonus are rare. Compared to morphine, methadone causes less constipation, sedation and nausea. Methadone causes histamine release and can exacerbate asthma. It also has an antidiuretic effect.

Drug addicts
Methadone should be considered early in the course of pain treatment of patients who have had chronic exposure to methadone e.g. through drug addiction programs.[693]

Topical opioids

Opioids can act peripherally as analgesics, and there are a number of reports of their successful use on painful ulcerated skin, relieving pain and possibly inflammation.[336,694-696] Morphine and diamorphine have been used most commonly, but fentanyl has also been reported.[669] Diamorphine has been mixed with metronidazole.[697] There have been no reports of systemic toxicity, and standard doses have been used, regardless of doses of systemic opioids taken simultaneously.

Morphine or diamorphine 10mg may be mixed with sterile aqueous gel, a hydrocolloid gel (e.g. *Intrasite*), or metronidazole gel, as appropriate. Apply once daily, and increase frequency if needed up to three times daily.

PRESCRIBING STATUS
Opioid analgesics used topically ••

Ketamine

Ketamine is a dissociative anaesthetic with strong analgesic properties. Its analgesic effect may be partly due to NMDA receptor blocking,[490] and may be useful clinically in sub-anaesthetic doses for treating neuropathic, inflammatory or ischaemic pain. In higher doses approaching anaesthetic doses, it may be useful for treating terminal uncontrolled overwhelming pain. It has been used by PO, CSCI and IV routes, and in a very wide range of doses.[698-706]

- CSCI in doses of 50-360mg/24h ± a loading dose of 10mg SC
- PO starting doses between 2mg and 25mg t.d.s. have been used, and up to 50mg q.d.s. or 240mg/day
- IV bolus doses of 0.1-0.5mg/kg (approx. 5-25mg)

Dysphoric effects including hallucinations are reported quite commonly in higher doses. They are more common in anxious patients, and small doses of benzodiazepines may help.[705] Anaesthetic experience suggests pre-treatment may help reduce the incidence.

Neuropathic pain

Use oral route if possible:
- Diazepam 2mg PO 2 hours before first dose then 2mg nocte for 3 days.
- Start ketamine 10mg q.d.s. PO
- Increase by 10mg increments once or twice daily, up to 50mg q.d.s. as appropriate.

If parenteral route appropriate:
- Ketamine 10mg SC stat. may be given if indicated for severe pain.
- Start infusion of ketamine 50-100mg/24h CSCI.
- Add midazolam 5mg/24h CSCI to reduce dysphoric effects, or higher dose if patient is very anxious.
- Increase ketamine dose by 50-100mg increments as indicated to maximum 400mg/24h CSCI.

Oral versus Parenteral doses

Ketamine is effective orally and in view of the wide dose ranges used, it is difficult to assess the potency ratio. It undergoes first-pass hepatic metabolism to an active metabolite, and one study suggests it may be more potent given orally than parenterally.[702] In general, equivalent daily doses should initially be used when changing route.

Ketamine for procedures

Ketamine can be used as an analgesic to allow patients to be positioned for epidural or certain procedures (e.g. dressing changes). It carries a high incidence of dysphoric effects at these doses.

- Ketamine 0.5mg/kg by slow IV injection (for 50kg man = 25mg), or
- Ketamine 1.5mg/kg IM (for 50kg man = 75mg)
- Pre-treatment with a benzodiazepine to reduce the incidence of dysphoric effects:
    - midazolam 2.5mg SC given 30 minutes before, or
    - midazolam 1-3mg slow IV immediately before

(N.B. Anaesthetic dose for 50kg man is 50-150mg IV over 1 min or 300-600mg IM)

Terminal overwhelming pain

- Give ketamine 25-50mg slow IV or SC for immediate effect if needed.
- Midazolam 5mg SC stat.
- Start ketamine 300-600mg/24h CSCI.
- Add midazolam at least 20mg/24h to prevent hallucinations.
- Increase ketamine to a maximum of 1,200mg/24h CSCI (up to 3.2g/24h have been given).[707]

PRESCRIBING STATUS
☼ Ketamine ●●

SEE ALSO
⇨ *Neuropathic pain (p.51), Mixing in syringe driver (p.173)*
📖 Reviews[698,708,709]
📖 NMDA receptor antagonists[489,710-713]

Drug preparations

KETAMINE ‡
Inj. 200mg/20mL, 500mg/10mL, 1000mg/10mL
TSD: 100mg/24h CSCI; 10mg PO 6-hourly
Ketamine can be given orally using the solution for injection. The taste is bitter and may be disguised by mixing with fruit cordials. It is normally a hospital-only drug, but can be obtained by community pharmacies on a named-patient basis if the GP contacts Parke Davis 01703 620500.[1]

Local Anaesthetic Infusions

Lidocaine (lignocaine) - IV or SC infusion

Infusions of lidocaine have been reported to help neuropathic pain of various aetiology, including cancer pain.[403,464,714-718]

Indications

- Neuropathic pain or ischaemic pain, not responding to opioids.

Single dose infusion

- Lidocaine as a single dose infusion IV or SC may produce analgesia lasting 12h or more; it may be useful to gain control of severe pain or to predict the likely benefit from the sodium channel blocker, mexiletine.[448]
- There is a risk of seizures and cardiac dysrhythmias with this treatment:
  - ideally given with ECG monitoring and resuscitation facilities available, or discuss potential risks with patient
  - reserve for patients with severe uncontrolled pain
  - relative contraindication in patients with known ischaemic heart disease
  - consider starting continuous infusion as alternative
- Single dose of 120mg or 2mg/kg (= 6mL 2% lidocaine) infused over 1h.
- A response may be expected by the end of the infusion.
- Continue treatment with either oral mexiletine or a continuous infusion of lidocaine given IV or CSCI.

Continuous infusion

- Start with 20mg/h lidocaine (24mL of 2% lidocaine/24h CSCI).
- Increase dose after 24-48h according to response and side-effects (max. 80mg/h[714] - 150mg/h.[715])

Side-effects

The side-effect profile of lidocaine is very predictable, with a wide margin of safety.[714]

Plasma conc. (μg/mL)	Side effects
4-6	Light-headedness, numb tongue, metallic taste increased blood pressure, dizziness
8	Visual and auditory disturbances, disassociation, muscle twitching, decreased blood pressure
12	Convulsions (very benzodiazepine sensitive)
16	Coma
> 20	Respiratory arrest and cardiovascular system collapse

Lidocaine is mainly metabolised in the liver, so reduced dose and caution should be taken in liver disease.

PRESCRIBING STATUS
☼ Lidocaine CSCI ●●●

SEE ALSO
📖 Reviews[479,719] & Systematic reviews[718]

Drug Preparations

LIDOCAINE

Inj. 0.5% 10mL; 1% 2mL, 5mL, 10mL, 20mL; 2% 2mL, 5mL

Inj. 4% and 10% are also available‡ ◌

TSD: 480mg/24h (20mg/h) by CSCI (1% = 10mg/mL)

Additional Information

A lidocaine patch has been licensed in the U.S. for post-herpetic neuralgia, applied directly to painful area. Little of the dose is absorbed systemically. Also used in other peripheral neuropathic pain states including thoracotomy scar pain.[720-722]

Entonox / Nitrous oxide

Entonox is a mixture of 50% nitrous oxide and 50% oxygen. Nitrous oxide is a gas which has both analgesic and anaesthetic properties. Even at sub-anaesthetic doses it has analgesic activity. It has occasional use in palliative care.[723,724] The cylinder head attachment used for self-administering Entonox has a valve in it that allows the gas out when negative pressure is created by the patient inspiring. The mask thus needs to be held over the face in an airtight fit. Some weak patients or those with respiratory difficulty will not be able to activate the valve.

Indications
Short-term analgesia for e.g.:
• painful dressings
• severe pain on movement
• spasms of pain - see caution below for colic

Contra-indications
• pneumothorax
• intestinal obstruction with abdominal distension
If breathed for any length of time, gas filled spaces in the body will expand due to nitrous oxide replacing the nitrogen. The main contra-indication is thus a pneumothorax. Theoretically, gaseous distension of the bowel in intestinal obstruction also contra-indicates its use, but it may have a place in treating severe colic spasms as long as it is for short periods of time and the patient is observed carefully for any worsening of the pain. An antimuscarinic would usually be much more appropriate.

Warning
If Entonox (which is a liquid due to the high pressure it is under) is allowed to go below -6°C, it may separate into two layers of the different gases. Initially 100% oxygen will be breathed, and then 100% nitrous oxide which could kill the patient. If Entonox has been stored outside, it should be kept above 10°C for 24h and then the cylinder inverted several times to mix the gases again.

Using Entonox
• Assess patient to exclude contraindications and note warning re. storage.
• Patient should have control of the mask or mouthpiece:
  – patients cannot overdose if they have control of the mask or mouthpiece, as it will fall away as they become sedated, wearing off quickly in a few minutes

Epidural & Intrathecal analgesia

Spinal analgesia (epidural or intrathecal) will normally be initiated by an anaesthetist or someone with specialist experience of this technique. A simple method using a Graseby syringe pump for an epidural that can be continued in the community has been described.[725] A mixture of opioid and local anaesthetic is most commonly used.

Indications
- neuropathic pain e.g. spinal cord compression or nerve root compression
- ischaemic leg pain
- movement-related incident pain[378]
- muscle spasticity

Contraindications
There are several contraindications to spinal analgesia; very few are absolute in a palliative care context:
- anticoagulation with warfarin (reversible with vitamin K)
- antiplatelet therapy e.g. aspirin (other NSAIDs can be stopped the day of the procedure ⇨ p.61)
- local infection at injection site
- tumour involvement of spine

Drugs used for spinal analgesia
- opioids
- local anaesthetic
- clonidine[726]
- midazolam
- baclofen[727-729]
- ketamine[730]

Bupivacaine, morphine, diamorphine, clonidine and midazolam are all compatible in combination.[731-734]

Adverse effects
Local anaesthetic
- hypotension - local anaesthetic causes vasodilation
- leg weakness
- urinary retention
- 'total spinal' - a profound block is caused if the needle accidentally and unknowingly punctures the dura into the cerebro-spinal fluid and an 'epidural' dose of local anaesthetic is given intrathecally. In this situation, a profound fall in blood pressure and complete paralysis of the legs will occur in a few minutes, which may spread to upper limbs, respiratory muscles, and ultimately brain. These changes will reverse with time, but the patient will need IV fluids or ephedrine to support the blood pressure, and may need ventilatory support. The physician inserting the epidural will be present and will be responsible for managing the situation.

Opioids
- all the typical adverse effects of systemic opioids may be seen e.g.
  - sedation
  - hallucinations
  - nausea

- urinary retention
- pruritus (more common than with systemic opioids)[735]

Non-drug related
- 'dural-tap' headache - develops in the 24h after procedure
- paraplegia - due to bleeding → epidural haematoma
- infection - epidural abscess or meningitis

Epidural fibrosis
Epidural fibrosis with indwelling epidural catheters has been described. Pain at injection or resistance to injection are initial manifestations, followed by poor, and eventually, no analgesic effect. Usually develops after 2-3 weeks.

Antibacterial filters
Antibacterial filters are usually used for continuous infusion, and can be changed weekly, but there is no evidence that the risk of infection is higher, even if left for up to a month.[736,737]

SEE ALSO
📖 Reviews[738-741] & Guidelines[742]

Drugs for hypotension from spinal analgesia
EPHEDRINE
  Inj. 30mg/1mL
    TSD: 30mg IV
  For hypotension associated with epidural sympathetic block. Dilute to 10mL with water and give 1-2mL IV; repeat every 3-4 minutes PRN

Additional Information

Doses
Diamorphine and morphine - 1/10th of the equivalent daily sc dose is often used as a starting dose given *epidurally*, but equianalgesic ratio may be more like 4:1[743,744] Use diamorphine 2.5-5mg/24h *epidurally* if opioid naïve.

Maximum dose of bupivacaine
Bupivacaine can cause seizures and cardiac dysrhthymias in overdose. The maximum recommended dose depends on the source:
- maximum single dose - 150mg (= 30 mL of 0.5%)
- maximum total daily dose - 400-600mg/24h (= 80-120 mL of 0.5%)

Ropivacaine
Ropivacaine is claimed to have a selective anaesthetic effect on pain fibres, and may be preferable to bupivacaine or lidocaine. It is approximately two-thirds as potent as bupivacaine (e.g. 1% ropivacaine ≅ 0.75% bupivacaine).

Post-dural puncture headache
An epidural blood-patch is the best treatment if anaesthetic support available. Caffeine for post-dural puncture headache 300mg gives short lived benefit.[745]

RESPIRATORY

Dyspnoea

Consider causes that may best be treated specifically:

Lung tumour	Radiotherapy (RT)
Bronchospasm	Bronchodilators
	Corticosteroids
Infection	Antibiotics
Pleural effusion	Pleural tap[746,747] *(p.205)*
	Pleurodesis
Anaemia	Blood transfusion[748]
Lymphangitis carcinomatosis	Corticosteroids
	Diuretics
	Bronchodilators
	Can only be diagnosed on X-ray, and even this may not be diagnostic; suspect when consistent severe dyspnoea at rest or on exertion, and widespread fine crepitations in lungs
Large airway obstruction	RT
	Stent[749]
	Laser treatment[750]
	Brachytherapy[751]
	Corticosteroids
	Diagnosed clinically by difficulty on breathing in, and inspiratory stridor
SVC obstruction	RT
	Corticosteroids
	Dilated veins over upper chest and neck, swollen face, neck and arms *(p.91)*
Ascites	Paracentesis *(p.37 and p.203)*
	Diuretics
Pulmonary embolism	Anticoagulation *(p.144 and 145)*
	Oxygen
Radiation-induced pulmonary fibrosis	Corticosteroids
Heart failure	Diuretic

Fatigue, muscle weakness (due to cachexia or steroid myopathy[752]), phrenic nerve palsy and restrictive chest wall tumours are common problems in cancer that can cause or exacerbate dyspnoea. Muscle weakness, fatigue and anxiety are the main factors that correlate with dyspnoea in cancer.[753,754]

Symptomatic treatment

1) Trial of oxygen if patient is hypoxic SaO_2 <90% *(p.92)*
2) Massage, aromatherapy or other relaxation methods.
3) Advise patient on non-drug measures:
   - position - sitting upright rather than lying
   - cool air from fan or open window
4) Consider a trial of bronchodilators e.g. nebulised salbutamol 2.5mg q.d.s.
   - bronchospasm is not always associated with wheeze, and

bronchodilators can improve dyspnoea without measurable changes in lung function;[755,756] a therapeutic trial is appropriate for any patient with advanced cancer

5) Morphine 2.5mg PO 4-hourly and titrate as for pain:
   – for patients already on regular opioids, a dose of 25-100% of the 4-hourly equivalent should be used[757-760]

6) Diazepam 2mg t.d.s or lorazepam 1mg sublingual PRN or midazolam 10-20mg/24h CSCI.

It is unclear whether opioids or benzodiazepines should be used first in preference.[761] They may help different patients, and can be used together.

PRESCRIBING STATUS
☼ Strong opioids, Benzodiazepines • (with special attention to precautions)
☼ Corticosteroids •

Think List

- nebulised furosemide •• 20mg/2mL q.d.s. may relieve dyspnoea even in the absence of LVF[762,763]
- nurse-led clinics providing counselling and breathing retraining have been shown to improve breathlessness and performance status[764]
- chlorpromazine • 25mg PR 4-hourly PRN has been used,[765] but there is no evidence of any benefit over benzodiazepines
- nebulised diamorphine ••• 5-10mg 4-hourly and other opioids have been used quite widely, but controlled trial suggests they are no more effective than nebulised saline or systemically administered opioids[766-772]
- nebulised local anaesthetics ••• have also been used for dyspnoea; an ultrasonic nebuliser is required to deliver drugs effectively into the lung,[773] and studies suggest they are of questionable benefit and may cause bronchospasm[768,774]
- acupuncture[775,776]
- helium 80%-oxygen 20% mixture ••• *(Heliox)* is less dense than air and can help dyspnoea in patients with large airways obstruction; usually used temporarily until definitive treatment can resolve obstruction[777,778]
- cannabinoids (dronabinol, nabilone) ••• [477]
- a rare presentation of neuroleptic-induced dystonia is supraglottic spasm causing acute airways obstruction[779] (↪ p.115)

SEE ALSO
↪ *Pleural aspiration (p.205), Oxygen (p.92)*
📖 Reviews[780-783]

Drugs used for Dyspnoea
BRONCHODILATORS
SALBUTAMOL
  Aerosol inh. 100μg *(Ventolin)*
    TSD: 2 activations q.d.s. inhaler
  Neb. soln. 5mg/mL[○] Nebules 2.5mg/2.5mL, 5mg/2.5mL
    TSD: 2.5mg q.d.s. via nebuliser
IPRATROPIUM BROMIDE
  Aerosol inh. 20μg, 40μg *(Atrovent)*
    TSD: 40μg q.d.s. inhaler
  Neb. soln. 250μg/1mL, 500μg/2mL *(Atrovent)*
    TSD: 250μg q.d.s. via nebuliser

CORTICOSTEROIDS
BECLOMETASONE
Aerosol inh. 50µg, 100µg, 200µg
TSD: 200µg b.d. inhaler
BUDESONIDE
Nebuliser solution 500µg/2mL, 1mg/2mL
TSD: 1mg b.d. via nebuliser

Additional Information
A Cochrane Library review is in preparation on opioids for dyspnoea in terminal illness.

Using morphine for dyspnoea
There is a 'therapeutic window' in which opioids (and benzodiazepines) can relieve the sensation of breathlessness, before respiratory depression occurs. Only in patients with severe ventilatory failure (such as advanced hypoxic COPD) is this therapeutic window very narrow. Oral or CSCI opioids given by the same rules as for pain control will not cause respiratory depression in most cancer patients. Starting doses for opioid-naïve patients are usually lower than for pain control e.g. morphine 2.5mg PO 4-hourly.

Terminal dyspnoea
Irreversible, severe dyspnoea in a dying patient can sometimes only be helped by increasing doses of opioid ± benzodiazepine up to doses that cause sedation. Sometimes these doses will cause respiratory depression and potentially hasten death. The ethical principle of 'double-effect' justifies this use, if the intention of treatment is to give only the necessary doses to relieve distress.

SVC obstruction

Obstruction of the superior vena cava by mediastinal compression from tumour can present acutely or chronically, resulting in dyspnoea. Venous distension over the neck and upper chest wall is visible, and the face and arms may be discoloured and swollen from venous congestion. Dexamethasone 16mg o.d. should be started to reduce oedema and relieve the compression, and an urgent oncology opinion sought. Diamorphine and midazolam may be used for the dyspnoea and accompanying distress as appropriate. Radiotherapy[784] is frequently helpful, but increasingly expandable metal stents are being used with more rapid relief of symptoms.[785-789] Thrombosis associated with a central venous catheter can be treated with antifibrinolytic therapy.[790]

PRESCRIBING STATUS
☼ Corticosteroids ●

SEE ALSO
⇨ *Corticosteroids (p.126)*
📖 Guidelines[791]

Oxygen

Oxygen may help dyspnoea (or confusion) in patients who are hypoxic,[792] either at rest, or who become so on exertion. It may help other dyspnoeic patients because of the effect of facial or nasal cooling,[793] or as a placebo. Hypoxic respiratory drive usually only starts with $PaO_2 < 8kPa$ (roughly equivalent to an oxygen saturation SaO_2 of 90%); hypoxic drive is often not significant until $PaO_2 < 5.3kPa$ (approx. SaO_2 75%). Most breathless cancer patients are not hypoxic to this degree and will not benefit from oxygen physiologically.

It is best to avoid *unnecessary* dependency on oxygen, which can limit mobility, may become a barrier between patient and family, and is expensive and inconvenient in the community. Much dependency is caused by injudicious use leading to habit.

However, it is difficult to predict those patients who will perceive benefit from oxygen purely from their oxygen saturation, because of the other potential benefits.[794]

Assessment

If available, a pulse oximeter should be used, and patients with an $SaO_2 \leq 90\%$ (after exertion if appropriate) *should* be offered a trial of oxygen. Those with an $SaO_2 > 90\%$ (or if pulse oximeter not available) *may* be offered a trial if desired.

Trial of oxygen

A trial of oxygen for a fixed period e.g. 15-30 minutes is recommended. After this time the patient should be reassessed, and a decision made as to its benefit. If it is agreed that it has not helped, the oxygen cylinder/mask should be removed from the patient. Explanation of the rationale for lack of benefit from oxygen, and offer of alternative strategies, such as a fan, open windows etc. will help.

Domiciliary oxygen

Intermittent or continuous domiciliary oxygen can be prescribed for palliation of dyspnoea in cancer patients.[795] An oxygen concentrator is generally more cost-effective for patients requiring oxygen more than 8 hours/day, unless it is only very short term. The 1,360L size of cylinder is the one usually dispensed in the community (3,400L is next largest) and at 2L/min this gives about 11 hours of use.

Oxygen concentration

Method	Flow rate	% O_2 delivered
Nasal cannulae	1L/min	24%
	2L/min	28%
Ventimask	2L/min	24%
	6L/min	35%

Severe COPD patients who are chronically hypoxic should not be given more than 28% oxygen unless properly monitored for respiratory depression. Flow rates of < 4L/min via nasal cannulae do not require humidification.[796]

SEE ALSO

⇨ *Dyspnoea (p.89)*
📖 Reviews[797-800] & Guidelines[795]

Cough

Treat underlying causes where possible and appropriate:

Infection	Antibiotics
Lung tumour	Radiotherapy, effective in 50% at reducing cough Awan, 1990 #2212]
LVF / Pulmonary oedema	Diuretics
Asthma / Bronchospasm	Bronchodilators Corticosteroids
Oesophageal reflux	*Frequent cause of chronic cough. Cough may be only symptom* [801,802] Metoclopramide **PPI**
Post-nasal drip	Antibiotic if sinusitis Nasal corticosteroid spray Nasal decongestant Ipratropium nasal spray
Aspiration	Speech therapist may be able to advise
Tracheo-oesophageal fistula	Covered metallic stent
ACE inhibitor	Change to an Angiotensin-II receptor antagonist e.g. losartan
Radiotherapy-induced pulmonary fibrosis	Corticosteroids

Symptomatic management of cough

The main distinction to be made is between a productive, or wet, cough and a dry cough. A wet cough is uncommonly due to massive over-production of mucus from alveolar lung cancer, called bronchorrhoea (see notes below).

Productive / Wet cough

- Promotion of an easy, effective cough to clear the mucus should be the aim, unless the patient is dying, and too weak to expectorate.
- Antibiotics may be appropriate even in very ill patients as symptomatic treatment for cough, even if they do not prevent death.

For patients still able to cough effectively with help:

- Nebulised 0.9% saline 2.5mL q.d.s. and PRN to loosen mucus.
- Treat any bronchospasm with nebulised salbutamol.
- Physiotherapist can teach patient to cough more effectively, or actively aid expectoration.
- For chronic persistent infection causing cough, nebulised gentamicin can be considered (see notes below).
- Antitussives should ideally be avoided, but may be helpful at night to aid sleep (see below for choice).

For patients who are dying and too weak to cough:

- antitussives (see below - usually diamorphine CSCI if dying), and
- antimuscarinic drug to dry secretions (⇨ *Death rattle p.98*)

Dry cough

A dry cough should be suppressed, once measures have been taken to exclude or treat an underlying cause.

- nebulised saline 0.9% 2.5mL q.d.s. may be helpful by reducing the irritation of dry airways (breathing oxygen or mouth-breathing) and helping loosen the normal bronchial secretions

Antitussive drugs:

1) Pholcodine 10mL t.d.s. is non-analgesic and causes less sedation or constipation than analgesic opioids; should be tried first for patients not already on opioids.

2) Codeine 30mg q.d.s. and increased if needed to 60mg q.d.s.[803]

3) Morphine 5mg 4-hourly PO, or morphine SR 10mg 12-hourly, or diamorphine 5-10mg/24h CSCI:
   – the dose should be titrated as for pain until either it is successful or side effects intervene
   – if a patient is already on opioids, a dose increment or two should be tried, but there is little evidence supporting the use of high doses of opioids for cough
   – the efficacy of hydromorphone, oxycodone and fentanyl is not well described; as the antitussive effect is not correlated to analgesic effect, consider a trial of morphine or diamorphine

4) Methadone is a little more potent than morphine; consider trial if a patient cannot tolerate morphine in low doses (e.g. ≤10mg 4-hourly); NB linctus strength is weaker than solution used for analgesia.

Comparable antitussive doses[804]

	Comparable antitussive doses	Antitussive/analgesic ratio
Pholcodine	10mg	No analgesic effect
Dextromethorphan	10-15mg	No analgesic effect
Dextropropoxyphene	10-12.5mg	(n/a)
Codeine	15mg	6.62
Dihydrocodeine	15mg	5.71
Morphine	2.5-5mg	2.87
Methadone	2mg	2.31
Benzonatate	100mg	No analgesic effect

PRESCRIBING STATUS

⚛ Antibiotics (gentamicin or colomycin) by nebuliser ●●●

ThinkList

- ipratropium bromide nebulised ● is an effective antitussive for persistent cough following clinical upper respiratory tract[805,806]
- inhaled sodium cromoglicate ●● 10mg q.d.s. has helped cough in lung cancer, usually acting within 48h[807]
- mucolytics e.g. carbocisteine 750mg t.d.s.●●● ◌ render sputum less viscid, but evidence of benefit is weak; a systematic review has confirmed that they do have some effect on reducing the number of exacerbations of COPD and the length of episode[808]
- baclofen●● inhibits cough experimentally; doses of 20mg/24h were required, and up to 2-4 weeks to achieve full effect[809]
- nifedipine ●● (calcium channel blockers) experimentally can be shown to potentiate the effect of opiate-like antitussives[810]
- nebulised local anaesthetics ●●● have been reported being used successfully, but have not been well evaluated[768,811] Lidocaine 2% 5mL or bupivacaine 0.25% 5mL t.d.s. are suggested;[3] care must be taken because of the risk of aspiration with pharyngeal anaesthesia
- interpleural bupivacaine infusion[812] ●●●
- benzonatate ●●● inhibits the excitation of pulmonary stretch-receptors (peripheral effect), in addition to a central effect;[813] not available in UK

Bronchorrhoea

Bronchorrhoea, voluminous amounts of clear frothy sputum, occurs in 6% of cases of alveolar cell cancer of lung (9% of lung cancers).[814] Radiotherapy should be considered, but other suggested symptomatic treatments are largely anecdotal:[4]

- antimuscarinic drugs (e.g. glycopyrronium) ••
- corticosteroids PO or nebulised ••
- octreotide ••
- macrolide antibiotics (erythromycin, clarithromycin) ••
- nebulised furosemide 20mg q.d.s.••• (⇨ *p.89*)
- nebulised indometacin 25mg/2mL 4-8hourly in saline pH adjusted with sodium bicarbonate ••• [815]

⇨ *(p.26)* for antimuscarinics and octreotide.

SEE ALSO
📖 Reviews[816,817]

Drugs used for Cough
⇨ *p.67* for preparations of morphine, *p.99* for benzodiazepines.
PHOLCODINE
    Linctus 5mg/5mL
    TSD: 10mL t.d.s. **PO**
CODEINE
    Tabs. 30mg, 60mg; Linctus 15mg/5mL; Syrup 25mg/5mL
    TSD: 25-30mg q.d.s. **PO**
METHADONE
    Linctus 2mg/5mL
    TSD: 2-4mg nocte **PO**
SIMPLE LINCTUS B.P.
    Liquid
    TSD: 10mL q.d.s. **PO**
    (Citric acid, anise water, syrup)
IPRATROPIUM BROMIDE
    Aerosol inh. 20μg, 40μg *(Atrovent)*
    TSD: 40μg q.d.s. inhaler
    Neb. soln. 250μg/1mL, 500μg/2mL *(Atrovent)*
    TSD: 250μg q.d.s. via neb.
SODIUM CROMOGLICATE
    Aerosol inhaler 5mg/dose; Breath-actuated inhaler (powder) 5mg/dose
    Nebuliser solution 20mg/2mL ⊘
    TSD: 10-20mg q.d.s.
    (Inhaled powder can cause bronchospasm)

DRUGS FOR POST-NASAL DRIP
BECLOMETASONE DIPROPIONATE
    Nasal spray 50μg/spray
    TSD: 2 sprays b.d.
PSEUDOEPHEDRINE HYDROCHLORIDE
    Tabs. 60mg; Liquid 30mg/5mL
    TSD: 60mg q.d.s.
EPHEDRINE HYDROCHLORIDE
    Nasal drops 0.5% 10mL, 1% 10mL
    TSD: 0.5% 1-2 drops 3-4 times daily
IPRATROPIUM BROMIDE
    Nasal spray 0.03%
    TSD: 2 sprays 2-3 times daily
    Helps watery rhinorrhoea of allergic and non-allergic rhinitis

Additional information

Nebulised antibiotics

Nebulised gentamicin is used quite frequently in cystic fibrosis. Purulent secretions colonised with gram negative organisms can be treated with nebulised gentamicin 80mg b.d. - t.d.s. with a significant reduction in the volume of secretions. Negligible systemic absorption has been shown.[818]

Haloperidol and antitussives

Studies on experimental models have shown that pre-treatment with haloperidol markedly reduces the antitussive effect of pentazocine and dextromethorphan. Haloperidol is a potent sigma-ligand and it is suggested that the antitussive effect is mediated by sigma-sites. Clinical relevance is unknown, but possibly a trial of alternative antiemetic is worth trying if a patient on haloperidol has intractable cough resistant to antitussives.[819]

Parenteral lidocaine

Intravenously administered lidocaine will suppress cough following tracheal intubation under general anaesthesia. The incidence of coughing decreased as the dose of lidocaine increased. A dose of 1.5 mg/kg or more of intravenous lidocaine suppressed the cough reflex significantly ($P < 0.01$). The cough reflex was almost entirely suppressed by plasma concentrations of lidocaine in excess of 4μg/mL. The results suggest that iv lidocaine••• is effective in suppressing cough reflex during tracheal intubation under general anaesthesia, but relatively high plasma concentrations of lidocaine, close to toxic levels, are required for complete suppression of coughing (high doses given - 1mg/kg or more repeated after 5 minutes).[820,821]

Haemoptysis

Assessment

Consider the commonest causes:
• tumour bleeding
• clotting disorders
• infection

Treatment

• Treat any evidence or signs suggestive of infection.
• Consider radiotherapy referral[822,823] (not if multiple lung metastases) or brachytherapy.[824-826]
• Consider and treat other systemic causes of bleeding - ⇨ *Bleeding and haemorrhage (p.147)*
    – blood tests for clotting screen and platelets
• Tranexamic acid 1g t.d.s. po:
    – stop if no effect after 1 week[295]
    – continue for 1 week after bleeding has stopped, then discontinue
    – continue long term (500mg t.d.s.) only if bleeding recurs and responds to second course of treatment
• Small bleeds can herald a larger massive haemorrhage; consider siting an iv cannula to administer emergency drugs ⇨ *Massive haemorrhage (p.184)*

Major bleeding

If patient's condition is not stable, with history of major haemorrhage or
ongoing bleeding:
- Consider if appropriate to transfer to an acute medical/endoscopy unit.
- Site an IV cannula to anticipate need for emergency drugs. *(p.184)*
- Treat anxiety or distress as needed:
    - midazolam 2-5mg initially by slow IV titration (10mg diluted to 10mL
      with 0.9% saline)
    - if no IV access, midazolam 5-10mg SC (give IM if shocked or
      vasoconstricted)

PRESCRIBING STATUS

☼ Tranexamic acid ®

ThinkList

- arterial embolisation[296-299,827]
- etamsylate ® ⇨ *Haemostatic drugs (p.150)*
- laser treatment - provides effective palliation for bronchial obstruction and
    haemoptysis in selected proximal endobronchial cancers[828]

SEE ALSO

⇨ *Bleeding & haemorrhage (p.147)*
▭ Review[829]

Drugs used for Haemoptysis

TRANEXAMIC ACID (CYKLOKAPRON) ☑

Tabs. 500mg; Syrup 500mg/5mL; Inj. 500mg/5mL
TSD 1g t.d.s. PO or by slow IV injection
Avoid if risk of ureteric obstruction e.g. renal haemorrhage. Discontinue if
disturbance in colour vision develops.

Additional Information

Tranexamic acid has been used successfully in treating haemoptysis in children
with cystic fibrosis.[830,831]

Death rattle

These guidelines are for patients who are imminently dying and develop
'rattling' or 'bubbly' breathing (the death-rattle). The following guidelines
should not be used as they stand if the patient is still aware enough to be
distressed by the dry mouth that will result from treatment.
1) Acute pulmonary oedema should be excluded, or treated with
    furosemide.
2) Try repositioning the patient on different sides.
3) Explain to any relatives present:
    - the noise is present because the patient is not coughing or clearing their
      throat as they normally would
    - if the patient is deeply asleep or unconscious, he/she will not be
      distressed by the rattling even though it may sound as though the
      breathing is difficult
    - despite best attempts at treating the rattle with medication, this does
      not always work

4) Give hyoscine hydrobromide 400µg stat subcutaneously, and
5) Start hyoscine hydrobromide 1.2-1.6mg/24h csci
6) Wait for half an hour and reassess the patient. If there is still an unacceptable rattle, and there has not been a marked improvement:
   – give a further dose of hyoscine hydrobromide 400µg stat sc.
7) Wait for half an hour and reassess the patient.
8) If the noise has been relieved, but recurs later, give repeat doses of hyoscine hydrobromide 400µg to a maximum of 800µg in any 4h.
9) Increase CSCI to 2.4mg/24h.
10) If the noise is not relieved:
    – If the respiratory rate is > 20 breaths per minute, the noise may be reduced by slowing the respiratory rate: give diamorphine 2.5-5mg sc (or a sixth of the 24h dose if already on csci). Repeat after 30 minutes if respiratory rate still above 20 per minute.
    – If the noise appears to be coming from the back of the pharynx, and the patient is deeply unconscious, try using suction.
    – Tip the bed 30 degrees 'head-up' allowing the secretions to drain back into the lungs from the throat or trachea.
11) Explanation and reassurance to the relatives are important, as medication will only stop the rattle in half of the patients.[832-834]
12) Ensure that the patient is not distressed, using sedative drugs such as midazolam if necessary.

Alternative drug treatment

Glycopyrronium may also be used for the death rattle.[834,835] It does not cause sedation or confusion, but lacks antiemetic effect, and sedation is often either required or irrelevant in the terminal stage. It is useful for the patient who is still conscious and wishes to remain as alert as possible. Equivalent doses are:
- glycopyrronium 200µg sc stat. repeated if necessary after 20-30 min.
- glycopyrronium 800µg/24h csci (max. 1.2mg/24h)

Hyoscine butylbromide *(Buscopan)* has also been used,[834] but appropriate dosage regimens are less well established. Hyoscine hydrobromide transdermal patch has also been reported.[836]

PRESCRIBING STATUS
☼ Hyoscine hydrobromide, Glycopyrronium •
☼ Hyoscine butylbromide *(Buscopan)* ••

Drugs for Death Rattle

GLYCOPYRRONIUM BROMIDE (GLYCOPYRROLATE)
  Inj. 200µg/1mL, 600µg/3mL ◎
  TSD: 800µg/24h CSCI
HYOSCINE HYDROBROMIDE (SCOPOLAMINE HYDROBROMIDE)
  Inj. 400µg/1mL, 600µg/1mL
  TSD: 1.2-1.6mg/24h CSCI
HYOSCINE BUTYLBROMIDE (SCOPOLAMINE BUTYLBROMIDE)
  Inj. 20mg/1mL *(Buscopan)*
  TSD: 40-160mg/24h CSCI

Additional Information

Only about 50% of patients respond to antimuscarinic drugs. The beta-blockers propranolol and metoprolol have been reported as helping thick tenacious secretions in drooling, as part of the salivary innervation is sympathetic.[371] No studies have yet reported any trials of beta-blockers in death rattle.

NEUROLOGICAL & PSYCHIATRIC

Anxiety

Anxiety may best be treated non-pharmacologically. Benzodiazepines are helpful, and concerns about addiction and tolerance are often irrelevant in terminal care.

Depression with anxiety symptoms should be excluded as well as akathisia, thyrotoxicosis, drug withdrawal (especially SSRIs and benzodiazepines), and alcohol or nicotine[837] withdrawal. Patients with 'panic attacks' should always be carefully assessed to exclude multiple pulmonary emboli, paroxysmal atrial fibrillation (PAF) or partial seizures. [838]

PRESCRIBING STATUS
☼ Midazolam •

SEE ALSO
⇨ SSRI withdrawal (p.101), Alcohol withdrawal (p.105)
📖 Reviews[839,840]

Drugs used for Anxiety

Diazepam is an appropriate first-line benzodiazepine. Lorazepam is shorter acting, and (taken sublingually) has faster onset, and is useful on a PRN basis. Midazolam can be used if a CSCI is required.

Propranolol is helpful, especially to control the somatic symptoms of anxiety e.g. tremor and palpitations.

The anxiolytic effect of buspirone develops over 1-3 weeks, and it probably has little place in palliative care. [839]

SSRIs can be used for panic attacks if benzodiazepines are ineffective.

DIAZEPAM
Tabs. 2mg, 5mg, 10mg; Oral solution 2mg/5mL, 5mg/5mL
TSD: 2mg t.d.s. PO or 5mg nocte
Rectal tubes 5mg/2.5mL, 10mg/2.5mL; Supps. 10mg
Inj. (emulsion) 10mg/2mL *(Diazemuls)* - IV use only
Inj. (solution) 10mg/2mL - IM use
Blood levels increased by omeprazole (increased sedation).

LORAZEPAM
Tabs. 1mg, 2.5mg; Inj. 4mg/1mL
TSD: 0.5- 1mg PRN t.d.s. PO or sublingual

MIDAZOLAM
Inj. 10mg/2mL, 10mg/5mL
TSD: 10-20mg/24h CSCI
Sedative effect markedly enhanced by itraconazole, ketoconazole and possibly fluconazole.

PROPRANOLOL
Tabs. 10mg, 40mg, 80mg, 160mg; Oral solution‡ 40mg/5mL; Tabs. SR 80mg, 160mg
TSD: 40mg o.d. PO, increased as needed to t.d.s. or 160mg daily total dose

Insomnia & Night Sedation

Causes of Insomnia to consider
- uncontrolled pain
- steroids, especially if taken late in the day
- depression - with anxiety symptoms stopping patients getting sleep, or early morning waking
- bladder or bowel discomfort
- hunger
- anxiety and fears

Night sedation
1) Regular or PRN night sedation should not be prescribed routinely.
2) If a patient is taking a regular benzodiazepine hypnotic e.g. temazepam, consider whether they need continue with night sedation:
   - tolerance to benzodiazepines usually develops within a few weeks
   - withdrawal nightmares and insomnia can occur
3) Insomnia due to depression should be treated with a sedative antidepressant e.g. dosulepin (dothiepin) starting at 50-75mg nocte (25mg if elderly and frail). Sleep improvement may occur within a few days, although the dose may have to be titrated up to 150mg/day for 2/52 for the antidepressant effect ⇨ *Antidepressants (p.101)*
4) Anxiety and fear may be most appropriately treated by sitting and talking to the patient, a hot drink etc. rather than medication.
5) If a night sedative is appropriate, temazepam 10mg nocte should be prescribed, increased to 20mg if needed.
6) If temazepam is effective but causes unacceptable 'hangover' effects, shorter acting zopiclone 7.5mg may be tried.
7) If temazepam is ineffective, or becomes tolerated, consider:
   - dosulepin 50-75mg nocte as a 2nd line night sedative - even in the absence of depression; may cause daytime drowsiness
   - clomethiazole may be effective in the elderly, especially if agitated or confused at night

ThinkList
- Give antidepressant or phenothiazine drugs at 7-8pm, as a bedtime dose will not start working until early hours of morning and there will be significant drowsiness early the next day.
- In extreme circumstances, a 'cocktail' of a benzodiazepine (temazepam or diazepam) and phenothiazine (chlorpromazine or levomepromazine) in high doses may be needed; daytime sedation is likely.
- Patients requiring only occasional use, may find an antihistamine• (chlorphenamine or promethazine) helpful. Tolerance to the hypnotic effect usually occurs quickly, and dependence does not therefore occur.

SEE ALSO
📖 Review[839]

Hypnotics
TEMAZEPAM
   Tabs. 10mg, 20mg; Elixir 10mg/5mL
   TSD: 10mg nocte PO (£0.95)

CLOMETHIAZOLE (CHLORMETHIAZOLE)
Caps. 192mg; Syrup 250mg/5mL *(Heminevrin)*
TSD: 2 caps. nocte PO (£4.05) - elderly 1 caps.; 10mL nocte PO (£3.39)
ZOPICLONE
Tabs. 3.75, 7.5mg
TSD: 7.5mg nocte PO (£4.43) - elderly 3.75mg
ZALEPLON ©
Tabs. 5mg, 10mg
TSD: 10mg nocte PO (£6.72) - elderly 5mg
Shortest acting hypnotic; may be useful if even zopiclone causes 'hangover'

ANTIDEPRESSANT (SEDATIVE)
DOSULEPIN (DOTHIEPIN)
Caps. 25mg; Tabs. 75mg *(Prothiaden)*
TSD: 25-75mg nocte PO

Depression

Asking "are you depressed?" will identify almost all dying patients with
substantial mood disorders.[841] Major depressive illness may then be diagnosed
using the DSM IV criteria *(p.220)*. There is good evidence that
antidepressants can be effective in terminal illness.[842]

Atypical presentations of depression
- irritability
- agitation and anxiety symptoms
- histrionic behaviour
- hypochondriasis
- psychotic features (delusions, paranoia) that are mood-congruent e.g.
    content of delusions consistent with depressive thoughts

Antidepressant treatment
A trial of at least 2 weeks, and preferably 4 or more, is needed to properly
assess response to an antidepressant. Discontinuation symptoms (withdrawal)
will not usually occur if stopped within 6 weeks of starting.
Use an SSRI unless other treatment specifically indicated:
- dose escalation is not usually needed, so more rapid control of symptoms
    may be possible
- side effects of SSRIs are generally better tolerated than tricyclics in ill cancer
    patients
Tricyclic antidepressants (TCA) indicated for:
- nausea & vomiting (may be exacerbated by SSRI)
- coincidental symptoms that may be helped by the antimuscarinic effect e.g.:
    – neuropathic pain
    – cancer-related sweats (or consider venlafaxine)
    – nocturnal urinary incontinence
    – sialorrhoea / drooling
- severe depression, when maximising efficacy is of overriding importance
    (more effective than SSRIs)
Venlafaxine, at a dose of 150mg or greater, may also be more effective than
SSRIs for major depression.[843,844]

ThinkList

- corticosteroids - may help mild depression and low mood by improving sense of well-being (can also induce psychosis or depression in others)
- psychostimulants ••• (methylphenidate or dexamfetamine) *(p. 103)*
- ECT (electro-convulsive therapy) - response can be very rapid; very occasionally appropriate e.g. severe depression developing during chemotherapy
- pathological crying may respond to citalopram[845]

SEE ALSO

⇨ *DSM Criteria for diagnosis (p.220)*

📖 Reviews[846-850] & Guidelines[851]

Antidepressants

TRICYCLICS & TETRACYCLICS

The original tricyclics (amitriptyline, clomipramine etc.) are used in low doses as co-analgesics, but they are poorly tolerated due to side effects in anti-depressant doses. The observation has been made that 'poor responders' to amitriptyline suffer more side-effects than good responders.[423]

Dosulepin (dothiepin) is a good first-line antidepressant, whilst lofepramine has a lower incidence of side effects, useful in the elderly. Usual treatment dose of most tricyclics is 150mg/day (perhaps less in elderly); lofepramine is 140-210mg/day.

Tricyclic antidepressants used concomitantly with amiodarone increase the risk of ventricular arrhythmias and should be avoided. The low doses of TCA's used for neuropathic pain probably carry a low risk.

DOSULEPIN (DOTHIEPIN)

Caps. 25mg; Tabs. 75mg *(Prothiaden)*
TSD: 50-75mg nocte PO

LOFEPRAMINE

Tabs. 70mg
TSD: 70mg o.d. - b.d. PO

SSRIs

There is little to choose between the **SSRIs**,[852] but fluoxetine has a slower onset of action and may cause more agitation than other **SSRIs**[853] and is therefore not recommended as first line, except for non-agitated, anergic patients.

SSRIs may cause nausea, vomiting and headaches. Extrapyramidal reactions can rarely occur with **SSRIs**.[854]

Antidepressant discontinuation syndromes occur with both **TCAs** and **SSRIs**.[855]

SSRI discontinuation symptoms include dizziness, light-headedness, insomnia, fatigue, anxiety/agitation, nausea, headache, and sensory disturbance.[856] **SSRIs** should be withdrawn gradually when possible, using alternate day dosing if needed. More common with paroxetine (short half-life), least with fluoxetine (half-life of weeks).

SSRIs may increase the risk of GI bleeding, especially in patients taking **NSAIDs**.[21-25]

Serious reaction with MAOIs, selegiline (serotonin syndrome).[857]
Increased serotonergic effects with St John's wort (avoid).
Fluoxetine and fluvoxamine increase blood levels of carbamazepine[858,859] and phenytoin (risk of toxicity).
Fluoxetine increases plasma levels of flecainide.

PAROXETINE ☑

Tabs. 20mg; Liquid 20mg/10mL *(Seroxat)*
TSD: 20mg mane PO increase by weekly increments of 10mg as necessary to max. 50mg o.d. (£16.58 at 20mg o.d.)

CITALOPRAM

Tabs. 10, 20, 40mg; Oral drops 40mg/mL *(Cipramil)*
TSD: 20mg mane PO; max. 60mg o.d. (£16.03 at 20mg o.d.)

SERTRALINE
  Tabs. 50, 100mg *(Lustral)*
    TSD: 50mg mane *PO*; max. 200mg o.d. (£16.20 at 50mg o.d.)

OTHER ANTIDEPRESSANT DRUGS

Venlafaxine is a serotonin and noradrenaline reuptake inhibitor (**SNRI**). It causes less side effects than the **SSRIs**. The **SR** capsules are preferable to use as they seem to be better tolerated. Mirtazepine is a **NaSSA** and is useful if there is marked anxiety/agitation.

VENLAFAXINE
  Tabs. 37.5, 50, 75mg
    TSD: 37.5mg b.d. *PO* increased to 75mg b.d. (£39.97 at 75mg b.d.)
  Caps. **SR** 75, 150mg
    TSD: 75mg o.d. *PO* increased to 150mg o.d. (£39.97 at 150mg o.d.)
  Dose should be increased gradually to usual dose 150mg, and higher
    according to response; maximum 375mg daily (225mg if **SR**)

MIRTAZEPINE
  Tabs. (scored) 30mg
    TSD: 15mg nocte *PO* increased to 30mg nocte (£22.92 at 30mg nocte)
  Dose should be increased gradually to usual dose 30mg, and higher according
    to response; maximum 45mg daily
  Risk of blood dyscrasias

Additional Information

St John's wort

A number of patients may be taking St John's wort[860] as an antidepressant. It is as effective as imipramine in mild to moderate depression,[861] but not in severe depression. It is not a licensed medication, but has a number of significant drug interactions:

- increases serotonergic effects with SSRIs (avoid)
- reduces anticoagulant effect of warfarin
- reduces plasma levels of carbamazepine, phenytoin, phenobarbital (risk of fits)
- reduces plasma levels of digoxin

Psychostimulants

Potential uses for psychostimulants

- depression
- opioid-induced sedation or cognitive impairment
- fatigue
- cognitive impairment due to brain tumours[862]
- hypoactive delirium[863,864]
- hiccups[248-250]

Psychostimulants for Depression

Psychostimulants have been shown effective in depression in medically ill patients including the terminally ill, although they do not seem to be effective in primary depression.[865] They are rarely prescribed for depression in the UK.[866] They are useful because of their rapid onset, and are generally well tolerated.[867] The beneficial effects of these drugs are reported to occur within 36-48h.[868,869] Drug habituation is generally not a problem.[868]

Methylphenidate appears to have been used more widely, but dexamfetamine is equally effective.[870]

Doses of methylphenidate as low as 1.25mg daily have been used successfully in patients over 90 years old.[871]

Methylphenidate (average dose after titration 30mg daily) is as effective as imipramine 150mg o.d. in significantly reducing depressive and anxiety symptoms.[872]

Opioid-induced sedation or cognitive impairment

Psychostimulants have been used as adjuvants to reduce opioid-induced sedation and potentiate analgesia.[873-876] In addition to methylphenidate and dexamfetamine, caffeine has also been shown to have a weak effect.[877] They may work by (1) reducing opioid-induced sedation or cognitive impairment and thus allowing dose escalation of the opioid, or (2) actually potentiating opioid analgesia.[878] Their effect on opioid-induced sedation may only be mild.[879]

Psychostimulants for fatigue

No trials have been published on psychostimulants in cancer-related fatigue, although their efficacy has been demonstrated in HIV and MS patients.[880] Observations on depression in advanced cancer also suggest they improve fatigue.

PRESCRIBING STATUS

Dexamfetamine, methylphenidate ●●●

SEE ALSO

⇨ *Depression (p.101), Opioid side effects (p.69)*

📖 Review[881]

Psychostimulant drugs

Side effects of agitation, dysphoria, insomnia and nightmares may occur,[882] and hypomania has been reported.[883]

METHYLPHENIDATE ☑

 Tabs. 5, 10, 20mg

 TSD: 5mg b.d. PO (8.00am and 12 noon); increase every few days up to 30mg b.d. according to response

DEXAMFETAMINE SULPHATE

 Tabs. 5mg

 TSD: 5mg b.d. PO (8.00am and 12 noon); increase every few days up to 30mg b.d. according to response

Delirium & Confusion

Treat cause of confusion if possible. Consider:

- hypercalcaemia
- hypoglycaemia
- hyponatraemia
- renal failure
- liver failure
- drug related, especially
  - opioids *(p.69)* N.B. opioids accumulate in renal failure
  - corticosteroids[884]
  - corticosteroid withdrawal
  - alcohol withdrawal (clomethiazole ± diazepam)
  - benzodiazepine withdrawal[885]
  - benzodiazepines and phenothiazines accumulate in liver failure
  - SSRI withdrawal (discontinuation syndrome) *(p.101)*
- nicotine withdrawal[837] (nicotine patch‡ ⊘)
- cerebral tumour
- CVA or TIA
- infection
- hypoxia
- disorientation of move to hospital in pre-existing dementia
- thiamine (vitamin B₁) deficiency[886] (see below)
- non-convulsive status epilepticus

Cause is often multifactorial.[887] Consider a primary anxiety state (see notes below - Benzodiazepines in agitation and restlessness).

Treatment of delirium & confusion with antipsychotics

	Non-elderly	Elderly
Confusion ± drowsiness, or where sedation undesirable / unnecessary	*Non-sedative antipsychotic* Haloperidol 1.5-3mg nocte or b.d. SC/CSCI (Risperidone 1mg b.d.[888,889])	*Non-sedative antipsychotic with lower risk of EPSE* Risperidone 0.5mg nocte or b.d. PO Haloperidol 0.5-1mg nocte SC/CSCI
Agitated confusion where sedative effects desired; mild - moderate agitation	*Sedative antipsychotic* Levomepromazine 25-50mg SC/CSCI/PO (Chlorpromazine 25-50mg b.d. - q.d.s. PO)	*Sedative antipsychotic with lower risk of EPSE* Promazine 25mg nocte or up to q.d.s. PO Levomepromazine 12.5-25mg/24h CSCI (Olanzapine 2.5mg nocte PO)
Acutely disturbed, violent or aggressive; at risk to themselves or others[890]	*Antipsychotic with proven safety record in repeated high doses for rapid titration; suitable for parenteral use* Haloperidol 5mg SC/IM ± lorazepam 1-2mg SC/IM repeated after 20-30 minutes.	Haloperidol 2.5mg SC/IM ± lorazepam 0.5-1mg SC/IM repeated after 30 minutes

- Drugs should only be prescribed if necessary; reassurance and helping to orientate the patient may be all that is required.
- Doses should be adjusted according to age and general condition, level of disturbance, and likely tolerance.
- Antipsychotics are considered to be the drugs of choice for delirium:
    - haloperidol is standard treatment for delirium
    - risk of extrapyramidal side-effects (EPSE) most marked in elderly; risperidone and promazine carry lower risk and are suggested except when rapid control is needed of acutely disturbed patient
    - chlorpromazine and levomepromazine (methotrimeprazine) are more sedative than haloperidol
- Benzodiazepines carry a risk of paradoxical agitation (disinhibition with worsening of behavioural disturbance) especially in the elderly:
    - used in conjunction with haloperidol, lorazepam improves the control of the acutely disturbed patient, but used alone is less effective than antipsychotics in delirium[891]

Benzodiazepines in agitation and restlessness

Although antipsychotics are considered the treatment of choice for delirium, agitation and restlessness in the patient with advanced cancer may often be primarily an anxiety state, with secondary cognitive impairment or clouded consciousness. In this condition, benzodiazepines are in the author's experience more effective than antipsychotics. A knowledge of the previous psychological state of the patient is vital in determining this. (An example is the frightened patient who develops hallucinations with opioids and presents with acute paranoia.) See also *Terminal agitation (p.108)*.

Alcohol withdrawal

The best treatment for alcohol withdrawal in palliative care is usually alcohol! Clomethiazole $\pm$ benzodiazepines are the usual drug treatment. Alcohol withdrawal has also been treated with 10-20ml absolute alcohol made up to 50mls with saline/24h IV using a syringe driver.

Wernicke's encephalopathy (thiamine/vitamin B_1 deficiency) classically presents with ophthalmoplegia, nystagmus, ataxia and confusion. Diagnosis can be confirmed by RBC transketolase estimation. May be more common than anticipated in terminally ill, present atypically and be associated with cognitive impairment.[886]

Patients with a history of alcohol misuse who develop unexplained -

- ophthalmoplegia
- ataxia (not due to intoxication)
- acute confusion (not due to intoxication)
- memory disturbance
- seizures
- coma/unconscious
    - a presumptive diagnosis of Wernicke's encephalopathy should be made and treated with high-dose parenteral B-complex vitamins[892]

Thioridazine & Droperidol

Note that thioridazine *(Melleril)* has had its licence for treating agitation in the elderly removed because of the risk of cardiac arrhythmias, and should not be prescribed except under guidance from a psychiatrist.

Droperidol has been withdrawn for the same reason (prolonged QT intervals).

PRESCRIBING STATUS
☼ Risperidone **●●**
☼ Olanzapine **●●**

SEE ALSO
⇨ *Terminal agitation (p.108)*
📖 Reviews[893-898] & Guidelines[899]

Drugs for confusion
ANTIPSYCHOTICS

Haloperidol and levomepromazine can be given by CSCI. Most antipsychotics can be shown to decrease the convulsive threshold, and may increase the risk of fitting in susceptible patients, but the actual risk is undetermined.
Promazine and the newer, atypical antipsychotics (risperidone and olanzapine) have a lower incidence of EPSE.

HALOPERIDOL

Caps. 0.5mg; Tabs. 1.5mg, 5mg; Liquid 2mg/mL; Inj. 5mg/1mL
Indometacin given with haloperidol can cause severe drowsiness.

LEVOMEPROMAZINE (METHOTRIMEPRAZINE)

Tabs. 6mg[‡◌] 25mg; Susp. 25mg/5mL[‡◌] ; Inj. 25mg/1mL *(Nozinan)*
TSD: 12.5mg nocte or b.d. PO; 12.5mg/24h CSCI
6mg tabs. available on named patient basis from Link Pharmaceuticals
Suspension available from Rhone-Poulenc Rorer (Canada); contact Idis World Medicines Ltd, Kingston-upon-Thames, Surrey[29]
Oral bioavailability of levomepromazine is approx. 40%.[1] Use half the daily oral dose by CSCI.
Avoid concurrent use with MAOIs (p.211)

PROMAZINE

Tabs. 25mg, 50mg; Liquid 25mg/5mL, 50mg/5mL; Inj. 50mg/1mL

RISPERIDONE

Tabs. 0.5mg, 1mg, 2mg, 3mg, 4mg, 6mg; Liquid 1mg/1mL

OLANZAPINE

Tabs. 2.5mg, 5mg, 7.5mg, 10mg; Oral lyophilisates 5mg, 10mg
Oral lyophilisates can be placed on the tongue to dissolve/disperse

BENZODIAZEPINES

Lorazepam is shorter acting than diazepam, and is therefore safer in repeated doses; can be given SC or sublingually for more rapid effect and in uncooperative patients. Midazolam can be given by CSCI.

LORAZEPAM

Tabs. 1mg, 2.5mg; Inj. 4mg/1mL
Dilute inj. with equal volume of water or saline for IM use

DIAZEPAM

Tabs. 2mg, 5mg, 10mg; Syrup 2mg/5mL; Rectal soln. 5mg/2.5mL, 10mg/2.5mL
Supps. 10mg
Blood levels increased by omeprazole (increased sedation).

MIDAZOLAM

Inj. 10mg/2mL, 10mg/5mL
TSD: 20-30mg/24h CSCI (maximum 100mg/24h)
Sedative effect markedly enhanced by itraconazole, ketoconazole and possibly fluconazole.

VITAMIN B PREPARATIONS
PABRINEX (VITAMINS B AND C)

Inj. Pair of ampoules containing 10mL
TSD:1 pair of ampoules daily for 3 days - for acute and severe and vitamin B deficiency states
Serious allergic reaction may rarely occur on IV administration (probably < 1 in 250,000, compared to incidence of 1-10% allergy with penicillin). Inject slowly over 10 minutes.

Terminal Agitation

Diagnosis of terminal agitation assumes that reversible conditions are excluded or failing to respond to treatment. Sedation is needed in many patients, but pain (especially from urinary retention) should be excluded or treated appropriately.

Most patients can be settled with midazolam by CSCI.[900] Tolerance is sometimes seen, and the addition of a sedative phenothiazine or barbiturate may be needed.

1) Midazolam 5-10mg SC stat. if needed and 20-30mg/24h by CSCI; increase by 10-30mg increments; if 60-100mg/24h not working, **add**
2) Levomepromazine (methotrimeprazine) 25mg SC stat. if needed and 50-100mg/24h by CSCI; increase by 50-100mg increments to 250mg/24h as required.
3) Phenobarbital 200mg stat. SC and 600-2400mg/24h by CSCI;[901] a second syringe driver is needed as phenobarbital in incompatible with most other drugs. *(p.173)*

PRESCRIBING STATUS
☼ Midazolam •
☼ Phenobarbital ••

ThinkList

- remember urinary retention, urinary retention and urinary retention!
- rising intracranial pressure in the terminal stages of cerebral tumours can cause a rapid and severe escalation of pain (headache), unlike most other pain states in cancer; if in any doubt of the cause of distress, use both generous doses of opioid analgesic and midazolam together
- haloperidol 5mg stat. and 10-20mg/24h by CSCI can be used as an alternative to methotrimeprazine if injection site irritation is a problem
- if a syringe driver is not available, alternative benzodiazepines ± phenothiazines may be used by sublingual or rectal routes e.g. chlorpromazine 25mg PR 4-6 hourly with escalation to response (up to 100-200mg 4-hourly),[765] diazepam rectally 10mg PRN, or clonazepam sublingually •• 0.5mg and titrate upwards[370]
- propofol ••• has been used in intractable cases - 20mg stat then 50-70mg/h[902,903]

SEE ALSO
📖 Reviews[904-906]

Drugs for Terminal Agitation

MIDAZOLAM
Inj. 10mg/2mL, 10mg/5mL
TSD: 5-10mg SC stat. PRN or 20-30mg/24h CSCI. Max. 100mg/24h
LEVOMEPROMAZINE (METHOTRIMEPRAZINE)
Inj. 25mg/1mL *(Nozinan)*
TSD: 25mg SC stat. PRN or 100mg/24h CSCI. Max. 250mg/24h. Note much smaller doses used as antiemetic.
PHENOBARBITAL
Inj. 60mg/1mL, 200mg/1mL; Elixir 15mg/5mL; Tabs. 15mg, 30mg, 60mg
Doses: see above

Convulsions & Seizures

General notes

- For patients with intracranial tumours, consider starting, or review dose, of corticosteroids.
- Remember to advise the patient about restrictions on driving. *(p.198)*
- Parenteral thiamine if alcohol abuse suspected. *(p.105)*
- Consider and treat hypoglycaemia in at-risk patients.
- Consider drug interactions that alter anticonvulsant levels:
  - corticosteroids (see below)
  - other anticonvulsants

Management of Status Epilepticus

1) Midazolam 5mg (dilute 10mg with water to 10mL) slow IV titration.
2) Midazolam is not licensed as an anticonvulsant, but is usually readily available in palliative care units; a number of alternative benzodiazepines can be used (lorazepam is recommended first choice if available):
   - lorazepam 4mg slow IV
   - *Diazemuls* 10mg slow IV
   - clonazepam 1mg slow IV (into large vein)
3) Repeat dose if needed after 10 minutes.
4) If the patient has not responded to a repeated dose of benzodiazepine or seizures recur, give phenobarbital 200mg (diluted in 10mL water) by slow IV injection, over minimum of 2 minutes.
5) Repeat phenobarbital if necessary up to a maximum of 10-15mg/kg (600mg - 1000mg) at maximum rate of 100mg/minute.
6) Once seizures have been controlled, review anticonvulsant therapy.

Initiating anticonvulsant therapy

- It is usually appropriate to initiate anticonvulsant therapy after one seizure in patients with terminal illness.
- Sodium valproate is an appropriate first line anticonvulsant for almost all types of convulsions or seizures, including focal and partial seizures, and those caused by intracranial tumours.
  - Aim to increase dose to lower end of quoted 'usual maintenance dose' unless side-effects occur, or frail elderly patient. Doses given below.
  - Carbamazepine and phenytoin are suitable alternatives.
- If the patient is unconscious or cannot take oral medication, see below.

Patients unable to take oral medication

- Patients who are unable to take oral medication due to dysphagia, vomiting or in terminal care, may need anticonvulsants by another route.
- The half-life of most anticonvulsants is quite long (> 24h), therefore no parenteral anticonvulsant is usually needed if
  - there is a low risk of seizures, and
  - only a single dose is missed, or
  - the prognosis is measured in days.
- The risk of seizures is higher if:
  - patient has decreased or stopped steroids (intracranial tumours)
  - recent rise in headache or vomiting or other signs suggesting rising ICP (intracranial tumours)

- myoclonus or other twitching is present
- history of poor control of seizures or recent seizures
- previously needing > 1 anticonvulsant to achieve control
- Because of the long half life of anticonvulsants, parenteral treatment can be started any time within 24h after the last oral dose.

Choice of non-oral anticonvulsant

Choice may be determined partly by availability:

Phenobarbital CSCI or daily SC☑	Well-proven anticonvulsant for all types of seizures. Experience suggests it is effective in doses of 200mg/24h. Phenobarbital is incompatible with most other drugs in a syringe driver therefore a second syringe driver may be necessary. The dose can also be given by daily SC or IM injection although this can sting.
Midazolam CSCI	Midazolam is more sedative than anticonvulsant. Anticonvulsant efficacy of 'standard' doses is unknown, but probably requires 20-30mg/24h minimum. Unlicensed use. If low risk of seizures, and midazolam indicated for e.g. terminal agitation, then additional anticonvulsant probably unnecessary. If higher risk of seizures, use phenobarbital in addition.
Clonazepam CSCI	Main advantage is that clonazepam is compatible with many other drugs used in CSCI *(p.173)*. Much less experience supporting its use in this way; doses recommended between 2-4mg/24h (4-8mg/24h if sedation acceptable or desired).
Carbamazepine or valproate⁺ suppositories	Occasionally suitable for patients well controlled on one of these drugs, who develop a temporary inability to take oral medication (e.g. vomiting and who would find rectal administration acceptable.

Dose of Phenobarbital as Anticonvulsant

- If a patient is dying, and sedation is acceptable, it is better to err on the generous side and give:
  - phenobarbital 200mg SC stat. as a loading dose - if there is > 24h interval since oral anticonvulsants last taken
  - phenobarbital 200mg/24h by CSCI, or
  - if high risk of seizures - phenobarbital 400mg/24h by CSCI
- If needing to minimise sedation, use 100mg SC stat. as a loading dose followed by 100-200mg/24h by CSCI.

Management of prolonged seizures

Most seizures are self-limiting and require only supportive care. For more prolonged seizures occurring at home, a number of measures can be arranged in anticipation which can avoid inappropriate emergency admission to hospital.

- Diazepam rectal solution 10mg PR - administered by district nurse or carer.
- Midazolam 5-10mg SC (or preferably IM) - administered by district nurse.
- Buccal midazolam 10mg/2mL can be administered by a carer if the rectal route for diazepam is unacceptable, and appears to be as effective and may be quicker-acting than rectal diazepam 10mg.[907,908] Oral solution is available as a 'special' or the injectable preparation can be used.

In an inpatient unit, midazolam 5-10mg SC (or preferably IM) may be given first before treating as status epilepticus as above.

PRESCRIBING STATUS
☼ Midazolam for seizures •

SEE ALSO
⇨ *Anticonvulsant blood levels (p.215)*

Anticonvulsants

Carbamazepine and phenytoin levels are decreased (risk of fits) by corticosteroids. Carbamazepine, phenytoin and phenobarbital can reduce the efficacy of corticosteroids. This two-way interaction[909,910] is common when managing patients with cerebral tumours. Carbamazepine, phenytoin or phenobarbital plasma levels reduced by St John's wort (risk of fits).

SODIUM VALPROATE ☑
Tabs. 200mg, 500mg; Syrup 200mg/5mL
TSD: 200mg t.d.s. PO
Increase 200mg/day at 3-day intervals. Usual maintenance 1-2g/24h. Max.
2.5g/24h in divided doses. Suppositories are available as special orders.

CARBAMAZEPINE
Tabs. 100mg, 200mg, 400mg; Liquid 100mg/5mL; Supps. 125mg, 250mg
TSD: 100mg b.d. PO
Increase from initial dose by increments of 200mg every week. Usual
maintenance dose 0.8-1.2g/24h in two divided doses. Max. 1.6-2 g/24h.
Equivalent rectal dosage: 125mg **PR** ≅ 100mg **PO**
Carbamazepine levels are increased (risk of toxicity) by clarithromycin, erythromycin, dextropropoxyphene[487,488] (co-proxamol), fluoxetine, fluvoxamine.

PHENYTOIN
Caps. 50mg, 100mg, 300mg; Susp. 30mg/5mL, 90mg/5mL
TSD: 90mg b.d. PO
Start 150-300mg daily. Usual maintenance dose: 300-400mg daily. Max.
600mg/24h. Single or two divided doses.
Phenytoin levels are increased (risk of toxicity) by clarithromycin, metronidazole, trimethoprim, fluconazole, miconazole, omeprazole, fluoxetine, fluvoxamine, aspirin, diltiazem, nifedipine, amiodarone.
Because phenytoin has a very long and variable half-life, it can take several
days and even up to 3-4 weeks for changes in dosage to take complete
effect; this should be borne in mind in determining the interval after dosage
is altered before measuring the plasma phenytoin concentration again.

GABAPENTIN
Caps. 100mg, 300mg, 400mg; Tabs. 600mg[○] 800mg[○]
TSD: Day 1 - 300mg nocte, day 2 - 300mg b.d., day 3 - 300mg t.d.s. PO
Used for neuropathic pain *(p.51)*]

BARBITURATE

PHENOBARBITAL (PHENOBARBITONE) ☑
Inj. 60mg/1mL, 200mg/1mL; Tabs. 15mg, 30mg, 60mg; Elixir 15mg/5mL
Elixir in various strengths can be made to order e.g. 10mg/mL, 90mg/mL‡
Phenobarbital is a barbiturate with sedative and anticonvulsant effects. It is
rarely used nowadays as a first line anticonvulsant, as it is too sedative. It
can be given by **CSCI**, but is incompatible with most other drugs *(p.173)* and
usually needs to be given in a separate syringe diver. It can be given by
daily **SC** or **IM** injection, but the preparation is very viscous and stings on
injection. *Doses: see above*

BENZODIAZEPINES
MIDAZOLAM
Inj. 10mg/2mL, 10mg/5mL
TSD: 30mg/24h CSCI
Oral solution available as special order, or use injection for buccal use.
Sedative effect markedly enhanced by itraconazole, ketoconazole and possibly fluconazole.

LORAZEPAM
   Tabs. 1mg, 2.5mg; Inj. 4mg/1mL
   Dilute inj. with equal volume of water or saline for **IM** use
DIAZEPAM
   Tabs. 2mg, 5mg, 10mg; Oral solution 2mg/5mL, 5mg/5mL
   Rectal tubes 5mg/2.5mL, 10mg/2.5mL; Supps. 10mg
   Inj. (emulsion) 10mg/2mL *(Diazemuls)* - **IV** use only
   Inj. (solution) 10mg/2mL - **IM** use
CLONAZEPAM
   Tabs. 500μg, 2mg; Inj. 1mg/1mL
   TSD: 1mg nocte for 4 nights
   Increase gradually to usual maintenance dose 4-8mg/24h. Oral solutions in
   various strengths are available from several sources.

Skeletal muscle spasm & Spasticity

1) Diazepam may be effective at reducing spasticity, and may be especially
   helpful for the acute treatment of severe spasms. Sedation is a
   disadvantage.
2) Baclofen should be used first-line as specific treatment.
   – tizanidine is a useful newer drug (recommended by the MS society for
   spasticity), causing less sedation, hypotonia or hypotension than
   baclofen
3) Dantrolene may be used in conjunction with baclofen, but the therapeutic
   effect may take a few weeks to develop.

ThinkList

- Gabapentin •• may help spasticity in MS.[911]
- Cannabinoids ••• may help painful spasticity in MS, although they are no
   more effective than codeine against most pain[477]

SEE ALSO
⇨ *Leg cramps (p.113), Cannabis (p.180)*
📖 Reviews[912]

Drugs for Spasm & Spasticity

DIAZEPAM ☑
   Tabs. 2mg, 5mg, 10mg; Oral solution 2mg/5mL, 5mg/5mL
   TSD: 2mg t.d.s. PO or 5mg nocte. Increase according to response.
   Blood levels increased by omeprazole (increased sedation).
BACLOFEN ☑
   Tabs. (scored) 10mg; Liquid 5mg/5mL
   TSD: 5mg t.d.s. PO. Increased gradually to max. 100mg/day in divided doses.
DANTROLENE
   Tabs. 25mg, 100mg
   *TSD: 25mg nocte PO. Increase at weekly intervals to usual dose 75mg t.d.s.
   Max. 100mg q.d.s.*
   **Care in liver impairment. It is recommended that LFTs should be tested
   before starting and monitored throughout treatment.**
TIZANIDINE
   Tabs. 2mg, 4mg
   *TSD: 2mg nocte PO. Increase according to response up to 24mg/day in 3-4
   divided doses. Max. 36mg/day.*

Leg cramps

Leg cramps

Most leg cramps are idiopathic. Conditions associated with leg cramps include:
- thyroid disease
- diabetes mellitus
- metabolic disturbances
  - hypoglycaemia
  - hyponatraemia
  - hypocalcaemia
  - hypomagnesaemia
  - hypo- and hyperkalaemia
- drugs
  - nifedipine
  - diuretics
  - alcohol
  - steroids[913]
- neoplastic peripheral nerve infiltration
- peripheral vascular disease or neuropathies

Management

1) Exclude or treat reversible causes.
2) Blood tests - glucose, calcium, U&E's (⇨ *Hypomagnesaemia p.134*), thyroid function.
3) Stretch calf muscles before going to bed.[914]
4) Quinine sulphate 200mg nocte:[915]
   - increase to 300mg nocte if no response after 2 weeks
   - may need up to 4 weeks treatment before effective
   - attempt withdrawal after 3 months to see if still needed

ThinkList

- naftidrofuryl oxalate •• 100mg nocte[916]
- vitamin E (alpha-tocopheryl) •• - conflicting evidence of efficacy[917,918]
- rutosides (oxerutins, *Paroven*) ••• 500mg b.d. - 50% advantage over placebo in cramps and restless legs associated with chronic venous insufficiency[919,920]

Drugs for Leg Cramps

QUININE SULPHATE

Tabs. 200mg, 300mg
Caution in cardiac conduction defects or dysrhthymias
Side-effects include tinnitus, visual disturbances, nausea & vomiting, thrombocytopenia.
Quinine used concomitantly with amiodarone or flecainide increases the risk of ventricular arrhythmias and should be avoided. Increases blood levels of digoxin.
   TSD: 200mg nocte PO

NAFTIDROFURYL OXALATE ⊘

Caps. 100mg
   TSD: 100mg nocte PO

Tremor

History, examination and investigations (TFTs) should exclude:
- parkinsonism or Parkinson's disease
- thyrotoxicosis
- cerebellar signs (tumour or paraneoplastic)
- drugs or alcohol - intoxication or withdrawal

Anxiety and agitated depression should be considered. Many cases are of unknown aetiology.

Tremor of parkinsonism is most prominent at rest ('pill-rolling' tremor), although it subsides during sleep. Cerebellar signs include 'intention' tremor, which improves at rest.

Symptomatic treatment if required:
- propranolol 40mg o.d. PO increased up to 40mg t.d.s. (maximum 160mg daily)

ThinkList
- gabapentin (maximum of 2,700mg/day) for benign essential/familial tremor ●● [921]
- ataxic tremor in MS may be helped by isoniazid ●●● [922], carbamazepine,●● clonazepam,●● or ondansetron ●●● [911]

SEE ALSO
⇨ Anxiety (p.99)

Restless legs syndrome

Restless legs syndrome affects 5% of the general population. It can lead to severe fatigue due to insomnia. Diagnostic criteria:[923]
- intense, irresistible urge to move the legs, associated with sensory complaints
- motor restlessness
- worsening of symptoms at rest, and relief with movement
- increased severity in evening or at night

Differential diagnosis includes akathisia and periodic leg movements of sleep, but these may all be part of a spectrum of conditions characterised by dopaminergic system dysfunction.[924-926]

Restless leg syndrome is associated with iron deficiency, and treatment with iron can improve symptoms.[927,928] It is also associated with renal failure, SSRI antidepressants[929,930] and mianserin.[931]

Levodopa or dopamine agonists, and opioids are most commonly used for treatment. Although levodopa is normally used first-line, there may be many situations in palliative care when an opioid is useful for other symptoms, in which case it may be used before levodopa.

Management

1) Exclude or treat iron-deficiency anaemia.
2) Review any dopamine antagonist medication (haloperidol, metoclopramide, phenothiazines) and SSRIs.
3) Levodopa[932-934] e.g.
   - co-beneldopa (*Madopar*) 12.5/50 or 25/100 nocte
   - higher doses ≥ 200mg levodopa may exacerbate symptoms[935]
4) Morphine SR 10mg nocte, increased if needed up to 30mg nocte.
   - various different opioids have been successfully used: morphine,[936,937] oxycodone,[938] codeine,[939] and propoxyphene.[940]
5) Pergolide may be used as an alternative to levodopa - titrated up to 0.4-0.5mg nocte ± domperidone for nausea.[941-943]

PRESCRIBING STATUS

☼ Levodopa, co-beneldopa ⊛
☼ Opioids ●
☼ Pergolide ●●

ThinkList

- gabapentin ●● (used up to max. 2,700mg/day)[921,944]
- clonazepam ●● [945]
- baclofen ●● [946]
- amitriptyline ●● [947]
- propranolol ●● [948]
- rutosides (oxerutins, *Paroven*) ●● 500mg b.d. - in restless legs associated with chronic venous insufficiency[919,920]
- alprazolam ●● [949]
- clonidine ●●● [950-952]

SEE ALSO

⇨ *Leg cramps (p.113)*
▢ Review[953]

Drugs for Restless Legs Syndrome

CO-BENELDOPA (MADOPAR) ☑

Caps. 12.5/50 (benserazide 12.5mg, levodopa 50mg)
Caps. 25/100 (benserazide 25mg, levodopa 100mg)
Caps. 50/200 (benserazide 50mg, levodopa 200mg)
Tabs. Disp. 12.5/50 (benserazide 12.5mg, levodopa 50mg)
Tabs. Disp. 25/100 (benserazide 25mg, levodopa 100mg)
   TSD: 12.5/50 nocte, increased if needed to 50/100 nocte for restless legs syndrome
Tabs. SR 25/100 (benserazide 25mg, levodopa 100mg) *Madopar CR*

Parkinsonism & Extrapyramidal side effects

Acute extrapyramidal side-effects (EPSE) can be caused by all antipsychotic drugs (e.g. haloperidol), other dopamine antagonists (e.g. metoclopramide) and SSRIs.[854] They may present in a number of forms.

- Stop, reduce dose, or change the causal drug(s) if possible:
  - domperidone may substitute for metoclopramide
  - a phenothiazine e.g. methotrimeprazine with antimuscarinic activity is better than haloperidol

– an atypical antipsychotic e.g. risperidone or olanzapine *(p.105)* may be better than conventional antipsychotics

Management of extrapyramidal effects

Parkinsonism	Rigidity Tremor Bradykinesia	Procyclidine 2.5mg t.d.s. increasing to 5mg t.d.s.
Acute dystonia	Spasm of neck or jaw Oculo-gyric crisis Dysphagia Tongue protrusion	Procyclidine 5mg IV (or IM) May need to be repeated after 20 minutes
Akathisia	Pacing, or rocking Restless and unable to sit still	Procyclidine 2.5mg t.d.s. increasing to 5mg t.d.s. Add diazepam 5mg nocte if needed. Change diazepam to propranolol 40mg b.d. if needed.
Tardive dyskinesia	Follows chronic drug-usage. Choreiform or athetoid writhing of the tongue, trunk or limbs	Alter causal drug if at all possible. Usually resistant to drug treatment. **Avoid antimuscarinic drugs which may exacerbate.**

Drugs for Extrapyramidal side effects

PROCYCLIDINE
Inj. 10mg/2mL *(Kemadrin)*
    TSD: 5-10mg IM or IV repeated once if necessary after 20 min. for acute dystonia
Tabs. 5mg *(Kemadrin)*
    TSD: 2.5-5mg t.d.s. PO

Drugs for Parkinson's disease

Co-careldopa *(Sinemet)* is the other commonly used levodopa preparation. Co-beneldopa is suggested if initiating treatment for newly-diagnosed Parkinson's disease in advanced cancer simply because dispersible tablets are available if dysphagia is/becomes a problem.

CO-BENELDOPA *(MADOPAR)* ☑
Caps. 12.5/50 (benserazide 12.5mg, levodopa 50mg)
Caps. 25/100 (benserazide 25mg, levodopa 100mg)
Caps. 50/200 (benserazide 50mg, levodopa 200mg)
Tabs. Disp. 12.5/50 (benserazide 12.5mg, levodopa 50mg)
Tabs. Disp. 25/100 (benserazide 25mg, levodopa 100mg)
    TSD: 12.5/50 t.d.s., increased by 12.5/50 twice weekly; usual maintenance dose 400-800mg levodopa daily
Tabs. SR 25/100 (benserazide 25mg, levodopa 100mg) *Madopar CR*

Additional Information

Neuroleptic malignant syndrome

Neuroleptic malignant syndrome has four classic signs: fever, rigidity, autonomic instability and altered consciousness. It has been described in patients taking antipsychotics (all currently used antipsychotics are implicated) and patients whose dopamine precursors have been stopped. It may also occur with SSRIs.[854] It may be one end of a range of effects produced by antipsychotics including dystonia and parkinsonism.[954]

INFECTIONS

Antibiotics

Use first choice as listed below unless infection has already proved resistant to recent treatment with that antibiotic, or allergy exists. Be guided by reported antibiotic sensitivities as soon as they are available.

First-line antibiotics for 'blind' empirical treatment

Urinary tract infections	1) Trimethoprim PO 2) Co-amoxiclav PO/IV 3) Cefalexin PO/Cefuroxime IV 4) Ciprofloxacin PO/IV Trimethoprim or nitrofurantoin are most suitable for long term prophylaxis, if required.
Cellulitis	Complicating lymphoedema ⇨ (p.163) Around pressure sores or fungating tumours: 1) Co-amoxiclav PO/IV 2) Cefalexin PO/Cefuroxime IV + Metronidazole PO/IV 3) Clarithromycin PO/IV 4) Doxycycline PO (for oral cavity)
Chest infections	1) Co-amoxiclav PO/IV 2) Cefalexin PO/Cefuroxime IV (+ metronidazole if aspiration or bronchial obstruction) 3) Clarithromycin (if atypical infection likely) PO/IV 4) Ciprofloxacin PO/IV To reduce chronic infected sputum production: 1) Cefalexin PO 2) Chloramphenicol PO 3) Nebulised gentamicin or colistimethate sodium (colistin)[818]
Conjunctivitis	1) Chloramphenicol eye drops 2) Fusidic acid eye drops
Cholangitis	Infection in obstructive jaundice: 1) Co-amoxiclav PO/IV 2) Ciprofloxacin + Metronidazole PO or IV
Clostridium difficile entero-colitis	(Pseudomembranous / antibiotic-associated colitis) 1) Metronidazole PO/IV 2) Vancomycin PO/IV
Epidural or Intrathecal line	Insertion site infection: 1) Flucloxacillin PO/IV 2) Vancomycin IV (or Teicoplanin) (Vancomycin is very expensive, but for suspected deeper epidural infection, Staph. epidermidis is resistant to Flucloxacillin)
Faecal fistula or pelvic abscess	To reduce odour (from anaerobic GI organisms): 1) Metronidazole PO/IV

Neutropenic patients

For neutropenic patients (neutrophils < 1.0) who are unwell or pyrexial, follow the current guidelines from the local oncology or haematology departments.

PRESCRIBING STATUS

🔅 Antibiotics (gentamicin or colistimethate sodium/colistin) by nebuliser •••

SEE ALSO

⇨ *Topical antibiotics with steroids (p.165)*

📖 Reviews of infections in cancer[955,956]

Antibiotics
PENICILLINS
PENICILLIN V
   Tabs. 250mg; Susp. 250mg/5mL
   TSD: 250-500mg q.d.s. PO
AMOXICILLIN
   Caps. 250mg, 500mg; Susp. 250mg/5mL
   TSD: 250mg t.d.s. PO
CO-AMOXICLAV
   Tabs. 375mg, 625mg; Tabs. Disp. 375mg; Inj. 600mg, 1.2g *(Augmentin)*
   TSD: 375-625mg t.d.s. PO or 1.2g t.d.s. IV
   Reduce dose in moderate renal failure.
FLUCLOXACILLIN
   Caps. 250mg, 500mg; Susp. 250mg/5mL: Inj. 250mg, 500mg, 1g
   TSD: 500mg q.d.s. PO or 1 q.d.s. IV

CEPHALOSPORINS
CEFALEXIN ☑
   Tabs. 250mg, 500mg; Susp. 250mg/5mL, 500mg/5mL
   TSD: 250-1000mg q.d.s. PO
CEFACLOR
   Caps. 250mg, 500mg; Tabs. SR 375mg; Susp. 250mg/5mL
   TSD: 250-500mg t.d.s. PO
   Dose does not need to be adjusted in renal failure.
CEFUROXIME
   Inj. 750mg vial
   TSD: 750mg t.d.s. IV
   Oral form is poorly absorbed. Reduce dose in any degree of renal failure.

TETRACYCLINES
DOXYCYCLINE ☑
   Caps. 50mg, 100mg
   Tabs. Disp. 100mg
   TSD: 200mg first day then 100mg o.d.-b.d. PO
   May be used in renal disease. Absorption unaffected by milk and antacids.
OXYTETRACYCLINE
   Tabs. 250mg
   TSD: 250-500mg q.d.s. PO
   Avoid in renal disease. Absorption decreased by milk and antacids.

QUINOLONES
Quinolone antibiotics may increase the anticoagulation effect of warfarin.
CIPROFLOXACIN
   Tabs. 250mg, 500mg, 750mg: Susp. 250mg/5mL
   Inj. 200mg/100mL, 400mg/200mL
   TSD: 250-750mg b.d. PO or 200-400mg b.d. IV (as infusion over 30-60 minutes)
   Increased risk of convulsions, especially with NSAIDs.

AMINOGLYCOSIDES
GENTAMICIN
Inj. 20mg/2mL, 40mg/1mL, 80mg/2mL
Dose via nebuliser (mix with 1mL saline): 80mg in 2mL b.d.[818]

MACROLIDES
***Clarithromycin and erythromycin increase blood levels of
carbamazepine***[858,859] ***(risk of toxicity) and may increase the anticoagulation
effect of warfarin.***
CLARITHROMYCIN ☑
Tabs. 250mg, 500mg; Granules 250mg/sachet; Susp. 250mg/5mL; Inj. 500mg
TSD: 250-500mg b.d. PO (£22.48-£44.98) or 500mg b.d. IV
Clarithromycin increases phenytoin blood levels (risk of toxicity).
Reduce dose in moderate renal failure. Fewer gastro-intestinal adverse effects
than erythromycin. Better tissue penetration than erythromycin.
ERYTHROMYCIN
Tabs. 250mg, 500mg[○] Susp. 250mg/5mL, 500mg/5mL[○]
TSD: 250-500mg q.d.s. PO (£12.32-£24.64)
Use of the succinate (in the suspension) reduces gastric intolerance
***Erythromycin (parenteral) used concomitantly with amiodarone increase
the risk of ventricular arrhythmias and should be avoided***

OTHER ANTIBIOTICS
CHLORAMPHENICOL
Caps. 250mg
TSD: 500mg q.d.s. PO
Rarely causes fatal aplastic anaemia. Acceptability of risk must be assessed
for each patient. Avoid in liver failure.
***Enhances effect of warfarin. Increases plasma concentration of
phenytoin.***
COLISTIMETHATE SODIUM (COLISTIN)
Inj. 500,000u; 1,000,000u *(Colomycin)*
*TSD (mix with 3mL saline): 500,000u b.d. via neb. < 40 Kg; 1,000,000u b.d.
via neb. > 40 Kg.*
METRONIDAZOLE
Tabs. 200mg, 400mg; Susp. 200mg/5mL; Supps. 500mg, 1g; Inj. 500mg
TSD: 400mg t.d.s. PO; 1 gram b.d. PR; 500mg t.d.s. IV
Gel 0.75%, 0.8% *(Metrotop)*
***'Antabuse' or disulfiram-like reaction with alcohol occurs in up to 25%
patients.***[1] ***Systemic absorption from topical gel is possible. All patients
should be warned about a possible interaction with alcohol, but if the
patient wishes to take a drink, advise cautious trial with small quantity
first. Enhances anticoagulation with warfarin. Increases phenytoin
blood levels (toxicity) and blood levels of fluouracil (5-FU) increasing
toxicity. Reduce dose in severe liver failure.***
NITROFURANTOIN
Tabs. 50mg, 100mg; Susp. 25mg/5mL
TSD: Treatment - 50mg q.d.s. PO ; Prophylaxis - 50mg nocte.
Avoid in renal failure.
TRIMETHOPRIM
Tabs. 100mg, 200mg; Susp. 50mg/5mL
TSD: Treatment - 200mg b.d. PO; Prophylaxis - 100mg nocte.
Trimethoprim increases phenytoin blood levels (risk of toxicity).
VANCOMYCIN
Caps. 125mg, 250mg; Inj. 250mg, 500mg, 1g
*TSD: Pseudomembranous colitis 125mg q.d.s. PO for 7-10 days; Systemic
infection 500mg over ≥60 minutes q.d.s. IV*
Oral form is poorly absorbed; only use for pseudomembranous colitis with
Clostridium difficile, not systemic infection.

EYE DROPS

CHLORAMPHENICOL ☑
Eye drops 0.5%; Eye ointment 1%
TSD: 1 drop t.d.s. (2-hourly if severe) and ointment at night is ideal treatment; alternatively used drops or ointment q.d.s.
Ointment remains in the eye longer, but can blur vision during the day.

FUSIDIC ACID
Eye drops m/r 1%
TSD: 1 drop b.d.
Gel basis, liquefies on contact with eye.

Fungal infections

Oral candidiasis is common in cancer patients. Oesophageal candidiasis may also occur after mediastinal radiotherapy, or in patients who have been treated with antibiotics, corticosteroids or PPIs;[957] 50% do not have signs of oral infection (but do have a classic appearance on barium swallow).[958] Funguria may also occur, often due to Candida species, and responds to systemic antifungals.[959] Candida infection has been described causing secretory-type diarrhoea,[155] and can be treated with oral nystatin.

SEE ALSO
⇨ *Oral candidiasis (p.44)*

Antifungal Drugs
Fluconazole and miconazole increases phenytoin blood levels (risk of toxicity).
Fluconazole, miconazole, itraconazole, and ketoconazole all enhance warfarin anticoagulation.
Fluconazole and miconazole increase sulphonylureas e.g. gliclazide, glibenclamide (risk of hypoglycaemia)
Fluconazole increases celecoxib levels[349] – halve celecoxib dose
Itraconazole, ketoconazole and possibly fluconazole increase sedation with midazolam

FLUCONAZOLE ☑
Tabs. 50mg; Susp. 50mg/5mL
TSD: 50mg o.d. PO

ITRACONAZOLE
Caps. 100mg; Liquid 10mg/mL
TSD: 100mg o.d. PO

KETOCONAZOLE
Tabs. 200mg; Susp. 100mg/5mL
TSD: 200mg o.d. PO

TOPICAL & ORAL ANTIFUNGAL TREATMENTS

NYSTATIN
Susp. 100,000U/mL; Pastilles 100,000U
TSD: 2-5mL q.d.s. PO; 1 pastille q.d.s. PO

MICONAZOLE
Oral gel 25mg/mL
Apply q.d.s. PO

AMPHOTERICIN
Lozenges 10mg *(Fungilin)*
TSD: 1 tabs. q.d.s. PO

Viral infections

Immunosuppression due to advanced malignancy and/or corticosteroids make patients more prone to varicella-zoster (shingles) and herpes simplex infections.

SEE ALSO
⇨ *Painful mouth (p.43), Flu vaccination (p.201)*

Antiviral Drugs

VALACICLOVIR ☑
  Tabs. 500mg
  TSD: 500mg b.d. PO for 5 days (£23.50)

ACICLOVIR
  Tabs. and Tabs. Disp. 200mg, 400mg, 800mg; Susp. 200mg/5mL; Cream 5%
  TSD: 400mg 4-5 times/day PO for 5 days (£40.44 - use 200mg disp. tabs.)

FAMCICLOVIR
  Tabs. 125mg, 250mg, 500mg
  TSD: 500mg b.d. PO for 7 days (£157.47)

Additional Notes

Amitriptyline ● 25mg o.d. started immediately upon diagnosis of herpes zoster infection and taken for 3 months may significantly reduce the incidence of post-herpetic neuralgia.[960,961]

In varicella-zoster infections - silver sulfadiazine *(Flamazine)* cream has some antiviral activity and may reduce pain within 24-72hrs.[962]

ENDOCRINE SYSTEM

Diabetes mellitus

Management of diabetes in palliative care

- A limited prognosis for a patient makes *close* control of blood glucose (aimed at reducing long term sequelae) unnecessary, thereby allowing a less invasive/interventional approach.
- Changes in the patient's condition (e.g. cachexia), infection or treatment (e.g. corticosteroids) commonly alter the diabetic treatment needed; changes may be quite rapid over time.

Aims of control

- to keep the patient asymptomatic
  - keeping a blood glucose < 15 is usually sufficient to prevent symptoms from hyperglycaemia
  - symptoms usually presenting : infections, polyuria, thirst, nausea & vomiting, 'feeling unwell'
  - note that a dry mouth is commonly due to drugs (morphine or antimuscarinics) and is not a good indicator of dehydration
- to prevent hypoglycaemia occurring
- to minimise intervention i.e.
  - frequency of testing
  - no. of injections

Hyperglycaemia in advanced malignancy

In addition to pre-existing diabetes mellitus (including previously undiagnosed cases, which may present in the terminal stages), there are two particular causes of hyperglycaemia that may present in patients with advanced malignancy:

- corticosteroid-induced diabetes
- insulin deficiency/resistance in pancreatic cancer[963,964]

Hypoglycaemia

Common changes in patients with advanced malignancy that lead to a reduced insulin or oral hypoglycaemic requirement in pre-existing diabetics are:

- cancer cachexia in advanced illness (reduced body mass)
- reduced food intake due to anorexia, dysphagia, 'squashed stomach' or nausea/vomiting etc.
- liver replacement by tumour causing low glycogen stores and limited gluconeogenesis

Corticosteroids

Corticosteroids are commonly used in advanced malignancy. Corticosteroid-induced hyperglycaemia is a dose-related effect in any patient, but there is wide variability between patients in their response to steroids.
Corticosteroids have a direct metabolic hyperglycaemic effect, but may also increase appetite - sometimes dramatically.

Treatment options for diabetes

Oral hypoglycaemic drugs

- Gliclazide is a short acting hypoglycaemic. It may be given once or twice daily. Starting dose 40-80mg mane.
- Increase as required to a maximum total dose 160mg b.d.
- Avoid metformin in patients with advanced cancer.

Insulin

- It is sensible to stick to two or three insulins, such as:
  - Human Insulin Zinc Suspension (mixed) *(Human Monotard)*
  - Human Isophane Insulin *(Human Insulatard ge* or *Humulin I)*
  - Human Soluble Insulin *(Human Actrapid* or *Humulin S)*
- Use either:
  - a single dose of *Human Monotard* daily (given at bedtime), or
  - Isophane insulin: 2/3 rd. daily dose mane, 1/3 rd dose nocte
- If converting from mixed insulin regime (e.g. Isophane + Human Soluble Insulin) to single daily *Human Monotard*:
  - calculate the total daily insulin requirement
  - reduce the dose by approximately 20-30% to account for the conversion
  - adjust the dose as necessary if blood glucose has been high or low
  - give this dose once daily as *Human Monotard*
- For a patient who has been uncontrolled on oral hypoglycaemics, start with *Human Monotard* 10u daily.

Initiating treatment in new diagnosis hyperglycaemia

- Restrict diet *if overeating:* do not impose a strict diet on a patient with advanced illness. It is more important to try and achieve a regular caloric input from one day to the next.
- Reduce dose of corticosteroids if appropriate.
- Consider infection as a factor causing the hyperglycaemia.
- Thin cachectic patients are less likely to respond to oral hypoglycaemic drugs, and insulin should be considered early, if not responding to simple measures e.g. gliclazide 80mg o.d.
- If the patient is peripherally vasoconstricted, give insulin by IM route, rather than SC.

Blood sugar	Action
11-17	Dietary advice. Reduce steroids if possible. Start gliclazide 40mg daily and increase as necessary every few days.
17-27	Start Gliclazide 80mg mane if no, or mild, ketonuria. If moderate or severe ketonuria the patient will need insulin - start *Human Monotard* 10u nocte. If ketonuria and symptomatic, consider reducing blood glucose more rapidly using Human Soluble Insulin 4-8u every 4h until glucose < 17, or IV regimen below.
>27	Consider if admission to acute medical unit is appropriate, especially if ketonuria present. Use IV regimen as below if intensive treatment appropriate, or Human Soluble Insulin 4-8u every 4h until glucose < 17.

Managing diabetes when vomiting or not eating

Diabetes type	Action
Oral hypoglycaemics	Reduce dose by 50% if oral intake reduced, or discontinue if no oral intake.
Insulin dependent	Insulin is required to prevent ketosis, even with no oral intake.
	Use IV regimen below if intensive control is appropriate, or use sliding scale of Human Soluble Insulin 8-hourly, together with IV 5% dextrose infusion 1L 8-12 hourly.

Managing diabetes in the terminal days

Diabetes type	Action
Oral hypoglycaemics	Discontinue when unable to take oral intake.
Insulin dependent	Insulin is required to prevent ketosis, even with no oral intake.
	1) If patient unconscious/unaware, discontinue insulin and monitoring.
	2) If the patient is still aware/conscious, several strategies may be appropriate, depending on the patient/relatives' attitude to burden of treatment (and monitoring) and prognosis:
	- Consider discussing with patient/relatives discontinuing insulin, as an unnecessary life-prolonging therapy (also stop monitoring).
	- Use sliding scale soluble insulin 8-hourly.
	- Give approximately half of the patient's recent insulin requirement as a single dose of *Human Monotard* as a single daily injection, with or without blood sugar monitoring.

Sliding scale Insulin regimen

Monitor blood glucose and give soluble insulin sc as indicated. Use 8-hourly if patient not eating, or t.d.s. before mealtimes. Adjust sliding scale doses according to response.

Fasting blood sugar	Soluble Insulin
10-14	4u
15-18	6u
19-22	8u
>22	10u

IV Insulin regimen

- Give insulin in a syringe pump (diluted with N/Saline), and 'piggy-backed' via a 3-way tap on to an IVI.
- Use soluble insulin 50u made up to 50mL with sodium chloride 0.9%
- Infusion rate according to scale below.
- Give IVI of Dextrose 5% or sodium chloride 0.9% ± potassium as below.
- Monitor blood sugar - initially 4-hourly if glucose > 17
- If the patient has cardiac failure, use 500mL dextrose 10% every 6-8h.
- Review sliding scale if:
    - glucose < 4 (and increase strength of dextrose)
    - glucose > 17 and no change in 2-4h - increase insulin on scale

IV insulin dose

Blood Glucose (mmol/L)	Infusion Rate Insulin units/hour	IV infusion
0 - 4	0.5	Dextrose 5%
> 4 - 7	1	1 litre 6-8 hourly
> 7 - 11	2	if glucose < 11
> 11 - 17	3	Sodium Chloride 0.9%
> 17 - 27	4	1 litre 6-8 hourly
> 27	6	if glucose > 11

Added potassium

Serum K^+	Potassium to add per litre
> 5.0 mmol/L (or unknown)	None
3.5 - 5.0 mmol/L	1.5g (20mmol)
< 3.5 mmol/L	3g (40mmol)

Using a Graseby MS16 or MS26

Syringe driver	MS16		MS26
Soluble Insulin (units)	20u	40u	60u
Dilute with saline 0.9% to syringe length:	40 mm	40 mm	40 mm
At maximum rate, syringe will last:	3.3h	6h	10h
Units insulin/hour	Set syringe driver to		
6	12 mm/h	6 mm/h	96 mm/24h
4	8 mm/h	4 mm/h	64 mm/24h
3	6 mm/h	3 mm/h	48 mm/24h
2	4 mm/h	2 mm/h	32 mm/24h
1	2 mm/h	1 mm/h	16 mm/24h
0.5	1 mm/h	-	8 mm/24hr

SEE ALSO
📖 Reviews & Guidelines[965,966]

Drugs for Diabetes

GLICLAZIDE ☑
Tabs. 80mg
TSD: 80mg mane PO
Blood levels increased by fluconazole and miconazole (hypoglycaemia)
HUMAN INSULIN SOLUBLE
Inj. 100u/mL *(Human Actrapid or Humulin S)*
HUMAN INSULIN ISOPHANE
Inj. 100u/mL *(Human Insulatard ge or Humulin I)*
HUMAN INSULIN ZINC SUSPENSION (MIXED)
Inj. 100u/mL *(Human Monotard)*

Drugs used in Hypoglycaemia

Glucagon may be ineffective in a starved patient, as it depends on adequate liver glycogen.
GLUCAGON
Inj. 1mg
Dose: 1mg IM (<12yrs 0.5mg)
Do not give by SC route, as the patient may be peripherally vasoconstricted.
GLUCOSE / DEXTROSE
Oral Gel 10g *(Hypostop Gel)*; Inj. 25% 25mL ⊘ 50% 25mL
Dose: 25mL of 50% IV or 10g PO

Corticosteroids

Uses of steroids in advanced malignancy
Average doses of dexamethasone

2-4mg/day	4-8mg/day	Up to 16mg/day
Increase appetite	Co-analgesic in:	Cerebral tumours
Sense of well-being	Nerve compression	Raised intracranial
Non-specific pain	pain	pressure
relief	Pain from	Spinal cord compression
Anti-emetic	hepatomegaly	SVC obstruction
Weakness		Large airways
		obstruction
		Intestinal obstruction
		Ureteric obstruction[967]

- Dexamethasone can be used for all these indications:
  - dexamethasone 1mg ≅ prednisolone 7.5mg
  - dexamethasone & betamethasone are equipotent
- Concurrent use of phenytoin (and some other enzyme-inducing anticonvulsants) may reduce plasma dexamethasone levels by up to 50%:
  - the dose of steroids may need to be increased (up to double) if starting one of these anticonvulsants

Principles of dexamethasone use
- Doses >4mg o.d. are likely to lead to side-effects after several weeks.
- Doses ≤4mg o.d. are often tolerated in someone with a prognosis of months.
- Doses ≤4mg daily can be stopped abruptly if used for less than 3 weeks.
- If used for longer, doses must be reduced slowly to avoid adrenal insufficiency due to adrenal suppression.
- Doses must be adjusted to individual patient's response: 0.5mg daily may have the same effect for one patient as another taking 4mg daily.
- When reducing doses, allow time on the new dose to assess whether there is any deterioration (3-4 days if there is a need for rapid reduction e.g. getting adverse effects, or 1-2 weeks if not).
- If used for more than 8 weeks, consider notes below on osteoporosis and proximal myopathy.

Specific guidelines for dexamethasone use
General tonic effects - appetite & well-being
- Dexamethasone 4mg o.d.
- Stop after 1 week if no benefit.
- Leave at this dose unless side effects develop or patient has a prognosis of more than a few weeks - if so, try reducing to 2mg o.d.

Co-analgesic
- Start at 8mg o.d. for rapid effect.
- Expect a result in 3-5 days.
- If no benefit then stop after this time.
- Once benefit is established, reduce dose in steps to minimum dose that maintains benefit (often ≤4mg o.d.).

High dose - Not currently taking steroids

- Dexamethasone 16mg o.d. (as 8mg b.d.)
- Expect effect in 2-3 days maximum.
- Consider referral for radiotherapy (urgently for cord compression).
- If no response at all, stop after 4-5 days.
- If beneficial, remain on high dose for 1-2 weeks until stable, then reduce by 2mg once or twice weekly to the lowest dose that maintains benefit.
- Check urine for sugar weekly while on doses above 4mg o.d.

Recurrence of symptoms from cerebral tumour

- Double the dose of steroids (if treatment is appropriate).
- 16mg daily is often the maximum appropriate dose in view of the increasing risk of side effects at higher dose; sometimes doses up to 32mg are appropriate especially if patient taking anticonvulsants (see above).
- If there is a response, try reducing the dose slowly after a week or two to minimum dose that maintains benefit.

Side Effects

- fluid retention
- Cushingoid changes to appearance
- increased risk of candida infection
- neuropsychiatric side-effects including insomnia (common), agitation, euphoria, hypomania, and paranoia[884,968]
    - avoid giving after 6 p.m. to reduce risk of insomnia
    - only need to be given once or twice daily (morning and noon) for beneficial effects
    - if psychiatric effects of high doses occur, dividing the dose (q.d.s.) may reduce these[969]
    - many patients feel emotionally labile on steroids without frank psychosis
- gastritis - corticosteroids alone are not proven to cause gastric ulcers, but definitely increase the risk when co-prescribed with NSAIDs;[18] patients taking both should have a gastro-protective drug ⇨ *Dyspepsia (p.16)*
- hyperglycaemia ⇨ *Diabetes (p.122)*
    - increase monitoring of known diabetics when starting, or changing dose of steroids
    - check blood or urine for sugar if any symptoms occur attributable to hyperglycaemia
- proximal myopathy[970] (see below)
- osteoporosis (see below)
- 'pricking' sensation/pain around anus (bolus IV administration only)

Proximal myopathy

Steroid-induced myopathy[971] can be very debilitating. It is most likely to occur in patients who have been taking ≥4mg dexamethasone daily for >8 weeks.[971,972] It can improve on stopping, or reducing the dose of steroids, although improvement may take months. If myopathy starts to develop, or the patient has been on steroids more than 6-8 weeks:

- Carefully weigh up the balance of benefit versus adverse effects.
- Reduce the steroid dose to the minimum possible.
- Consider changing to prednisolone (non-fluorinated steroid; lower risk of developing myopathy than fluorinated steroids e.g. dexamethasone).[973,974]
- Consider use of a progestagen in selected severe cases. *(p.129)*

Corticosteroid-induced osteoporosis

Patients taking at least dexamethasone 1mg (prednisolone 7.5mg) for 6 months are at risk of corticosteroid-induced osteoporosis. Any patient who has been taking steroids for this long, *or who is anticipated to do so*, should be considered for preventive treatment.[975] Bisphosphonates are effective for the prevention[976] and treatment[977] of corticosteroid-induced osteoporosis, and are probably the treatment of choice in most patients with cancer.

Options:

- bisphosphonates ⇨ *(p.141)*
- hormone replacement (if not contraindicated for specific cancer)
    - postmenopausal women or premenopausal with low oestradiol levels
    - men with demonstrable hypogonadism (testosterone replacement)
- consider use of a progestagen in selected cases *(p.129)*
- other options rarely indicated:
    - calcitonin 100u sc alternate days[978] (also shown to reduce pain)
    - raloxifene - if postmenopausal and not contraindicated for an oestrogen sensitive cancer
    - calcium & vitamin D supplementation if dietary insufficiency
    - calcitriol

SEE ALSO

⇨ *Anorexia (p.35), Diabetes (p.122)*

📖 Reviews[979,980] & Guidelines on osteoporosis prevention[975]

Corticosteroids

Dexamethasone (and betamethasone) cause less fluid retention than prednisolone as they have less mineralocorticoid effect. Prednisolone causes less proximal myopathy than dexamethasone as it is a non-fluorinated steroid. *Carbamazepine and phenytoin levels are decreased (risk of fits) by corticosteroids. Carbamazepine, phenytoin and phenobarbital can reduce the efficacy of corticosteroids. This two-way interaction[909,910] is common when managing patients with cerebral tumours.*

DEXAMETHASONE ☑

Tabs. 0.5mg, 2mg; Inj. 4mg/1mL, 8mg/2mL, 120mg/5mL
Susp. 2mg/5mL‡ (available from Rosemount)
Dexamethasone is up to twice as potent given sc as by the oral route
TSD: 4mg o.d. for anorexia (£4.84)

BETAMETHASONE

Tabs. sol. 0.5mg *(Betnesol)*; Inj. 4mg/1mL
TSD: 4mg o.d. for anorexia (£8.13)
Soluble tablets are useful alternative if cannot manage tablets. Equipotent to dexamethasone. 8mg will dissolve in <=10mL water.

PREDNISOLONE

Tabs. 1mg, 2.5mg, 5mg, 25mg; Tabs. sol. 5mg
TSD: 30mg o.d. for anorexia (£4.02)

Drugs for prevention of steroid-induced osteoporosis

RISEDRONATE ☑

Tabs. 5mg
TSD: 5mg o.d. PO (only licensed for post-menopausal) (£21.83)

DISODIUM ETIDRONATE (WITH CALCIUM CARBONATE)

Tabs. etidronate 400mg & tabs. calcium carbonate 1.25g *(Didronel PMO)*
TSD: 1 tab. etidronate o.d. for 14 days, 1 tab. calcium 76 days (£12.50 28d)

ALENDRONATE (ALENDRONIC ACID)

Tabs. 5mg⁰ 10mg
TSD: 5mg o.d. PO (10mg o.d. if post-menopausal, not on HRT) (£23.12 either dose)

Additional Information

Phenytoin may give some protection against the development of steroid-induced proximal myopathy.[971]

Conventional doses of corticosteroids are often empirical. Studies suggest than 4mg/day may be as effective as 16mg/day for cerebral metastases.[981]

Progestagens

Progestagens

Megestrol acetate and medroxyprogesterone have beneficial effects on appetite, sense of well-being, pain and nausea similar to corticosteroids.[982-985] Side effects of progestagens include muscle cramps and sweating, but in general they are well tolerated. Corticosteroid-type side effects of Cushingoid facies and oedema may occur. Weight gain occurs in most patients - unlike dexamethasone, which can increase appetite without affecting weight. The effect is not noticeable until 4 weeks after treatment, after which a steady increase in weight is seen. Very much more expensive than corticosteroids (see below).

Megestrol acetate

- Megestrol 800mg daily is as effective as dexamethasone 3mg daily, improving appetite in up to 60-70% patients, but with different side effects.[985]
- Reduces the incidence of nausea and vomiting compared with placebo.[984]
- Causes non-fluid weight gain measurable at 4 weeks.[985]
- Causes a measurable increase in well-being compared to placebo.[986]
- Appetite usually increases after a few days, and by 10 days.[987,988]
- Appetite stimulation and weight gain with megestrol acetate are dose dependent between 160 and 800mg per day.[989,990]
- Lower incidence than corticosteroids of proximal myopathy, Cushingoid changes, peptic ulcer, and insomnia.[985]
- Higher incidence than corticosteroids of thromboembolic events.[985]
- May cause secondary adrenal suppression; abrupt withdrawal may lead to adrenal insufficiency after prolonged administration.[991-994]
- Very much more expensive than dexamethasone (£136 vs. £5 per month)
- 800mg/day requires 5 tablets daily (5 x 160mg)

Indications

An alternative to corticosteroids for anorexia, well-being, fatigue, and non-specifically for nausea, in certain circumstances:

- weight gain, as opposed to just improving appetite, is the main aim (minimum prognosis of a few months)
- steroid-induced proximal myopathy

SEE ALSO
⇨ *Corticosteroids (p.126)*

Progestagens
MEGESTROL ACETATE
   Tabs. 40mg, 160mg *(Megace)*
   TSD: *800mg daily (£136.73)*

Hormone replacement therapy

Uses of HRT

- sweats & hot flushes (⇨ *Sweats & Hot flushes p.166*)
- osteoporosis prevention (⇨ *Corticosteroids p.126*)
- atrophic vaginitis

Menopausal symptoms may occur in patients due to:

- natural menopause
- ovarian ablation or dysfunction
    - surgery
    - radiotherapy
    - chemotherapy
- anti-oestrogen drugs e.g. tamoxifen

Risks of HRT in cancer

When oestrogen cream is used for atrophic vaginitis, a significant amount of oestrogen is absorbed through the vaginal mucosa. Contra-indications therefore apply as for systemic HRT.

HRT and cancer type

Hormone replacement therapy for menopausal symptoms women is clearly contra-indicated in patients who have oestrogen-dependent cancer e.g. oestrogen-receptor positive breast cancer.

There is no consensus on the risk of HRT in patients with other cancers that are active.[995] Most information is from epidemiological studies of patients after treatment for cancer ('cured'). In studies, HRT has been shown not to affect disease-free survival in women with ovarian cancer,[996] or in women who have been previously treated for melanoma.[997]

Cancer	Suggested action
Any cancer - taking hormone treatment e.g. tamoxifen	HRT contra-indicated. Discuss with oncologist, as treatment may be altered if causing symptoms.
Oestrogen-receptor +ve Breast Ca. Endometrial Ca. Adenocarcinoma cervix	Contra-indicated
Oestrogen-receptor -ve Breast Ca.	Probably contra-indicated. Discuss with oncologist.
Squamous cell Ca. cervix, vulva, and vagina	Unlikely to be affected by HRT[996]
Other female genital tract cancers	Uncertain effect. Discuss with oncologist.
Renal tumours	Some are oestrogenreceptor +ve.[998] Discuss with oncologist.
Other cancers	Unlikely to be affected by HRT

HRT and Venous thromboembolism

Although HRT increases the risk of venous thromboembolism (VTE) i.e. deep venous thrombosis or pulmonary embolism, current CSM advice for patients without other risk factors is that the medical benefits (e.g. on osteoporosis, coronary disease) outweigh the risk.

All patients with active cancer may be considered to have a risk factor for VTE. Combined oestrogen and progestagen HRT increases the risk of VTE three-fold,[999] [1000] (an excess risk of 4 per 1000 woman-years). Amongst women with cancer, the relative risk of VTE on HRT is four-fold.[1000] Whether this increased risk in cancer is still outweighed by the medical benefits is unclear. In many patients with incurable cancer, quality of life issues (symptomatic control of menopausal symptoms) are likely to outweigh the relatively finely balanced risk/benefit ratios for medical events.

Cancer patients Additional risk factors for VTE	Suggested action
History of VTE during current cancer illness	Avoid HRT unless anticoagulated.
Past history of VTE Prolonged immobility/bed-rest Obesity	Increased risk of VTE - must be carefully balanced against potential benefits if using HRT
Cancer as only risk factor	Small additional risk. Benefits of symptomatic control from HRT will usually outweigh risks.

METABOLIC DISORDERS

Hypercalcaemia

Significant symptoms that may be caused by hypercalcaemia
- drowsiness or confusion
- nausea & vomiting
- pain (usually bone) that is difficult to control
- dehydration

Tumours commonly associated with hypercalcaemia
- squamous cell tumours of - breast, bronchus, head & neck, oesophagus
- renal and genito-urinary tract tumours
- myeloma and lymphoma
- NB prostate is surprisingly rare[1001]

Treatment
- Treatment should only be given if symptomatic.
- Symptoms are unlikely unless the **corrected** calcium is > 2.8 mmol/L (⇨ p.214 for formula).
- For choice of bisphosphonate, and route of administration ⇨ p.141
1) Give 0.9% saline IVI 1L every 6h for 24h before bisphosphonate if calcium > 3.5 or clinically dehydrated.
2) If symptoms very severe or progressing rapidly, give calcitonin 800u/24h by CSCI for a more rapid effect, in addition to the bisphosphonate for 48h.[1002,1003]
3) Pamidronate IV infusion (see below for dose), or clodronate IV 1500mg.
4) Continue 0.9% saline IVI 1 litre every 6-8h for further 48h, then as clinically indicated.

Doses of pamidronate in hypercalcaemia

Corrected Calcium (mmol/L)	Dose	Min. volume of dilution	Min. duration of infusion Normal renal	Renal failure
<= 3.5	60mg	250mL	1h	3h
> 3.5	90mg	375mL	1½ h	4½ h

- In renal failure, the maximum rate of infusion should be 20mg/h.
- Rehydration is an important part of the treatment of hypercalcaemia, therefore unless a short infusion is necessary e.g. day case, dilute all doses in 1 litre of 0.9% saline over 6-8h.

Further management
- Check calcium after 3-4 days if symptoms have not significantly improved:
  – normocalcaemia should be achieved in 3-7 days
  – if calcium is not falling, repeat dose of bisphosphonate
- Be aware that mean length of response is 2-4 weeks.
- Arrange for serum calcium to be checked every 2 weeks.
- If symptoms of hypercalcaemia recur, or there is a general deterioration in the patient's condition after a few weeks, recheck serum calcium.
- Institute maintenance therapy after two episodes of hypercalcaemia.

Maintenance treatment to prevent recurrence

- pamidronate 90mg IV every 4 weeks, or
- clodronate 1500mg IV every 3 weeks, or
- oral clodronate 800mg b.d.

Treatment-Resistant Hypercalcaemia

Pamidronate may progressively less effective when hypercalcaemia recurs (90% response to first treatment, 15% response to third treatment).[1004] This is observed mainly in patients with hypercalcaemia of humoral origin i.e. usually without bone metastases, or tumours other than breast. The usefulness of pursuing further therapy has been questioned, although resistance can sometimes be overcome by the use of increasing doses of pamidronate,[1005] or by a more potent bisphosphonate e.g. zoledronic acid.[1006] See notes below for octreotide, which has been reported to control bisphosphonate-resistant hypercalcaemia of humoral origin.

PRESCRIBING STATUS

☼ Calcitonin by CSCI ●●

ThinkList

- corticosteroids ●● (e.g. dexamethasone 8mg o.d.) are no longer used routinely for hypercalcaemia, but may be effective for tumours that are steroid-responsive e.g. lymphomas and myeloma
- newer bisphosphonates that are longer-acting and more potent, are becoming available *(⇨ p.141)*
- octreotide ●●● [1007-1009]
- gallium ●●● [1010-1012]
- mithramycin °°° - hypercalcaemia recurs rapidly after discontinuation[1001,1013,1014]
- calcitonin has been used as a suppository ●●● [1015,1016]
- phosphate depletion has been described as a reason for failure of calcitonin therapy[1017] - relevance to bisphosphonates unknown

SEE ALSO

⇨ *Bisphosphonates (p.141)*

📖 Reviews[1018-1021]

Drugs for Hypercalcaemia

DISODIUM PAMIDRONATE ☑

Inj. 15mg, 30mg ⓢ 90mg (dry powder for reconstitution)
 TSD: *See relevant sections (90mg £155.80)*

SODIUM CLODRONATE

Inj. 300mg/5mL ⓢ 300mg/10mL
 TSD: *See relevant sections (1500mg £68.90)*
Caps. 400mg ⓢ 520mg *(Loron)* ⓢ Tabs. 800mg
 TSD: *800mg or 520mg b.d. PO (£162.55)*

CALCITONIN (SALMON)

CSCI may reduce side effects of nausea & vomiting, and stinging at **SC** injection sites[497]
Inj. 100u/1mL ⓢ 400u/2mL
 TSD: *200u q.d.s. SC, or 800u/24h CSCI (for 2 days £102.48)*

Hypomagnesaemia

Hypomagnesaemia occurs in 7-11% hospital patients. Serum magnesium < 0.65mmol/L (although there is not a clear relationship with intracellular magnesium). Hypokalaemia, hypocalcaemia, and/or hyponatraemia are usually found in association.

Serum magnesium should be checked in any patient with a low calcium, potassium, or sodium, who has any of the following symptoms:

Symptoms
- anorexia
- nausea and vomiting
- muscle weakness and paraesthesia
- twitching or tremor
- irritability
- ataxia
- depression
- confusion

Causes / Risk factors
- reduced dietary intake (including IV fluids > 3 weeks)
- malabsorption (small intestinal absorption)
- diuretics
- nephrotoxic drugs (especially chemotherapy e.g. cisplatin)
- chronic vomiting/gastric suction/diarrhoea

Intravenous treatment
Oral magnesium is poorly absorbed and large doses cause diarrhoea. Symptomatic hypomagnesaemia is associated with a body deficit of 0.5-1mmol/kg which may need to be replaced over several days. Renal failure and dehyration are contraindications to oral or intravenous use.

1) Rehydrate if clinically or biochemically dehydrated.
2) Magnesium sulphate 20mmol (5g) in 250mL N saline over 1h.[1022]
3) Repeat daily, checking magnesium levels after 2 or 3 treatments.

Oral maintenance treatment
- Magnesium glycerophosphate 1-2g t.d.s. PO

PRESCRIBING STATUS
☼ Oral magnesium ®

SEE ALSO
Reviews[1022-1025]

Drugs for Hypomagnesaemia
MAGNESIUM SULPHATE
Inj. 50% 20 mmol/10mL (5g/10mL)
TSD: 20 mmol in 250 mL normal saline IV infusion over 1 hour (1g = 4mmol)
Side effects: flushing, hypotension, neuromuscular or respiratory depression - rare. Loss of patellar reflexes, drowsiness, slurred speech and blurred vision may indicate toxicity; treated with calcium gluconate IV.
Magnesium given to patients on calcium channel blockers (e.g. nifedipine) can cause profound hypotension.
MAGNESIUM GLYCEROPHOSPHATE
Tabs. 4mmol (1g)
TSD: 1-2g t.d.s. PO
Unlicensed, but recommended in BNF - available from IDIS

Hyponatraemia & SIADH

Common finding in advanced cancer. If sodium ≥125mmol/L treatment is rarely indicated. Symptoms include confusion, fits, cardiac failure, oedema and weakness. Mortality & morbidity are high if sodium ≤110mmol/L.
If appropriate to investigate, send FBC for haematocrit (PCV), U&E, glucose, plasma and urine osmolality, and urinary sodium.

Causes of hyponatraemia

Dehydrated / hypovolaemic	Urinary Na >20mmol/L	*(Renal water and Na loss)*
		Diuretics
		Osmolar diuresis - renal failure (urea) hyperglycaemia
	Urinary Na <20mmol/L	*(Non-renal water and Na loss)*
		diarrhoea
		vomiting
		fistulae
Not dehydrated	Oedema	Liver cirrhosis
		Cardiac failure
		Renal failure
	No oedema Urine osmolality >500mmol/kg	SIADH
	No oedema Urine osmolality <500mmol/kg	Water overload excessive drinking IV fluids

- Specific causes should be addressed as appropriate.
- If not dehydrated and good renal function, water restriction to ≤ 1 litre/day, if tolerated, can be tried.
- If dehydrated and good renal function, 0.9% saline can be given. Plasma sodium should be corrected **slowly** to about 125mmol/L; rapid changes can cause heart failure or acute central pontine myelinosis (potentially fatal brainstem demyelination).

Syndrome of Inappropriate ADH (SIADH)

Accounts for approximately one third of cases of hyponatraemia in cancer patients.[1026] Causes include: any malignancy, but especially small cell lung; numerous drugs including carbamazepine, opioids, tricyclic antidepressants and SSRIs.[1027]

Diagnosis is made by finding concentrated urine (sodium >20mmol/L) in presence of hyponatraemia (<125mmol/L) or low plasma osmolality (<260mmol/kg), and absence of hypovolaemia, oedema or diuretics.
Water restriction to ≤ 1 litre/day, if tolerated may suffice. Alternatively, demeclocycline may be used in doses of 600-900mg daily (150mg q.d.s.-300mg t.d.s.) without water restriction.

Dugs for SIADH
DEMECLOCYCLINE
  Caps. 150mg
  TSD: 150mg q.d.s. PO

Diabetes Insipidus

Differential diagnosis of causes for hypernatraemia includes hypercalcaemia and fluid loss without water replacement e.g. diarrhoea, vomiting, fistulae. In diabetes insipidus, the patient is unable to concentrate urine, even if fluid restricted.

Diagnosis
- Restrict fluid to <0.5L 1hr before to 8h after desmopressin 20µg nasally.
- Measure urine concentration in the period 5-9 h after spray:
  - ≥700 mOsm/kg → cranial diabetes insipidus
  - <700 mOsm/kg → nephrogenic diabetes insipidus

Drugs for Diabetes Insipidus

DESMOPRESSIN

Tabs. (scored) 100µg[⊘] 200µg

TSD: 100µg t.d.s.

Nasal spray 10µg/activation

TSD: Nasal spray 1 activation nocte

Maintenance dose desmopressin usually between 10µg nocte - 20µg b.d.

Risk of hyponatraemia and fluid retention, especially in the elderly.
Monitor blood pressure and U&E's.

SIADH & Diabetes Insipidus

	Diabetes Insipidus	SIADH
Causes	Head trauma incl. post-surgical. Pituitary or hypothalamus tumours. (Breast Ca esp.)	Any malignancy especially: Small cell lung Mesothelioma Brain Drugs incl. carbamazepine tricyclic antidepressants and SSRIs[1027]
Body water	Dehydrated	Water retention
Serum Sodium	> 150 mmol	< 130 mmol (<120 usually if symptomatic)
ADH	Reduced	Increased
Serum Urea	↑	↓
Urine output	↑	↓
Urine concentration	Dilute	Concentrated or Normal
Symptoms	Thirst Lethargy Weakness Confusion	Nausea Lethargy Weakness Anorexia Confusion Coma
Signs	Polyuria	Convulsions Myoclonus
Treatment	Desmopressin	Fluid restriction Demeclocycline

URINARY TRACT DISORDERS

Bladder spasms

Common causes
- urinary tract infection
- tumour infiltration of bladder or rectum
- urinary catheter
- radiation cystitis

Treatment
1) Treat UTI if present.
2) Change catheter for a smaller one.
3) Partially deflate the balloon (the inflated balloon can cause spasm by irritation of the bladder neck).
4) Use bladder washouts for debris in bladder (saline, or *Suby G*).
5) Strap catheter to leg to avoid traction on the bladder trigone area.
6) Oxybutynin 2.5-5mg PO t.d.s.
   - if ineffective or poorly tolerated, try tolterodine 2mg b.d.
7) Lidocaine (lignocaine) bladder instillation 20mL 2% lidocaine (diluted if required in saline) - clamp if possible for 20min-1h, repeated as necessary.[1028-1030]
8) Antimuscarinic drugs e.g. propantheline 15mg nocte-t.d.s. PO, or glycopyrronium 0.2-0.4mg/24h by CSCI, or hyoscine butylbromide 40-120mg/24h by CSCI

PRESCRIBING STATUS
- 🔅 Lidocaine bladder instillation •
- 🔅 Propantheline ®
- 🔅 Glycopyrronium, Hyoscine butylbromide •

Think List

- NSAIDs • are recognised treatment for unstable bladder, and are as effective as opioids at treating renal colic;[1031] ketorolac has been used for postoperative bladder spasms[1032]
- corticosteroids • may be helpful if tumour-related inflammation may be irritating the bladder
- intravesical bupivacaine •• may be more effective than lidocaine[1033]
- spinal analgesia may be appropriate in severe cases
- intravesical oxybutynin ••• 5mg in 30mL 1-3 times a day[1034-1036]
- intravesical capsaicin ••• [1037,1038]
- opioids ••• have historically been instilled into the bladder[1039]

Drugs for Bladder Spasms

OXYBUTYNIN ☑
  Tabs. 2.5mg, 3mg, 5mg; Liquid 2.5mg/5mL
  TSD: 5mg t.d.s. (£14.89) 2.5mg in elderly
TOLTERODINE TARTRATE
  Tabs. 1mg, 2mg
  TSD: 2mg b.d. (£27.50)

Dysuria

Causes
- infection
- tumour infiltration of bladder
- radiotherapy cystitis
- chemotherapy (cyclophosphamide)

Consider bladder spasms if pain follows micturition or occurs at other times.

Treatment
- Treat UTI if present with antibiotics.
- Alkalinisation of the urine with potassium citrate helps relieve urethral pan from UTIs.
- NSAIDs or corticosteroids may help if inflammation present e.g. tumour infiltrating bladder or urethra, radiation cystitis.
- Lidocaine gel in an appropriate syringe (as *Instillagel*) may be used PRN.

Drugs for Urethral pain
POTASSIUM CITRATE
Mixture 1.5 g/5mL
TSD: 10mL t.d.s. **PO**
LIDOCAINE AND CHLORHEXIDINE GEL *(INSTILLAGEL)*
Gel (lidocaine 2% + chlorhexidine 0.25%) 6mL, 11mL

Haematuria

Assessment
Consider the commonest causes:
- tumour bleeding
- clotting disorders *(p.147)*
- infection

Treatment
1) Treat any evidence or signs suggestive of infection.
2) Encourage good urine output (to avoid clot retention).
3) Consider radiotherapy referral.[1040]
4) Consider and treat systemic causes of bleeding *(p.147)*
   - blood tests for clotting screen and platelets
5) Tranexamic acid 1g t.d.s. PO:
   - avoid if bleeding is renal in origin because of risk of ureteral obstruction
   - stop if no effect after 1 week[295]
   - continue for 1 week after bleeding has stopped, then discontinue
   - continue long term (500mg t.d.s.) only if bleeding recurs and responds to second course of treatment
6) Consider transfusion for symptomatic anaemia.

PRESCRIBING STATUS
☼ Tranexamic acid ®

ThinkList

- arterial embolisation[1041-1043] [296-299]
- tranexamic acid bladder instillation ●●● [295]
- alum installation into the bladder;●●● [1044-1046] possible side-effect encephalopathy[1047,1048]
- sodium pentosan polysulphate ●●● ‡☉ [1049,1050]
- conjugated oestrogens ●●● ‡☉ (see below)
- cutaneous ureterostomy has been successfully performed for severe intractable haemorrhagic cystitis following radiotherapy[1051]
- formalin installation into bladder ●●● - carries high risk of serious adverse effects[1052-1058]
- Maalox for hemorrhagic radiation-cystitis: 50-100mL of original or 1/2 diluted Maalox instilled into bladder ●●● and catheter clamped for 30 min. to 1 hr. after sufficient irrigation with 500 ml of 100 times diluted iodine; haematuria should cease within 2 to 8 days[315]
- etamsylate ® ⇨ *Haemostatic drugs (p.150)*

SEE ALSO
⇨ *Bleeding & haemorrhage (p.147)*

Drugs for Haematuria

TRANEXAMIC ACID *(CYKLOKAPRON)* ☑
  Tabs. 500mg; Syrup 500mg/5mL; Inj. 500mg/5mL
    TSD 1g t.d.s. PO or by slow IV injection
  Avoid if risk of ureteric obstruction e.g. renal haemorrhage (see below).
    Discontinue if disturbance in colour vision develops.

Additional Information
Tranexamic acid
Tranexamic acid has been shown to reduce blood loss after prostatectomy. It is contraindicated in patients with bleeding from the upper urinary tract because of the risk that clots will be retained in the ureter and bladder causing renal damage.[287,1059-1063]

Alum bladder instillation
A 1% alum solution can be made using 400g potash of alum in 4L hot sterile water. 300mL of this is added to 3L 0.9% sodium chloride through a sterilising filter. The bladder is irrigated via 3-way catheter with up to 10-30L in 24h. Haematuria should cease within 4 days. [1046,1064-1066]

Conjugated oestrogens
Severe hemorrhagic cystitis induced by radiation and/or cyclophosphamide has been treated with conjugated oestrogens. Doses of 1mg/kg b.d. for 2 days followed by 5mg/24h PO decreased haematuria after 6-8h. Patients treated with 5mg/24h conjugated oestrogen cleared the haematuria within 4 to 7 days. Long term treatment up to 12-22 months has been used successfully. Complications, including thromboembolism, have not been observed.[1067]

Pentosan polysulphate
Administration of pentosan polysulphate sodium by mouth controlled haemorrhage in 5 patients with radiation cystitis.[1050] Not available in UK. Oral, parenteral or topical use.

Urinary Incontinence & Enuresis

Urinary incontinence may be caused by non-specific conditions (general debility, cerebral tumours, confusion), neurological or pelvic problems.
Consider especially:
- constipation (small bladder expansion capacity and frequency)
- exclude or treat underlying UTI
- spinal cord compression - other neurological signs often present
- vesico-vaginal fistula
- over-use of hypnotics or sedation causing nocturnal incontinence
- causes of polyuria e.g. hypercalcaemia, diabetes

Management
1) For frequency or unstable bladder, consider treatment as for bladder spasms ⇨ *(p.137)*
2) NSAIDs can help with an unstable bladder.
3) Antimuscarinic drugs at night for nocturnal incontinence:
   – amitriptyline 25mg nocte, or
   – dosulepin 50-75mg nocte if more sedation required
4) Desmopressin (licensed only for primary nocturnal enuresis up to 65yr)[1068]

PRESCRIBING STATUS
Nocturia/nocturnal incontinence
☼ Amitriptyline ®
☼ Desmopressin ®®

SEE ALSO
⇨ *Antidepressants (p.102), Bladder spasms (p.137)*

Drugs for Urinary Incontinence
AMITRIPTYLINE
   Tabs. 10mg, 25mg, 50mg; Syrup 25mg/5mL, 50mg/5mL
   TSD: 25mg nocte PO
DESMOPRESSIN
   Tabs. (scored) 100µg[⊙] 200µg
   TSD: 200-400µg nocte
   Nasal spray 10µg/activation
   TSD: Nasal spray 10-40µg nocte
   ***Risk of hyponatraemia and fluid retention, especially in the elderly.
   Monitor blood pressure and U&E's.***

MALIGNANCY & IMMUNOLOGY

Bisphosphonates

Uses
- hypercalcaemia *(p.132)*
- bone pain *(p.58)*
- prevention for morbidity from bone metastases
- corticosteroid-induced osteoporosis - prevention

Prevention of morbidity from bone metastases
Over a period of more than a few months, regular bisphosphonates will reduce progression of bone metastases, and thus reduce the incidence of pathological fractures, spinal cord compression, and pain.

Indications
- bone metastases from any carcinoma or myeloma (see below), and
- prognosis of more than a couple of months, and
- already had one pathological fracture, or
- at risk of significant morbidity e.g.
  - large lytic lesion in neck of femur
  - partial collapse of vertebra (which may progress to cord compression)

Use of bisphosphonates should not prevent appropriate referral for radiotherapy, but should be considered *in addition*.

Treatment should be continued until the burden of treatment becomes unacceptable, or prognosis is measured in weeks.

Treatment options
Intravenous therapy is recommended as first-line, with oral clodronate used for patients with difficult venous access etc. Intravenous therapy is more effective, and better tolerated;[492,1069] it is also more predictable, as oral bisphosphonates are poorly and variably absorbed.

- pamidronate 90mg IV every 4 weeks
  - dilute to 500mL 0.9% N saline (minimum 375mL)
  - infuse over 2hr (minimum 1½hr, or 4½hr in renal failure)
- clodronate 1500mg IV every 3 weeks
- clodronate 800mg b.d. PO

(Clodronate, but not pamidronate can be given by subcutaneous hypodermoclysis in 1000mL saline if venous access is not possible.[1018,1070,1071])

Corticosteroid-induced osteoporosis - prevention
Preventive measures should be considered for patients who take corticosteroids for more than 6 months, *or who are anticipated to do so.* Bisphosphonates are effective for the prevention and treatment of corticosteroid-induced osteoporosis.[976,977]

- For patients with bone metastases, consider options as above for *Prevention of morbidity from bone metastases.* These drugs are not licensed for this specific use, and optimum doses are not determined; it is probable that doses used are *more* than adequate for prevention of osteoporosis.

- For patients with primary cerebral tumours, use etidronate with calcium - as *Didronel PMO* (no/low risk of hypercalcaemia).
- For other patients with malignancy (with risk of hypercalcaemia), use risedronate 5mg o.d. PO.

⇨ *Corticosteroids (p.126)*

Side effects of bisphosphonates

- hypocalcaemia[1072,1073]
  - if treating hypercalcaemia, adjust dose; if treating for pain or skeletal effects, calcium supplements may be needed
- fever (up to 39°C) and myalgia for 1 to 3 days after first IV use, in up to 10% patients; resembles a typical acute-phase response[511,517,1074]
  - reported with pamidronate, but not with clodronate
- uveitis or scleritis occurs sporadically; occasionally severe[1074,1075]
  - recurs after repeat administration
  - reported with pamidronate, but not with clodronate
- transient increase in bone pain can occur after first use in up to 10% patients[511]
- renal failure due to renal calcinosis - rehydrate first, and follow minimum recommended infusion durations
- gastric irritation; amino derivatives (e.g. pamidronate) may induce dose-related serious gastrointestinal lesions when taken orally, with the sporadic appearance of erosive oesophagitis

PRESCRIBING STATUS
Reduce morbidity from metastatic bone disease - Ca Breast & myeloma:
☼ Bisphosphonates •
Reduce morbidity from metastatic bone disease - other solid tumours:
☼ Bisphosphonates ••
☼ Clodronate via hypodermoclysis ••

SEE ALSO
⇨ *Hypercalcaemia (p.132), Bone pain (p.58)*
📖 Guidelines[510,1075-1077] & Reviews[1078-1081] - Systematic review[1082]
📖 Review & Guidelines[1083]

Bisphosphonate Preparations
TREATMENT OF HYPERCALCAEMIA & PAINFUL BONE METASTASES
DISODIUM PAMIDRONATE ☑

  Inj. 15mg, 30mg○ 90mg (dry powder for reconstitution)
    TSD: See relevant sections (90mg £155.80)
SODIUM CLODRONATE
  Inj. 300mg/5mL○ 300mg/10mL
    TSD: See relevant sections (1500mg £68.90)
  Caps. 400mg○ 520mg *(Loron)*○ Tabs. 800mg
    TSD: 800mg or 520mg b.d. PO (£162.55)
ZOLEDRONIC ACID ○
  Inj. 4mg/5mL
    TSD: 4mg IV diluted in 50mL saline or dextrose over 5-15 mins. (£195.00)

PREVENTION & TREATMENT OF STEROID-INDUCED OSTEOPOROSIS
Etidronate (with calcium, as *Didronel PMO*), risedronate and alendronate are
licensed for this use. The other bisphosphonates are probably equally effective,
but are not licensed, and dose regimens have not been determined for this use.
Doses to prevent osteoporosis are probably less than those used for bone
metastases.
Didronel PMO is best avoided in patients at potential risk of hypercalcaemia i.e.
most cancer patients. Alendronate can cause serious oesophagitis. Risedronate
appears to cause fewer adverse effects.[1084]

DISODIUM ETIDRONATE (WITH CALCIUM CARBONATE) ☑
   Tabs. etidronate 400mg & tabs. calcium carbonate 1.25g *(Didronel PMO)*
      TSD: 1 tab. etidronate o.d. for 14 days, 1 tab. calcium 76 days (£12.50 28d)

RISEDRONATE SODIUM ☑
   Tabs. 5mg, 30mg
      TSD: 5mg o.d. PO (only licensed for post-menopausal) (£21.83)

ALENDRONATE (ALENDRONIC ACID)
   Tabs. 5mg ⊘ 10mg
      *TSD: 5mg o.d. PO (10mg o.d. if post-menopausal, not on HRT) (£23.12 either
      dose)*

Additional Information

Optimum dose regimens have not been determined for the prevention of
morbidity from bone metastases. Evidence supports the use of intravenous
clodronate 1500mg every 3 weeks as well as various doses of pamidronate
from 60-90mg 3-4 weekly. Cost and other factors will dictate local
guidelines.

Some guidelines have recommended bisphosphonates for all patients with
metastatic (breast) cancer who have imaging evidence of lytic destruction of
bone and who are concurrently receiving systemic therapy with hormonal
therapy or chemotherapy. For women with only an abnormal bone scan but
without bony destruction by imaging studies or localized pain, there is
insufficient evidence to suggest starting bisphosphonates.[1076]

Although there is most evidence supporting treatment to reduce skeletal
events and pain in multiple myeloma and in breast cancer patients with
metastatic bone disease, there is also level I evidence for their use as part of a
pain management program for bone metastases from carcinoma of the lung
and prostate.[1082]

There is some evidence that bisphosphonates may also have an anti-tumour
effect, but more evidence is needed.[1085,1086]

Zoledronic acid has recently been introduced; it has a longer-lasting effect,
requiring less frequent administration, and can be given over a shorter infusion
duration.[1006]

Bone anti-resorption potency[1076]	
Etidronate	1
Clodronate	10
Pamidronate	100
Risedronate	1,000
Alendronate	10,000
Ibandronate	50,000
Zoledronic acid	100,000

HAEMATOLOGY & CARDIOVASCULAR SYSTEM

Venous thromboembolism (DVT & PE)

Cancer patients carry a high risk of venous thromboembolism overall.[1087]
However, poorly controlled anticoagulation with warfarin is a particular
problem in palliative care.[1088-1091]

Decisions about management of venous thromboembolism in cancer must be
made on an individual basis weighing up the benefits and risks, and taking
individual circumstances into account. Increased bleeding risk should be taken
into account e.g. thrombocytopenia or liver failure.

Management of DVT or PE

Treatment goals should be:

- Symptomatic relief of acute event :
  - DVT: consider leg elevation, compression garment and analgesia for
    swelling and tenderness.
  - PE: consider oxygen, opioids $\pm$ benzodiazepine for dyspnoea and fear.
- Resolution of thrombus, if possible:
  - If pelvic DVT due to external tumour compression or infiltration, this
    may not be achievable.
  - Low molecular weight heparin treatment for 7-14 days can be given
    quite safely, even as an outpatient, without blood monitoring.
  - Fibrinolytic therapy (e.g. streptokinase) may be appropriate for selected
    patients e.g. with central venous catheter-related SVC thrombosis.[790]
- Prevention of further DVT or more serious PE's. Warfarin anticoagulation is
  the standard treatment ($\Rightarrow$ p.145) but note:
  - It is unknown whether a DVT due to external tumour compression or
    infiltration is more or less likely to predispose to a PE.
  - Warfarin anticoagulation may be too high risk in patients with advanced
    disease (especially liver disease or on multiple other medications) and
    the burden of monitoring too great.
  - Consider continuing low-molecular weight heparin in 'prophylaxis' dose
    by daily SC injection for a further 4 weeks or until the terminal stages.
  - Aspirin 75-150mg PO daily may be an appropriate compromise for
    other patients, probably affording a degree of protection against
    further events.
  - Vena caval filters are used to treat recurrent pulmonary emboli when
    anticoagulation is contra-indicated or ineffective; vena cava
    thrombosis can occur in up to 20% patients, therefore in the absence
    of bleeding or high bleeding risk, anticoagulation need be
    continued.[1092,1093]

SEE ALSO

$\Rightarrow$ *Anticoagulation (p.145)*
📖 Reviews[1094-1098]

Anticoagulation

See previous section on *Venous thromboembolism (p.144)* for decision-making about anticoagulation.

Initiating oral (warfarin) anticoagulation
1) Confirmation of diagnosis should not delay starting therapy.
2) Commence low molecular weight heparin in treatment dose.
3) Commence warfarin when diagnosis confirmed, 10mg daily (6pm) for day 1 and day 2.
4) Check INR on day 3 and adjust subsequent doses of warfarin as below.
5) Continue heparin for a minimum of 4 days, and at least 2 days after INR in therapeutic range (initial period of warfarin treatment causes. hypercoagulant state); in large thromboses give heparin up to 10 days.
6) When INR in therapeutic range, continue to check INR weekly until stable.

Warfarin schedule[1099]

Day	INR (9 am)	Warfarin dose (6 pm)
1	-	10mg
2	-	10mg
3	< 2.0	10mg
	2.0 - 2.1	5mg
	2.2 - 2.3	4.5mg
	2.4 - 2.5	4mg
	2.6 - 2.7	3.5mg
	2.8 - 2.9	3mg
	3.0 - 3.1	2.5mg
	3.2 - 3.3	2mg
	3.4	1.5mg
	3.5	1mg
	3.6 - 4.0	0.5mg
	> 4.0	0mg
		Predicted maintenance dose
4	< 1.4	> 8mg
	1.4	8mg
	1.5	7.5mg
	1.6 - 1.7	7mg
	1.8	6.5mg
	1.9	6mg
	2.0 - 2.1	5.5mg
	2.2 - 2.3	5mg
	2.4 - 2.6	4.5mg
	2.7 - 3.0	4mg
	3.1 - 3.5	3.5mg
	3.6 - 4.0	3mg
	4.1 - 4.6	Miss next day's dose then 2mg
	> 4.5	Miss 2 days' doses then give 1mg

If INR on day 4 is < 2.0, continue heparin

Target INRs[1092]

Target INR	Indication
2.0 - 2.5	DVT prophylaxis
2.5	Treatment of DVT and PE (or recurrence in patients not on warfarin)
3.5	Recurrent DVT and PE in patients receiving warfarin, Mechanical prosthetic heart valves

INR should be within 0.5 of the target INR.

SEE ALSO
⇨ Haemorrhage whilst anticoagulated - *Bleeding & haemorrhage (p.147)*
📖 Guidelines[1092]

Anticoagulants

WARFARIN

Tabs. 0.5mg, 1mg, 3mg, 5mg

Anticoagulation effect may be increased by: dextropropoxyphene (co-proxamol), NSAIDs, amiodarone, erythromycin, clarithromycin, quinolone antibiotics (e.g. ciprofloxacin), metronidazole, imidazole antifungals (e.g. fluconazole), stanozolol, and omeprazole.
Anticoagulant effect reduced by St John's wort.

DALTEPARIN

Inj. 2500u/0.2mL, 5000u/0.2mL, 10000u/0.4mL, 12500u/0.5mL, 15000u/0.6mL, 18000u/0.72mL

Dose for treatment of DVT or PE: 200u/kg SC o.d. - 10000u (body weight 46-56kg);12500u (57-68kg); (69-82kg); 18000u (> 82kg) (£49.42 for 7 days for 60kg man)

Dose for prophylaxis: 5000u SC o.d. (£78.96 for 28 days)

ENOXAPARIN

Inj. 20mg/0.2mL, 40mg/0.4mL, 60mg/0.6mL, 80mg/0.8mL, 100mg/1mL, 150mg/1mL

Dose for treatment of DVT or PE: 1.5mg/kg SC o.d. (£50.33 for 7 days for 60kg man)

Dose for prophylaxis: 40mg SC o.d. (£126.56 for 28 days)

1mg = 100u

TINZAPARIN

Inj. 3500u/0.35mL, 4500u/0.45mL

Inj. 2500u/0.25mL[○] 10000u/0.5mL[○] 14000u/0.7mL[○] 18000u/0.9mL[○] 20000u/2mL[○] 40000u/2mL[○]

Dose for treatment of DVT or PE: 175u/kg SC o.d. (£67.55 for 7 days for 60kg man)

Dose for prophylaxis: 3500-4500u SC o.d. (£107.24 for 28 days)

HEPARIN (UNFRACTIONATED)

Inj. 1000u/mL 1mL, 5mL

Inj. 5000u/mL 1mL, 5mL

Inj. 25,000u/mL 1mL, 5mL

Bleeding & haemorrhage

Bleeding in cancer may be due to local pathology e.g. tumour, peptic ulcer, haemorrhoids or varices.

Systemic causes of bleeding may exacerbate local factors, or present as more diffuse mucosal bleeding:

- thrombocytopenia
- liver disease or jaundice
- anticoagulant medication
- renal failure
- vitamin C deficiency (scurvy)

General measures

Radiotherapy, which causes a radiation thrombosis, can be helpful to reduce bleeding from tumour sites, including ulcerating skin tumours, haemoptysis, and haematuria.

General medical management will include assessment of blood loss, appropriate fluid replacement or transfusions.

If bleeding tendency is present, attention should be paid to optimise:

- oral hygiene
- skin care
- avoid constipation

Thrombocytopenia

Continuous bleeding due to low platelet count (rare unless < 20) may occur in pancytopenia from bone marrow infiltration, leukaemia, chemotherapy etc.

- platelet transfusions[1100]
    - may be appropriate if bleeding is distressing
    - will only raise the platelet count in the patient for a matter of days
    - only indicated if active bleeding
    - 5 units IV over 1 hour
    - may need to be repeated every few days
- tranexamic acid (or aminocaproic acid) can control mucosal bleeding (nose, uterus, GI tract) in thrombocytopenia of various aetiologies.[1101-1109]

Liver Disease & Jaundice

Clotting factors may be reduced in advanced liver disease and lead to bleeding from mucosal surfaces.

Obstructive jaundice will lead to fat malabsorption and thus reduced vitamin K absorption. Abnormal clotting may be normalised by giving vitamin K:

- vitamin K given IV or orally
- needs to be water soluble (Menadiol) if given orally
- 10mg PO or by slow IV injection daily

Hepatocellular damage will prevent many clotting factors being manufactured; this may only be reversed by fresh frozen plasma.

Fresh frozen plasma needs to be given daily, but may very rarely be appropriate in late stage disease to reduce severe distress from oral bleeding, haemoptysis, etc.

Haemorrhage on warfarin

Poorly controlled anticoagulation with warfarin is a particular problem in cancer patients.[1088-1090] However these patients also carry a higher risk of venous thromboembolism.[1087]

British Society for Haematology Guidelines:[1092]

- Major bleeding - stop warfarin. Phytomenadione (vitamin K_1) 5mg by slow IV injection; FFP 15mL/kg
- INR > 8.0, no bleeding or minor bleeding - stop warfarin, restart when INR < 5.0. If other risk factors for bleeding give Phytomenadione (vit K_1) 0.5mg by slow IV injection or 5mg orally. Repeat phytomenadione after 24h if INR still > 5.0
- INR 6.0-8.0, no bleeding or minor bleeding - stop warfarin, restart when INR < 5.0

Haemorrhage on heparin

If bleeding occurs on heparin, it is usually sufficient to stop the heparin. Protamine is a specific antidote, but is only partially effective against low molecular weight heparins.

Heparins (unfractionated and low molecular weight) can cause thrombocytopenia. Immune reaction, seen after 5 days or more of treatment. Stop heparin if this occurs.

Chronic renal failure

Renal failure causes complex disturbances of blood clotting.

- Tranexamic acid shortens bleeding time in chronic renal failure.[1110]
- Conjugated oestrogens[‡] shorten prolonged bleeding times in renal failure. Daily IV infusion 0.6mg/kg daily for 4-5 days, or 50mg daily for 7 days (duration of effect 10-15 days).[1111]

Vitamin C deficiency (scurvy)

Scurvy is usually due to dietary insufficiency and is most common in elderly people, living alone, or dependent on alcohol. Its frequency is probably underestimated in cancer patients.[1112]

It should be suspected in cases of unexplained haemorrhage, especially with intramuscular haemorrhage or haemorrhagic gingivitis, ecchymoses and purpura. 'Corkscrew hairs' due to failure of hair follicle eruption may be seen. Diagnosis is made on a mixture of clinical findings and serum vitamin C level (though these reflect recent dietary intake). Treatment is with vitamin C 1g daily for 2 weeks, then 60-100mg daily. Clinical signs should resolve within 1-2 weeks. ⇨ *Vitamins (p.157)*

PRESCRIBING STATUS

☼ Tranexamic acid ●
☼ Conjugated oestrogens ●●●

ThinkList

- tranexamic acid mouthwash ● (1g every 6h) for oral bleeding[1113-1116]
- desmopressin ●●● (intranasal 300µg or IV or SC 0.3µg per kg) has been used in a number of acquired bleeding disorders, including platelet disorders, von Willebrand's, and renal failure - it produces supra-normal levels of certain clotting factors. Peak effect 30 -60 mins after IV, 60-90 mins after SC or intranasal. Duration of effect 6-8h. Repeat doses 12-24h. Tachyphylaxis may occur after 3-4 doses.[1111] One report demonstrated synergy between desmopressin and etamsylate.[1117]

Bleeding & haemorrhage **149**

SEE ALSO
⇨ *Emergencies: Massive haemorrhage (p.184)*
⇨ *Haematuria (p.138), Haemoptysis (p.96)*
⇨ *Gastrointestinal bleeding (p.39), Haemostatic drugs (p.150)*
📖 Reviews[309,1118]

Drugs for treating Bleeding & Haemorrhage
VITAMIN K PREPARATIONS
MENADIOL PHOSPHATE (WATER SOLUBLE VITAMIN K)
> Tabs. 10mg
>
> Water soluble. Suitable for clotting disorders due to fat malabsorption e.g. biliary obstruction or hepatic disease.

PHYTOMENADIONE (VITAMIN K₁)
> Tabs. 10mg
>
> *TSD: 10mg o.d. PO*
>
> Fat soluble. Suitable for reversing warfarin anticoagulation, but not for clotting disorders due to fat malabsorption e.g. biliary obstruction or hepatic disease.

PHYTOMENADIONE (VITAMIN K₁) COLLOIDAL FORMULATION *(KONAKION MM)*
> Inj. 10mg /1mL
>
> *Konakion MM* is a colloidal formulation to reduce anaphylaxis on IV injection. Give by slow IV injection or infusion in glucose 5%

ANTIFIBRINOLYTIC DRUGS
TRANEXAMIC ACID *(CYKLOKAPRON)*
> Tabs. 500mg; Syrup 500mg/5mL; Inj. 500mg/5mL
>
> *TSD 1g t.d.s. PO or by slow IV injection*
>
> Avoid if risk of ureteric obstruction e.g. renal haemorrhage. Discontinue if disturbance in colour vision develops.

Haemostatic drugs

Tranexamic acid

Tranexamic acid works by inhibiting fibrinolysis and the consequent stabilisation of clots. It has been used (unlicensed) successfully for many different causes of bleeding, both in cancer and non-cancer patients. It is licensed for menorrhagia or 'local fibrinolysis'.

For specific sites ⇨ *Haematuria (p.138), Haemoptysis (p.96), Gastrointestinal bleeding (p.39).* Other reported uses:

- cancer patients with melaena, PV, PR bleeding, haematuria and haemoptysis[295]
- intraperitoneal haemorrhage (aminocaproic acid) in ovarian carcinoma.[1119]
- haemothorax in malignant mesothelioma.[1120]
- mucosal bleeding (nose, uterus, GI tract) in thrombocytopenia of various aetiologies.[1101-1109]
- chronic renal failure.[1110]
- topical tranexamic acid for superficial fungating tumour[295]
- mouthwash (1g every 6h) for oral bleeding[1113-1116]

Average time until significant improvement in bleeding is 2 days and average time for complete cessation, 4 days.[295]

Etamsylate

Etamsylate is licensed for menorrhagia. In this, it has been found less effective than tranexamic acid.[1121,1122] Other studies have looked at post-surgical bleeding, various bleeding disorders, and aspirin-induced gastric bleeding. More published studies seem to report negative findings than positive ones.[1123-1134]

SEE ALSO
⇨ *Bleeding & haemorrhage (p.147)*
📖 Reviews[1111]

Haemostatic drug preparations

TRANEXAMIC ACID *(CYKLOKAPRON)* ☑

Tabs. 500mg; Syrup 500mg/5mL; Inj. 500mg/5mL
TSD 1g t.d.s. PO or by slow IV injection
Avoid if risk of ureteric obstruction e.g. renal haemorrhage. Discontinue if disturbance in colour vision develops.

ETAMSYLATE (ETHAMSYLATE)

Tabs. 500mg *(Dicynene)*
TSD: 500mg q.d.s. PO

Additional Information

Aminocaproic acid work in the same way as tranexamic acid, by inhibiting fibrinolysis and the consequent stabilisation of clots. Tranexamic acid is more potent and has a longer half-life than aminocaproic acid, which is not available in the UK.[1111,1135,1136] Studies quoted showing benefit from aminocaproic acid are indirect evidence of likely benefit from tranexamic acid.

Anaemia

Commonest causes of anaemia

- leukaemia (normocytic)
- bone marrow involvement causing pancytopenia (normocytic)
  - myeloma
  - prostate
  - breast
- bleeding (microcytic if chronic)
  - gastro-intestinal
  - haematuria
- bone marrow suppression from chemotherapy
- general reaction to advanced malignancy, anaemia of chronic disease (usually normocytic)
- iron deficiency (microcytic)

Management of clinical anaemia

- Treat mild iron-deficient (microcytic) anaemia with ferrous sulphate
- Transfusion is unlikely to give benefit if the Hb is 10 g/dl or more, but symptoms may be better predictors of response[748,1137]
- Transfusion must be considered to be likely to help
  - dyspnoea (more often due to lung pathology) or
  - weakness (more often due to tumour cachexia)
  - and thus improve quality of life
- It is important to document if the transfusion has been effective in the notes. This helps plan future transfusions.
- If repeated transfusion is required, the frequency of transfusion, symptomatic benefit, and patient's desires regarding prolonging life need to be carefully reviewed.

ThinkList

- macrocytic anaemia due to vitamin B12 or folic acid deficiency, related to gastrectomy, or poor dietary intake

SEE ALSO
📖 Review[1138,1139]

Drugs for Anaemia

FERROUS SULPHATE
Tabs. 200mg
TSD: 200mg t.d.s. PO
FERROUS FUMARATE *(FERSAMAL)*
Syrup 140mg/5mL
TSD: 10mL b.d. PO
HYDROXOCOBALAMIN (VITAMIN B12)
Inj. 1mg/1mL
TSD: 1mg 3 times a week for 2 weeks IM; then 1mg every 3 months
FOLIC ACID
Tabs. 5mg; Syrup 2.5mg/5mL
TSD: 5mg o.d. PO for 4 months
Never give alone in megaloblastic anaemia that may be associated with vitamin B12 deficiency.

Erythropoietin

Erythropoietin is licensed for anaemia of chronic renal failure, and for patients undergoing chemotherapy. It may also be effective in improving the chronic anaemia of cancer, and cost is a major reason for not using it more widely as an alternative to intermittent transfusions. It may be appropriate for use in Jehovah's witnesses.

In iron deficient anaemia, erythropoietin should increase. In cancer anaemia erythropoietin is much less increased (relative deficiency). Patients with marrow failure therefore do not respond (reduced leucocytes and platelets). Erythropoietin levels < 100 predictive of good response. If after 1 month response of HB not >0.5 then probably will not respond.[1140] Maximum benefit occurs after about 2 months. Iron deficiency will stop response so iron supplements should be given as required.

PRESCRIBING STATUS
⚗ Erythropoietin ●●●

SEE ALSO
📖 Review[1141]

Erythropoietin preparations
EPOETIN ALFA (ERYTHROPOIETIN)
Pre-filled syringes Inj. 1000u/0.5mL, 2000u/0.5mL, 3000u/0.3mL, 4000u/0.4mL (Eprex)
TSD: 50u/kg three times weekly SC (£301.68)
EPOETIN BETA (ERYTHROPOIETIN)
Pre-filled syringes Inj. 500u/0.3mL, 1000u/0.3mL, 2000u/0.3mL, 3000u/0.3mL, 4000u/0.3mL, 5000u/0.3mL, 6000u/0.3mL, 10,000u/0.3mL (NeoRecormon)
TSD: 60u/kg weekly in 1-7 divided doses SC (£134.08)

Blood transfusion

Giving a blood transfusion
Concentrated red cells/whole blood transfusion
Target a blood transfusion level of 10 g/L e.g. two units if haemoglobin is 8, four units if haemoglobin is 6. Packed cells should be given at the rate of 1 unit over 2h.

Give 3-4 units during the day. If more are needed, the IVI can be taken down overnight and recommenced next day. Whole blood is rarely provided nowadays, but should be given at 1 unit over 4-6h.

Prophylactic furosemide 20-40mg IV with the first unit should be given when:
• significant history of CCF or LVF
• signs of fluid retention

Observations
The level of observation should be adjusted to suit the patient and their risk-status. Frequent blood pressure measurements are much less use than regular observation of respiratory rate, pulse and the patient's feeling of comfort.

Blood transfusion reactions

Pyrexia
- pyrexia up to 38.5°C $\pm$ mild flu-like symptoms
- can be reduced by using blood filter
- develops slowly over hours
- treat with paracetamol
- observe patient for any deterioration
- no other action required if patient otherwise well
- further transfusions are not contra-indicated

Rarely these reactions can cause higher pyrexias with rigors and marked systemic effects. Depending how important it is to continue with the transfusion, either stop the transfusion, or treat with chlorphenamine (chlorpheniramine) 10mg IV and hydrocortisone 100mg IV.

If a previous reaction has occurred these drugs should be given prophylactically before any further transfusions.

Major Allergic Reactions
Blood cross-matching can never ensure that antibodies in the patient will not react to any of the antigens on the given blood. An allergic type of reaction (releasing histamine) can lead to more serious reactions: bronchospasm, circulatory collapse or both.
- stop transfusion
- chlorphenamine (chlorpheniramine) 10mg IV & hydrocortisone 100mg IV
- adrenaline (epinephrine) 0.5-1mL of 1:1,000 IV or deep IM if severe

Bronchospasm
- usually develops within 30 minutes of starting that unit of blood
- distinguish from dyspnoea due to LVF (see below)
- stop the blood transfusion
- give salbutamol nebuliser 2.5mg
- then give chlorphenamine 10mg IV and hydrocortisone 100mg IV

If a patient has had a serious transfusion reaction on a previous occasion, then there is a significant risk on further transfusions, which should only be carried out with adequate back up i.e. as an in-patient in hospital.

Fluid Overload
In severe heart disease or renal failure the patient may become fluid overloaded and show signs of left $\pm$ right heart failure.
- raised BP initially
- rapid pulse of good volume
- dyspnoea with basal crepitations from left ventricular failure
- raised JVP may be present
- stop the transfusion
- give furosemide (frusemide) 40mg IV

Blood transfusion may continue under careful observation with further diuretic cover, if a good response is obtained to the first dose.

Further blood transfusions should be preceded by prophylactic diuretic, and closely supervised.

Difficult veins
Emla cream 1 hour before cannulation will reduce pain, and secondary venous spasm on insertion. If the infusion is slow due to venous spasm, a GTN patch on the skin over the vein will help dilate the vein.[1142-1146] Chlorphenamine (chlorpheniramine) can also be given IV slowly to reduce venous spasm.

Diuretics

Diuretics

Furosemide PO is the standard loop diuretic. Given orally in heart failure, cirrhosis, and probably any hypoalbuminaemic state, it is rendered less effective (mechanism unclear).[1147] It is also absorbed less well orally than bumetanide, and is more affected by food intake.[1148,1149]

Continuous infusion of furosemide in refractory oedema is safe and effective[1150,1151] and causes a greater diuresis than the same daily dose given by intermittent bolus.[1152,1153] It has been given successfully by CSCI.

Alternatively, bumetanide is more effective orally than furosemide in heart failure and probably other hypoalbuminaemic conditions.

Spironolactone is the preferred diuretic for ascites, steroid-induced fluid retention, and possibly heart failure.[1154] ⇨ (p.38) for more information.

Metolazone is a weak thiazide diuretic used alone, but has a very potent synergistic effect with furosemide: 2.5-5mg twice weekly

FUROSEMIDE (FRUSEMIDE)
  Tabs. 20mg, 40mg, 500mg; Liquid 1mg/mL, 40mg/5mL 50mg/5mL
    TSD: 40mg PO
  Inj. 20mg/2mL, 50mg/5mL, 250mg/25mL
    TSD: 100mg/24h CSCI
CO-AMILOFRUSE 5/40
  Tabs. *(Frumil)*
    TSD: 1 tab. mane PO
BUMETANIDE
  Bumetanide 1mg is approximately equivalent to 40mg furosemide
  Tabs. 1mg, 5mg; Liquid 1mg/5mL
    TSD: 1mg mane PO
  Inj. 1mg/2mL, 2mg/4mL
SPIRONOLACTONE
  Tabs. 25mg, 50mg, 100mg; Susp. 10mg/5mL, 25mg/5mL, 50mg/5mL
    TSD: 100mg mane PO
METOLAZONE
  Tabs. 5mg
    TSD: 2.5-5mg mane PO twice weekly

SEE ALSO
⇨ *Ascites (p.37), Lymphoedema (p.163)*

Additional Information

New York Heart Association heart failure classification

1	Asymptomatic	
2	Mild	Symptoms only on exercise
3	Moderate	Symptoms on mild exercise
4	Severe	Symptoms at rest

Angina

All patients with angina should receive aspirin 75-150mg daily.

Drugs used for Angina

NITRATES
Isosorbide mononitrate (generic, standard release) administered twice daily at 8am and 2pm is the preferred choice for maintenance therapy. Once daily modified release preparations are expensive and no more effective. GTN patches are expensive; if used, patients should be advised to remove them for a minimum of 8 hours a day (overnight) to avoid nitrate tolerance.

GLYCERYL TRINITRATE
Tabs. 500µg; Sublingual spray 400µg/activation
Transdermal patches 5mg/24h, 10mg/24h

ISOSORBIDE MONONITRATE
Tabs. 10mg, 20mg
TSD: 10mg b.d. 8am and 2pm

ADRENERGIC BETA-BLOCKERS

PROPRANOLOL
Tabs. 10mg, 40mg, 80mg, 160mg; Syrup[‡] 40mg/5mL
Caps. SR 80mg, 160mg; Inj. 1mg/1mL

ATENOLOL
Tabs. 25mg, 50mg, 100mg; Syrup 25mg/5mL; Inj. 5mg/10mL

Atrial fibrillation

Atrial fibrillation may occur in advanced cancer as an coincidental problem, or may be related to cardiac infiltration by adjacent lung tumour or cardiomyopathy. AF may be persistent or paroxysmal.

Aims of treatment
• symptomatic control of symptoms e.g. hypotension, pulmonary oedema
• prevention of thromboembolism

Treatment options
Immediate anticoagulation and then cardioversion for persistent AF is the treatment of choice in an otherwise healthy person, but is rarely indicated in palliative care. Drug treatment of AF can be complex,[1155,1156] and drugs such as amiodarone can cause a lot of toxicity.

Digoxin will not aid reversion to sinus rhythm, nor prevent recurrence of AF. Nevertheless it is often the appropriate option for symptomatic control in palliative care.

Beta-blockers (e.g. propranolol or atenolol *p.155*) may be used, or added to digoxin, to reduce ventricular rate.

Paroxysmal AF may be treated with sotalol starting 80mg o.d. PO. ECG monitoring of QT interval is advised.

Anticoagulation with warfarin carries increased risks in advanced cancer patients *(⇨ p.145)*. Aspirin is arguably as effective in preventing thromboembolism, although possibly not as much as warfarin in older patients.[1157,1158]

Drugs for Atrial Fibrillation

DIGOXIN

Tabs. 62.5µg, 125µg, 250µg; Liquid 50µg/mL

Inj. 100µg/1mL, 500µg/2mL

> *TSD: 500µg twice at 12h intervals as loading dose; then commence predicted maintenance dose - 62.5µg o.d. very frail/elderly to 250µg o.d. for fitter/younger patients*

SOTALOL

Tabs. 40mg, 80mg, 160mg

> *TSD: 80mg o.d. PO, increased every 2-3 days to usual dose 80-160mg b.d.*
> *ECG monitoring of QT interval is advised.*

AMIODARONE

A number of patients will be taking amiodarone for pre-existing **AF**. Amiodarone has a long half-life of several weeks, and many potential drug interactions and toxicity. Consider stopping in patients with advancing disease.

Tabs. 100mg, 200mg

Several drugs used concomitantly with amiodarone increase the risk of ventricular arrhythmias and the advice is to avoid them: tricyclic antidepressants (amitriptyline etc.), phenothiazines, haloperidol, flecainide, quinine, erythromycin (parenteral). The low doses of haloperidol (antiemetic) and TCA's (neuropathic pain) used in palliative care probably carry a low risk. Amiodarone may increase the anticoagulation effect of warfarin; also increases phenytoin blood levels (risk of toxicity).

NUTRITION & HYDRATION

Mineral supplements & Vitamins

Mineral preparations

POTASSIUM

Liquid or effervescent tablets should be used rather than modified-release tablets. Potassium chloride 25-50mmol is needed daily for the **prevention** of hypokalaemia; higher doses are required for treatment.

SANDO-K
Tabs. Effervescent 12 mmol K^+
  TSD: *2 tabs. t.d.s. PO (for treatment of hypokalaemia)*

KAY-CEE-L
Syrup 1mmol/1mL K^+
  TSD: *20mL t.d.s. PO (for treatment of hypokalaemia)*

CALCIUM

SANDOCAL-400
Tabs. Effervescent Ca^{2+} 10mmol
SANDOCAL-1000
Tabs. Effervescent Ca^{2+} 25mmol
CALCICHEW
Tabs. (chewable) Ca^{2+} 12.5mmol
CALCIUM-SANDOZ
Syrup Ca^{2+} 2.5mmol/5mL
  TSD: *up to 40mmol/day in divided doses*
CALCIUM GLUCONATE
Inj. 10% 10mL (Ca^{2+} 2.25mmol)
  TSD: *10mL 10% by slow IV injection for hypocalcaemic tetany or severe hyperkalaemia*

ZINC

Zinc deficiency may result in lethargy, anorexia, loss of taste, and delayed wound healing.[1159-1161] The evidence for symptomatic zinc deficiency in cancer is mixed and generally weak.[1162-1164] Use dietary measures unless marked deficiency or continuing loss.

ZINC SULPHATE
Tabs. Effervescent 125mg *(Solvazinc)*
  TSD: *1 tab. o.d. - t.d.s. PO*

Vitamin preparations

Vitamin B_1 deficiency usually occurs in alcoholics, and can present with confusion or dementia *(⇨ p.105).* Vitamin B_{12} deficiency is usually due to gastrectomy (may take years to deplete body stores), but may be more common than previously recognised in elderly patients.[1165] Diverse neuropsychiatric symptoms may occur, sometimes in the absence of macrocytosis or anaemia.[1166] Paraesthesia or ataxia were the most common first symptoms, but muscle weakness, diminished or hyperactive reflexes, spasticity, urinary or faecal incontinence, orthostatic hypotension, loss of vision, dementia, psychoses, and disturbances of mood may occur.

VITAMIN B_{12}

HYDROXOCOBALAMIN (VITAMIN B_{12})
Inj. 1mg/1mL
  TSD: *1mg IM 3 times a week for 2 weeks (treatment), then 1mg every 3 months*

VITAMINS B AND C
PABRINEX (VITAMINS B AND C)
IV High potency Inj. Pair of ampoules containing 10mL
TSD: 1 pair of ampoules daily for 3 days
Indications: coma or delirium from alcohol, Wernicke's encephalopathy and Korsakoff's psychosis.
Serious allergic reaction may occur on IV administration. Inject slowly over 10 minutes.

VITAMIN C
ASCORBIC ACID (VITAMIN C)
(High dose vitamin C has been proposed to acidify the urine and prevent urinary tract infection and blockage; evidence suggests it is ineffective[1167])
Tabs. 100, 200, 500mg
TSD: 500mg b.d. PO for 2 weeks (treatment), then 100mg PO daily (prevention)

MULTIVITAMINS
VITAMINS B.P.C.
Caps.
TSD: 1 cap. t.d.s. PO

VITAMINS, MINERALS & TRACE ELEMENTS
FORCEVAL
Caps.
TSD: 1 cap. o.d. PO (£4.81)

SEE ALSO
⇨ *Anaemia (p.151)* for iron, vitamin B12 and folic acid.
⇨ *Hypomagnesaemia (p.134)* for magnesium supplements.
⇨ *Bleeding & haemorrhage (p.147)* for vitamin K preparations & scurvy.
▢ Review of vitamins and nutritional support in cancer.[1168]

Hypodermoclysis

Subcutaneous fluid administration (hypodermoclysis) can be used as an alternative to IV infusion in patients unable to take oral fluids.[1169,1170]
Normal saline is infusion of choice, at a maximum rate of 1,500mL/24h.
If dextrose is required, use 2:1 mixture of 5% dextrose and N/saline, as plain dextrose can cause pain and inflammation. Up to 40mEq potassium can be added to each litre if needed.[1171,1172]
Hyaluronidase has often been added to improve absorption from the infusion site, but there is no good evidence that it helps, and should not be added routinely. There is no evidence that doses greater than 300u/L give greater benefit,[1173,1174] but 750u/L has often been used.[1169,1172]
Average duration of infusion site is around 4-5 days.[1169,1172]
NB Proctoclysis has also been described.[1175]

Dug additive for Hypodermoclysis
HYALURONIDASE
Inj. 1500u amp
TSD: 750u added to each litre of IV fluid

SKIN

Pruritus (itching)

Generalised pruritus **in the absence of a skin rash** may be due to:
- cholestatic jaundice
- renal failure
- opioids
- anaemia (iron deficiency)
- thyroid disease
- myeloma, lymphoma and polycythaemia rubra vera
- diabetes

The commonest cause in advanced malignancy is probably cholestatic jaundice, although there is not a clear association between the level of bilirubin and severity of pruritus.

There is often dry, scaling skin, which will itself cause pruritus through the itch/scratch cycle. Topical treatment with aqueous cream or emulsifying ointment is an essential part of the treatment, and is sometimes sufficient on its own.[1176]

Management

General measures for any pruritus should include cutting nails to avoid trauma, emulsifying ointment or aqueous cream instead of soap, loose cotton clothing, and an emollient after bathing.

1) Exclude dermatoses, especially scabies.
2) Treat underlying cause if possible e.g.
   - consider biliary stenting or percutaneous drain for obstructive jaundice
   - consider changing to alternative opioid if morphine-induced pruritus[605,606] *(p.69)*
3) Chlorphenamine (chlorpheniramine) 4mg nocte - t.d.s.
   - commonly used, but pruritus from renal failure or cholestasis is rarely relieved by antihistamines[1177]
   - the sedation may at least allow a night's sleep
   - newer, non-sedating antihistamines are probably ineffective for pruritus
4) Topical calamine lotion or menthol may be helpful.
5) For pruritus associated with cholestatic jaundice:
   - colestyramine (cholestyramine) is recommended as first-line but is usually poorly tolerated by patients with advanced cancer
   - stanozolol☑ 5mg daily is usually effective within 3-5 days;[1178,1179] see cautions below - an alternative is:
   - rifampicin 150mg b.d.[1180,1181]
   - corticosteroids are effective in some hepatobiliary disease[1181]
6) Ondansetron (and probably other 5-HT₃ antagonists) is effective against opioid-induced and uraemic pruritus, with conflicting reports in cholestatic pruritus;[1182-1192] relief of symptoms may follow single dose:
   - if pruritus is severe, ondansetron 4-8mg IV stat. then
   - ondansetron 4mg b.d. orally increased to 8mg b.d. if required
7) Paroxetine 20mg mane - reported to help pruritus of various cancer-related aetiologies;[1193] benefit is apparent within 4-7 days.

Ondansetron & Paroxetine

Serotonin (5-HT) is implicated in the pathogenesis of pruritus. Ondansetron is a direct 5-HT₃ antagonist, and paroxetine is thought to work by rapidly down-regulating the 5-HT receptors after an initial release of 5-HT. In view of the cost of ondansetron, if ondansetron is found effective:

• commence paroxetine, continuing both drugs for 7 days
• try stopping the ondansetron after 7 days

PRESCRIBING STATUS
☼ Stanozolol, Rifampicin, Corticosteroids, Ondansetron, Paroxetine ●●

Think List

• doxepin is a tricyclic antidepressant with potent antihistamine action (H_1 and H_2); it has been found effective for atopic dermatitis[1194,1195] both orally ●● and as a cream,●●● sometimes used in combination with corticosteroid cream;[1196] also reported use for generalised pruritus of unknown origin[1197]
• the effect of antihistamines (H_1) may be augmented by use of H_2 antagonists[1198]
• olanzapine ●● is probably the most potent antihistamine in clinical use;[1199] there are no reports of its use for pruritus
• phototherapy UVB for uraemic pruritus;[1200,1201]
• erythropoietin ●●● for uraemic pruritus[1202]
• parenteral lidocaine ●●● for cholestatic or uraemic pruritus[1198,1203]
• thalidomide ●●● for cholestatic or uraemic pruritus[1204,1205]
• opioid antagonists ●●● (nalbuphine, naltrexone, naloxone) are effective in opioid-induced, cholestatic and uraemic pruritus,[1206-1209] but have little role in advanced cancer because they may antagonise analgesia
• propofol ●●● (in sub-hypnotic doses) for opioid-induced or cholestatic pruritus[1181,1207,1210,1211]
• droperidol ●● for opioid-induced (spinal) pruritus[1212]

SEE ALSO
📖 Reviews[1177,1213-1215]

Drugs for Pruritus

TOPICAL ANTIPRURITICS
Despite common use, Crotamiton has been shown ineffective against pruritus.[1216]
CALAMINE LOTION
OILY CALAMINE LOTION
MENTHOL 2% IN AQUEOUS CREAM

OTHER DRUGS USED FOR PRURITUS
CHLORPHENAMINE (CHLORPHENIRAMINE, *PIRITON*)
    Tabs. 4mg; Syrup 2mg/5mL
    TSD: 4mg nocte PO (£0.42)
STANOZOLOL
    Tabs. 5mg
    TSD: 5mg o.d. PO (£12.54)
    Dose: 5-10mg daily. Usually well tolerated.
    Can enhance the hypoglycaemic effect of insulin. Avoid in diabetes, or consider lowering the dose of insulin by up to a third.[537] Increases the anticoagulant effect of warfarin. Avoid in prostate cancer. Possible risk of hypercalcaemia in breast cancer. Can cause a paradoxical increase in jaundice, therefore long-term safety uncertain.

RIFAMPICIN
 Caps. 150, 300mg; Syrup 100mg/5mL
 TSD: 150mg b.d. PO (£10.19)
 ***Can cause increase in hepatic dysfunction. Increases metabolism of
 many drugs including corticosteroids, anticonvulsants and
 anticoagulants. Discolours soft contact lenses, and urine coloured
 orange-red.***
PAROXETINE
 ⇨ *p.102* for preparations etc.
 TSD: 20mg mane PO (£16.58 at 20mg o.d.)
ONDANSETRON
 ⇨ *p.23* for preparations etc.
 TSD: 8mg IV then 8mg/24h CSCI, or 8mg b.d. PO (£433.22)

Additional Information
Aquagenic urticaria
Aquagenic urticaria is not uncommon in haematological malignancy. Contact
with water, or water based products (including aqueous cream) causes
irritation and itching. The skin should be kept dry, and oily preparations used.

Malignant ulcers & Pressure sores

Pressure sores (decubitus ulcers), superficial fungating tumours, and other
non-healing wounds and ulcers can cause:
- infection
- mal-odour[1217]
- pain
- bleeding

Wound healing
Control of these problems is often a more appropriate goal in palliative care
than wound healing. Nevertheless, attention should be paid to factors which
may reduce wound healing, if only to minimise extension of the ulcer:
- *Eusol*, povidone-iodine or hydrogen peroxide may inhibit wound healing,
 and should generally be avoided
- vitamin C deficiency[1218,1219]
- zinc deficiency[1220-1222]
- corticosteroids inhibit wound healing
Patients with non-malignant ulcers who have had poor nutrition over
preceding months, may be treated with zinc and vitamin C supplementation
e.g. *Forceval* 1 caps. daily.

Infection & Odour
- Topical metronidazole gel (applied once or twice daily) is effective for
 anaerobic infections, reducing odour, discharge, and pain.[1223-1226]
- Systemic administration of metronidazole 200-400mg b.d. PO is indicated
 if there is surrounding cellulitis, or if the wound is deep and topical
 application will not penetrate. ⇨ *Antibiotics (p.117) - NB warnings
 about alcohol.*
- Other methods that have been used to reduce bacterial growth include live
 yoghurt, chlorophyll, honey and icing sugar.[1217]

Pain

- Infection should be treated with topical or systemic antibiotics (see above).
- Barrier preparations will protect from irritation in perineal wounds or around fistulae *(p.164)*.
- Systemic analgesics including opioids and NSAIDs should be tried, but are often only partially effective.
- Topical anaesthetic or analgesic applications are useful
    - topical opioids *(p.83)*
    - lidocaine gel
    - benzydamine cream[1227]

Metronidazole and diamorphine gel have been used mixed together.[697]

Bleeding

⇨ *Bleeding & haemorrhage (p.147)*

- radiotherapy can be helpful to reduce bleeding
- haemostatic dressings e.g. *Kaltostat*
- oral tranexamic acid
- topical tranexamic acid[295]
- adrenaline (epinephrine) - 10mL 1 in 10,000 soaked on gauze is useful to control bleeding especially when dressings are being changed
- topical sucralfate has been used for fungating rectal tumour[1228]

PRESCRIBING STATUS

✲ Tranexamic acid oral or topical ®
✲ Adrenaline (epinephrine) topical ®
✲ Strong opioids (morphine, diamorphine, fentanyl) topically ••
✲ Benzydamine cream topical ••

SEE ALSO

⇨ *Topical opioids (p.83), Bleeding & haemorrhage (p.147)*
📖 Reviews[1229]

Drugs used in Wound Care

METRONIDAZOLE
Gel 0.75%, 0.8%
Apply PRN topical
ADRENALINE (EPINEPHRINE)
1 in 10,000 (dilute) 0.1mg/mL 10mL amp.
Apply 10mL PRN topical
LIDOCAINE AND CHLORHEXIDINE GEL
Gel (lidocaine 2% + chlorhexidine 0.25%) 6mL, 11mL
Other preparations of lidocaine and viscous lidocaine can be made to order.
BENZYDAMINE *(DIFFLAM)*
Cream 3%, 100g °
Apply PRN topical

Additional Information
Phenytoin & Wound healing

Phenytoin has been used topically••• mixed with sterile KY jelly to aid wound healing; the well-recognised side-effect of hyperplasia may promote tissue regeneration and healing once debridement has occurred and healthy tissue is present. It has been mixed with morphine for pain control.[370]

Lymphoedema

Lymphoedema is best managed by physical means: skin care, compression bandaging, compression garments, and massage techniques such as manual lymphatic drainage (MLD).

Diuretics

Diuretics *(p.154)* are not effective in pure lymphoedema, but may be helpful if there is associated non-lymphatic oedema:

- heart failure
- severe anaemia (hypoproteinaemia) → transfusion
- hypoalbuminaemia
- corticosteroid- or NSAID-induced fluid retention
- tamoxifen - may occur up to 6 weeks after starting[1230]
- venous obstruction

Venous obstruction

Mixed venous and lymphatic obstruction is quite commonly seen; venous thrombosis should be considered, especially if development has been rapid. If an element of venous obstruction is present:

- fingers or toes may be swollen, and skin creases less marked
- lymphorrhoea is more likely
- superficial venous distension may be present, especially on standing
- ulceration more common
- trunk oedema more likely

Acute inflammatory episodes / Cellulitis

Episodes of cellulitis are common in lymphoedema. It may be difficult to isolate the responsible pathogen, but antibiotic treatment should be started early to prevent further damage to the limb. Streptococci are probably the most common pathogens, but staphylococci should always be considered.

- Penicillin V 500mg q.d.s. PO for 2 weeks if skin intact, or flucloxacillin 500mg q.d.s. PO if skin broken
  (clarithromycin 500mg b.d. PO if mild penicillin allergy e.g. rash)
  – change to co-amoxiclav 625mg t.d.s. PO if not resolving
    (cefalexin 500mg q.d.s. PO if mild penicillin allergy)
- If systemic upset e.g. fever, flucloxacillin 2g q.d.s. IV for 1 week
  (cefuroxime 1.5g t.d.s. IV if mild penicillin allergy)
  – cefuroxime 1.5g t.d.s. + metronidazole 500mg t.d.s. IV if not resolving
  – then change to oral antibiotics for a second week

ThinkList

- Corticosteroids •• may occasionally reduce lymphoedema (or venous obstruction) by reducing peri-tumour oedema; fluid retention and skin thinning may however exacerbate the problem longer term; if recent onset of lymphoedema, consider trial of dexamethasone 4-8mg o.d. for 5 days, and stop if there is not a clear-cut, significant improvement.
- Anecdotal reports of gauze soaked in Epsom salts and wrapped around the legs for approximately 30 minutes (the concentrated salt is thought to draw out excess fluid); also used for associated scrotal oedema; applications are usually done 3-4 times a day, depending on the patient's tolerance and outcome.[370]

SEE ALSO
⇨ *Antibiotics (p.117)*
📖 Reviews[1231,1232] - Lymphorrhoea[1233] & Guidelines[1077]

Additional Information

Benzopyrones (coumarin, warfarin, oxerutins) have been suggested in lymphoedema,[1234] but recent evidence suggests they are ineffective.[1232,1235]

Emollients & Barrier skin preparations

Emollients

Emollients are used to soothe and hydrate the skin. Greasy preparations (ointments versus creams) are probably more effective, but less acceptable to patients; patient preference is important in determining the best choice.

Suitable preparations include:
AQUEOUS CREAM
WHITE SOFT PARAFFIN/LIQUID PARAFFIN (WSP/LP) 50/50
EMULSIFYING OINTMENT
OILATUM SHOWER EMOLLIENT
WHITE SOFT PARAFFIN
DIPROBASE CREAM
DIPROBASE OINTMENT
UNGUENTUM M

Emollient bath additives / Soap substitutes

OILATUM EMOLLIENT BATH ADDITIVE
BALNEUM BATH OIL
BALNEUM PLUS BATH OIL
ALPHA KERI BATH OIL

Barrier preparations

Barrier preparations protect the skin around stomas, fistulae, and pressure sores.

ZINC AND CASTOR OIL OINTMENT
CONOTRANE CREAM
SUDOCREM
METANIUM OINTMENT
CAVILON

Cavilon[175] is available as a spray or stick applicator, drying to leave a protective membrane over the skin - applied once every few days.

Topical corticosteroids

Mild
HYDROCORTISONE
Cream 1%, 2.5%; Ointment 1%, 2.5%

Moderately potent
EUMOVATE
Cream or Ointment (clobetasone butyrate 0.05%)

Potent
BETNOVATE
Cream or Ointment (betamethasone valerate 0.1%)
SYNALAR
Cream, Ointment or Gel (fluocinolone acetonide 0.025%)
LOCOID
Cream, Ointment or Lipocream (hydrocortisone butyrate 0.1%)

Topical antibiotic - antifungal - corticosteroid preparations

Mild
VIOFORM-HYDROCORTISONE
Cream or Ointment (hydrocortisone + clioquinol)
CANASTEN HC
Cream (hydrocortisone + clotrimazole)
DAKTACORT
Cream or Ointment (hydrocortisone + miconazole)
TIMODINE
Cream (hydrocortisone + nystatin + benzalkonium chloride)

Moderately potent
TRIMOVATE
Cream (clobetasone + oxytetracycline + nystatin)

Potent
LOCOID C
Cream or ointment (hydrocortisone butyrate + chlorquinaldol)

Steroid potency	Antibiotic	Antifungal	Antibiotic & antifungal
Mild	VioformHC	Canasten HC Daktacort	Timodine
Moderate			Trimovate
Potent	Locoid C		

MISCELLANEOUS SYMPTOMS

Sweats & Hot Flushes

Excessive sweating (hyperhydrosis or diaphoresis) may be caused by:
- infection
- hormonal treatment for cancer including tamoxifen and LHRH analogues
    e.g. goserilin *(Zoladex)*, or iatrogenic menopause by RT or chemotherapy
- neoplastic fever
    - Hodgkin's lymphoma
    - renal cell carcinoma
    - any solid tumours, but most commonly with liver metastases[1236]
- opioid analgesics (relatively uncommon side-effect)
- hypoxia
- pain
- anxiety
- thyrotoxicosis
- hypoglycaemia

Hormonal, menopausal-like, sweats are usually associated with hot flushes
('hot flashes' in the USA), but either symptom may occur alone.
Patients with cancer-related sweats ('neoplastic fever') may not have
measurable pyrexia, even though small febrile pulses may precede the
sweats.[1237]

Treatment of hormonally-induced hot flushes ± sweats
(Hormonally-induced vasomotor symptoms in men or women)
1) Hormone replacement therapy for women if not contraindicated *(p.130).*
2) Megestrol acetate 20mg o.d. - b.d. (i.e. low-dose);[1238] maximal effect
    takes 2 to 3 weeks; hot flushes may become more severe for a few days
    after initiating treatment - this is only seen in women taking tamoxifen.
3) Venlafaxine SR 75mg o.d.[1239,1240]
4) Paroxetine 20mg o.d.,[1241] or sertraline 50mg o.d. increased if needed to
    100mg o.d.[1242]
5) Antimuscarinic drug (see below).

Sweating ± hot flushes - other causes
1) Take appropriate steps to diagnose and treat infection; consider empirical
    course of antibiotics if infection suspected.
2) Review dose of opioid and consider reducing if appropriate or try
    alternative opioid *(p.71).*
3) Exclude thyroid or hypoglycaemic causes.
4) NSAID e.g. diclofenac 50mg t.d.s.
    - change to an alternative NSAID if unsuccessful e.g. naproxen 250-
        500mg b.d.[1243-1245]
5) Antimuscarinic drug (see below)
6) Consider trial of dexamethasone 4mg o.d., or venlafaxine or paroxetine as
    above.

Antimuscarinics

Any drug with antimuscarinic effects can block sweating under parasympathetic control (not all sweating); glycopyrronium,[1246] hyoscine butylbromide 40mg/24h CSCI or hyoscine hydrobromide transdermal patch,[1247] and propantheline PO 15mg nocte or t.d.s.[1248] have all been used.
⇨ *Sialorrhoea/Drooling p.47* for discussion of options.

Propantheline PO 15mg nocte is suggested as first-line for most patients.

PRESCRIBING STATUS
☼ NSAIDs •
☼ Venlafaxine, Sertraline, Megestrol acetate, Antimuscarinic drugs ••

ThinkList

- clonidine •• for hot flushes in women on tamoxifen,[1249] or men on LHRH antagonists;[1250] oral clonidine 0.1-0.2mg/day increased in increments of 0.1-0.3mg/day every two weeks as needed gave partial response; other studies have found it ineffective[1251]
- cyproterone acetate •• 100mg t.d.s. for hot flushes following orchidectomy[1252]
- diethylstilbestrol •• 1/3mg o.d. for post-orchidectomy prostate cancer patients[1253]
- acupuncture / acupuncture studs for hot flushes[1254]
- thalidomide ‡◎ ••• 100-200mg nocte for night sweats[192,193,1255-1257]

SEE ALSO
📖 Reviews - Hot Flushes[1258] and Sweats[1259]

Drugs for Sweats

(⇨ *Sialorrhoea/Drooling p.47* for antimuscarinic drugs)
MEGESTROL ACETATE
   Tabs. (scored) 40mg, 160mg *(Megace)*
   TSD: 20mg daily (£3.56)
VENLAFAXINE
   Tabs. 37.5, 50, 75mg; Caps. SR 75, 150mg
   TSD: 37.5mg b.d. PO (£19.99) or 75mg SR o.d. PO (£19.99)
PAROXETINE ☑
   Tabs. 20mg; Liquid 20mg/10mL *(Seroxat)*
   TSD: 20mg mane PO increase by weekly increments of 10mg as necessary to max. 50mg o.d. (£16.58 at 20mg o.d.)
SERTRALINE
   Tabs. 50, 100mg *(Lustral)*
   TSD: 50mg mane PO; max. 200mg o.d. (£16.20 at 50mg o.d.)

Additional Information

Thioridazine 10-30mg/day has been used effectively.[1260,1261] Recent restrictions on its use due to risk of QT prolongation mean that it should no longer be routinely used. Mechanism of action is unknown, but thought to be due to its antimuscarinic effect.

Venlafaxine can also *cause* sweats, which have been treated with benzatropine.[1262-1265]

'Gustatory' sweating i.e. sweat on the forehead, lips and nose after eating, occurs in diabetics, and following parotid gland surgery nerve damage. It has been treated with 0.5% topical glycopyrronium.[1266-1268]

Fatigue

Management

1) Consider differential diagnoses e.g.
   - depression *(p.101)*
   - renal or hepatic failure
   - drowsiness or sedation from drugs, brain tumour, hypercalcaemia
   - recent chemotherapy or radiotherapy
   - localised muscle weakness e.g. steroid-induced proximal myopathy, spinal cord compression etc.
   - Lambert-Eaton myasthenic syndrome[1269]

2) Exclude or treat reversible causes, including:
   - anaemia (p.151)
   - hyponatraemia (p.135)
   - hypomagnesaemia (p.134)
   - hypokalaemia
   - hypothyroidism

3) Cancer-related fatigue may respond to corticosteroids or progestagens:
   - dexamethasone 4mg o.d. *(p.126)*

PRESCRIBING STATUS

✿ Corticosteroids •

✿ Progestagens (medroxyprogesterone & megestrol acetate) ••

ThinkList

- psychostimulants ••• i.e. methylphenidate, dexamfetamine *(p.103)*

SEE ALSO

📖 Reviews[880,1270-1272]

Additional Information

Amantadine ••• 200mg b.d. has been shown to have a modest beneficial effect on fatigue in multiple sclerosis,[1273-1275] although ineffective in post-polio fatigue.[1276]

SYRINGE DRIVER MEDICATION

Syringe Drivers

Continuous subcutaneous infusion using a syringe driver is a proven, reliable method of delivering medication. Once familiar with syringe drivers, they are found to be simple to use and highly acceptable to both patient and staff.

Indications
• persistent nausea and vomiting
• severe dysphagia (including carcinoma of mouth, tongue & jaw)
• unable to swallow
• patient too weak for oral drugs (reduced conscious level)
• poor alimentary absorption (rare unless intestinal obstruction)
• doubts about, or problems with compliance

The use of opioids in a syringe driver will **not** give better analgesia than the oral route, unless there is a problem with absorption or administration.

Advantages of syringe driver
• constant drug levels (no peaks or troughs)
• reloaded only once in 24h
• cost effective
• ease of use and reliability
• comfort and confidence (no repeated injections)
• mobility of patient maintained
• absorption of drugs ensured

Types of syringe driver
There are a number of syringe drivers in use. Care should be taken especially when setting the rate of administration if an unfamiliar driver is being used.
Two of the most commonly used syringe drivers are the Graseby MS16 (blue) and the MS26 (green).
The MS16 is set at **mm / hour** whilst the MS26 is set at **mm / day**.
The MS16 is usually set at **02**mm / hr, the MS26 at **48**mm / 24hr.
At this rate, the volume contained in 48mm of the syringe (usually 9-10mL in a 10 or 12mL syringe) is that required for 24hrs.

Setting up a syringe driver

For a Graseby MS16 or MS26 pump.
1) Explain procedure to patient and relatives:
   – some people associate a syringe driver with 'the end' and may need reassurance
2) Draw up the prescribed medication.
3) The drugs prescribed should be diluted with water or normal saline to give 48mm in length of fluid in the syringe - this can be measured against the rule on the side of the driver.
4) A 10mL or 12mL syringe is most commonly used, but if the volume of fluid exceeds 48mm in length, a 20mL or 30mL syringe can be used.

5) Approximately 0.5mL of fluid is needed to prime the tubing; when a new tubing set is used, either:
   - prime the tubing with the contents - the syringe driver will stop approximately 1 hour earlier the next day, or
   - draw up an extra 0.5mL of diluent so that once primed, the syringe contents are 48mm in length

6) Set pump to the correct rate - usually 02mm/hr for the MS16, 48mm/24h for the MS26.

7) Insert a paediatric 'butterfly' needle with 1 metre tubing attached at an angle of 45 degrees to the skin:
   - a common site for the needle is an intercostal space
   - outer upper arm, upper thigh or abdomen are alternative sites
   - avoid oedematous areas

8) Place a square of gauze under the wings of the butterfly to maintain the 45 degree angle.

9) Make a loop of the tubing, and secure with a semi-permeable dressing.

10) Insert the battery.

11) Attach syringe to pump, making sure that the syringe plunger is in contact with the barrel of the syringe.

12) Press the start / check button and ensure that light starts flashing.

13) Consider giving a loading dose of analgesic or antiemetic, as the medication from a syringe driver will take several hours to reach stable levels:
    - for a loading dose of opioid, give an equivalent 4-hourly dose (i.e. 1/6th the 24-hour dose in the syringe driver)

Equipment required for domiciliary syringe driver

- syringe driver & holster
- 2 batteries
- prescribed medication
- water for injection or normal saline 10ml amps.
- needle to draw up medication
- syringes 10ml or 20ml
- butterfly giving set - paediatric 25G needle with 100mm tubing
- alcohol swabs
- semi-permeable dressing - *Opsite* or *Tegaderm*
- gauze square
- sharps box
- controlled drug prescribing and record sheets

Sunlight

Drugs in solution tend to become inactivated, and this may be speeded up by ultraviolet light.[1277] Syringes should be covered with the plastic cover provided and kept out of direct sunlight, preferably in a light-proof container.

Mobile telephones

The risk of radio-frequency emissions from mobile phones causing an error in the circuitry of a syringe driver has probably been overstated. The power of RF emissions reduces proportional to the fourth power (r^4) of the distance from the phone, and a phone would probably have to be held within centimetres of the driver to risk any problem. It is worth advising patients not to carry phones in a jacket pocket close to a holster containing a syringe driver.

It is worth remembering that ambulance men' and hospital porters' radios emit much more powerful radio waves than a mobile telephone!

Commonly used drugs

Diamorphine

Indications:	Pain
	Dyspnoea or cough
Starting dose/24h:	10-20mg (if not already taking opioids)
Ampoules available:	10, 30, 100, 500mg
Notes:	If converting from oral morphine, use 1/3rd of the 24h oral morphine dose.
	(60mg/24h oral morphine ≅ diamorphine 20mg/24hr by CSCI)

Cyclizine

Indications:	Intestinal obstruction
	Nausea and vomiting of various causes
Starting dose/24h:	100-150mg (Range 50-200mg)
Ampoules available:	50mg/1mL
Notes:	Some sedation which often wears off after 2-3 days. Tendency to crystallise. Moderately irritant to skin. Use water as diluent.

Haloperidol

Indications:	Drug induced nausea
	Metabolic causes of nausea
Starting dose/24hrs:	2.5mg (Range 1-10mg)
Ampoules available:	5mg/1mL (or 20mg/2mL)
Notes:	Tendency to crystallise. Extrapyramidal side-effects and sedation may be seen in higher doses

Metoclopramide

Indications:	Impaired gastric emptying
Starting dose/24hrs:	40mg (Range 40-80mg)
Ampoules available:	10mg/2mL
Notes:	Use with care in intestinal obstruction as it may increase colic or vomiting

Midazolam

Indications:	Terminal agitation
	Myoclonic jerking
	Anticonvulsant
Starting dose/24hrs:	10-30mg (Range 30-120mg)
Ampoules available:	10mg/2mL (or 10mg/5mL)
Notes:	Short-acting benzodiazepine. Useful for anxious restlessness

Hyoscine hydrobromide

Indications:	1) 'Death rattle'
	2) Colic
	3) Reducing salivation
Starting dose/24hrs:	1) 1.2-2.4mg
	2) 0.8-1.2mg
	3) 0.2-0.8mg
Ampoules available:	0.4mg/1mL or 0.6mg/1mL
Notes:	Also has antiemetic activity. Sedative

Levomepromazine (Methotrimeprazine)

Indications:	1) Nausea and vomiting
	2) Sedation for confusion/terminal agitation
Starting dose/24hrs:	1) 12.5-25mg (Range 6.25-50mg)
	2) 100-150mg (Range 50-250mg)
Ampoules available:	25mg/1mL
Notes:	Moderately irritant to skin. Use saline as diluent. Similar to chlorpromazine but twice as sedative. Useful for confused agitation

Contraindicated
Too irritant for subcutaneous use

- diazepam
- prochlorperazine
- chlorpromazine

Mixing drugs
For compatibility on mixing these drugs in a syringe driver ⇨ *p.173.*

Mixing drugs in a syringe driver

General
Combinations of drugs mixed in Subcutaneous Infusions (CSCI)

The mixing of drugs prior to administration, unless specifically mentioned in the product licence, constitutes 'off-label' prescribing. Many patients receiving palliative care will need an analgesic, one or more antiemetic, an anxiolytic / sedative, and possibly an antimuscarinic drug. Profound weakness or vomiting often necessitates a non-oral route; the concurrent use of up to 5 syringe drivers is impractical. Therefore drugs are commonly used in combination as subcutaneous infusions via a syringe driver.

Potential problems include degradation of the drug(s) and therefore reduced efficacy, and precipitation/crystallisation. Degradation rate may be increased by other drugs which alter the pH of the mixture. Crystallisation can occur either through formation of an insoluble product of drug interaction, or because a drug alters the pH of the solution rendering a second drug insoluble. The more drugs mixed, the greater is the potential for interaction. Drugs which have a high or low pH in solution are more likely to interact with others.

Data from compatibility studies are only available for a few combinations. Turbidometers (or similar) detect crystallisation or precipitation by optical means. HPLC methods determine drug stability as e.g. the percentage of original drug present after 24h.

The possibility exists of two drugs chemically interacting to form a new - potentially toxic - compound. Neither turbidometry nor HPLC will detect this. Therefore, even 'gold-standard' studies using HPLC will not prove that a combination is 'safe'. Simple visual inspection of a mixture before and during administration will detect most problems of crystallisation/precipitation, although fine particles may not be visible to the naked eye. However, some combinations have been shown to interact without any visible change, e.g. dexamethasone, which inactivates glycopyrronium without causing precipitation.

Doctors wishing to prescribe a combination of drugs they have not previously used, should:

- Be aware of the risks (see above).
- Refer to appropriate sources of evidence:
  - local Palliative Care Centres
  - Palliative Care Formulary[1]
  - *www.pallmed.net* (database of drug mixtures for syringe drivers)
  - SIGN cancer pain guidelines[377]
  - 'The syringe driver in palliative care' (Dickman, 1998)[131]
  - Drug Information Centres & hospital pharmacists
- Have considered the use of more than one syringe driver.
- Use as few drugs in combination as possible.
- Carefully inspect the mixture before use for any signs of crystallisation/precipitation.
- Continue to inspect regularly during its use - preferably 4-hourly for the first 24h.
- Monitor the patient carefully, especially for evidence of reduced efficacy of any of the drugs.

Diluent

Water for injection should be considered the standard diluent for drug mixtures for use in a syringe driver.

Saline is recommended as the diluent for levomepromazine used alone, to make the solution isotonic and reduce site inflammation.[1278] Many centres use saline for all drug combinations containing levomepromazine, but there is no evidence to support this.

Saline has also been recommended for granisetron, ketamine, ketorolac, octreotide and ondansetron,[1] but water may be better when these drugs are used in combination with others.

Cyclizine tends to precipitate if saline is used as diluent,[131] so water is recommended for any mixture containing cyclizine.

Commonly used drugs

- diamorphine
- haloperidol
- metoclopramide
- cyclizine
- levomepromazine
- hyoscine hydrobromide (HBr)
- midazolam

Chemically stable and compatible

The following drug mixes have been shown to be physically compatible and chemically stable, although there are limits on the maximum concentrations of each drug, especially diamorphine and cyclizine.[1]

Cyclizine, Diamorphine[1279-1282]
Diamorphine, Haloperidol[1279-1282]
Diamorphine, Hyoscine HBr[1279,1280]
Diamorphine, Levomepromazine[1280]
Diamorphine, Metoclopramide[1279,1280]
Diamorphine, Midazolam[1283]
Cyclizine, Diamorphine, Haloperidol[1282]

Incompatibility

There are no consistent incompatibilities between any of these 7 drugs, even in combinations of up to five drugs; however cyclizine and metoclopramide have occasionally caused precipitation (this is not a combination of antiemetics usually recommended).

Compatible (visually) - common drugs

The following drug mixes have been used successfully in palliative care units, and are visually compatible.

Cyclizine, Diamorphine, Haloperidol, Hyoscine HBr (water)[1284]
Cyclizine, Diamorphine, Haloperidol, Midazolam (water)[1284]
Cyclizine, Diamorphine, Hyoscine HBr (water)[1284]
Cyclizine, Diamorphine, Hyoscine HBr, Midazolam (diluent not stated)[1285]
Cyclizine, Diamorphine, Midazolam (water)[1284,1285]
Diamorphine, Haloperidol, Hyoscine HBr (water)[1284]
Diamorphine, Haloperidol, Hyoscine HBr, Levomepromazine (saline)[1284]
Diamorphine, Haloperidol, Hyoscine HBr, Midazolam (water)[1284,1285]
Diamorphine, Haloperidol, Levomepromazine (saline)[1284]
Diamorphine, Haloperidol, Levomepromazine, Midazolam (water)[1284]
Diamorphine, Haloperidol, Midazolam (water)[1284-1286]
Diamorphine, Hyoscine HBr, Levomepromazine (saline or water)[1284,1287]
Diamorphine, Hyoscine HBr, Levomepromazine, Midazolam (saline)[1284]

Diamorphine, Hyoscine HBr, Metoclopramide, Midazolam (water)[1284]
Diamorphine, Hyoscine HBr, Midazolam (water)[1284,1285]
Diamorphine, Levomepromazine, Metoclopramide (saline)[1284]
Diamorphine, Levomepromazine, Metoclopramide, Midazolam (saline or water)[1284]
Diamorphine, Levomepromazine, Midazolam (saline or water)[1284]
Diamorphine, Metoclopramide, Midazolam (water)[1284,1285]

Less commonly used drugs

The following drugs, amongst others, have also been used in palliative care units by CSCI. Refer to the Palliative care formulary,[1] 'The syringe driver in palliative care' (Dickman, 1998),[131] or on-line database[1284] for further details.

Drug	Notes
Alfentanil	Compatible with commonly used drugs (except cyclizine in certain mixes)
Clonazepam	Compatible with commonly used drugs and glycopyrronium
Dexamethasone	Inactivates glycopyrronium although no precipitation seen. Precipitation seen quite commonly, but unpredictably. If used, dilute dexamethasone before adding other drugs
Fentanyl	Compatible with commonly used drugs (except cyclizine in certain mixes), and also: ketamine, ketorolac, octreotide, ondansetron and glycopyrronium.
Glycopyrronium	Compatible with commonly used drugs, ketamine and octreotide. Inactivated by dexamethasone although no precipitation seen
Hyoscine butylbromide	Compatible with commonly used drugs (except cyclizine in certain mixes); also compatible with octreotide and fentanyl
Ketorolac	Compatible with diamorphine and fentanyl; incompatible with cyclizine, haloperidol, and levomepromazine; mixed reports with midazolam.
Ketamine	Compatible with commonly used drugs; also compatible with fentanyl, lidocaine, glycopyrronium, ondansetron, hyoscine butylbromide and ketorolac
Octreotide	Incompatible with cyclizine or dexamethasone. Compatible with commonly used drugs except cyclizine; also compatible with hyoscine butylbromide, fentanyl, glycopyrronium and ondansetron
Ondansetron	Compatible with diamorphine, hyoscine hydrobromide, metoclopramide, midazolam; also compatible with fentanyl, alfentanil, glycopyrronium, octreotide, and dexamethasone
Phenobarbital	Compatible with diamorphine and fentanyl otherwise incompatible.

Chemically stable and compatible - less common drugs

The following drug mixes have been shown to be physically compatible and chemically stable.
Diamorphine, Hyoscine butylbromide[1279]
Diamorphine, Ketorolac[561]
Diamorphine, Octreotide[1288]

Incompatible mixes
Cyclizine, Hyoscine butylbromide[1284]
Cyclizine, Ketorolac[1]
Cyclizine, Octreotide[92]
Dexamethasone, Octreotide[92]
Dexamethasone, Glycopyrronium[131]
Haloperidol, Ketorolac[1289]

Compatible (visually) - less common drugs
The following drug mixes have been used successfully in palliative care units, and are visually compatible.

Cyclizine, Diamorphine, Glycopyrronium, Haloperidol, Midazolam (water)[1284]
Cyclizine, Diamorphine, Glycopyrronium, Midazolam (water)[1284]
Cyclizine, Diamorphine, Haloperidol, Octreotide (water)[1284]
Dexamethasone, Diamorphine (diluent not stated)[1290]
Dexamethasone, Diamorphine, Ketamine, Metoclopramide (water)[1284]
Diamorphine, Fentanyl, Levomepromazine, Metoclopramide (saline)[1284]
Diamorphine, Glycopyrronium (water)[1284]
Diamorphine, Glycopyrronium, Haloperidol (water)[1284]
Diamorphine, Glycopyrronium, Haloperidol, Ketamine, Midazolam (water)[1284]
Diamorphine, Glycopyrronium, Haloperidol, Levomepromazine, Midazolam (saline)[1284]
Diamorphine, Glycopyrronium, Haloperidol, Midazolam (water)[1284]
Diamorphine, Glycopyrronium, Ketamine, Midazolam (water)[1284]
Diamorphine, Glycopyrronium, Levomepromazine (saline)[1284]
Diamorphine, Glycopyrronium, Levomepromazine, Metoclopramide (saline)[1284]
Diamorphine, Glycopyrronium, Levomepromazine, Metoclopramide, Midazolam (saline)[1284]
Diamorphine, Glycopyrronium, Levomepromazine, Midazolam (saline or water)[1284]
Diamorphine, Glycopyrronium, Metoclopramide, Midazolam (water)[1284]
Diamorphine, Glycopyrronium, Midazolam (water)[1284]
Diamorphine, Haloperidol, Hyoscine butylbromide, Midazolam (water)[1284]
Diamorphine, Haloperidol, Hyoscine butylbromide, Octreotide (water)[1284]
Diamorphine, Haloperidol, Ketamine, Midazolam (water)[1284]
Diamorphine, Haloperidol, Octreotide (diluent not stated)[1291]
Diamorphine, Hyoscine butylbromide, Levomepromazine (water)[1284]
Diamorphine, Hyoscine butylbromide, Levomepromazine, Midazolam (water)[1284]
Diamorphine, Hyoscine butylbromide, Levomepromazine, Octreotide (saline)[1284]
Diamorphine, Hyoscine butylbromide, Midazolam (water)[1284]
Diamorphine, Hyoscine butylbromide, Octreotide (water)[1284]
Diamorphine, Hyoscine HBr, Levomepromazine, Octreotide (saline)[1284]
Diamorphine, Hyoscine HBr, Midazolam, Octreotide (water)[1284]
Diamorphine, Hyoscine HBr, Midazolam, Ondansetron (water)[1284]
Diamorphine, Ketamine, Levomepromazine (saline)[1284]
Diamorphine, Ketamine, Levomepromazine, Midazolam (water)[1284]
Diamorphine, Ketamine, Metoclopramide, Midazolam (water)[1284]
Diamorphine, Ketamine, Midazolam (water)[1284]
Diamorphine, Ketorolac, Midazolam (water)[1284]
Diamorphine, Levomepromazine, Midazolam, Octreotide (saline or water)[1284]
Diamorphine, Levomepromazine, Octreotide (saline or water)[1284]
Diamorphine, Metoclopramide, Midazolam, Octreotide (water)[1284]
Diamorphine, Metoclopramide, Octreotide (water)[1284]
Diamorphine, Midazolam, Octreotide (water)[1284,1291]
Diamorphine, Ondansetron (water)[1284]
Diamorphine, Phenobarbital (water)[1284]

Problems with Syringe Drivers

Syringe driver checks

Syringe drivers should be checked four-hourly on an in-patient unit, and daily in the community.

- syringe driver
  - light is flashing
  - correct volume of fluid remaining
  - correct rate set
  - no leakage
- injection site
  - pain
  - swelling
  - erythema
- mixture
  - crystallisation/precipitation

Syringe driver errors

There have been occasional reports of syringe drivers discharging their load over too short a period of time, and overdosing the patient. One cause of this has been found to be water ingression into the pump causing an electrical short in the timing mechanism. Care should be taken not to spill fluid on the pumps, or allow them in the bath.

Irritation at injection site

Most commonly due to cyclizine or levomepromazine (methotrimeprazine). A nickel allergy is not uncommon; patient may have a history of being unable to wear certain types of jewellery.

Sites should last on average about 3 days.[1292]

Absorption of drugs may be impaired, causing poor symptom control.

- Ensure needle tip is not too shallow.
- Try plastic cannula[1293,1294] (⇨ *Special equipment p.236*).
- Try a different diluent (saline or water) unless specifically recommended.
- Dilute drugs to a larger volume using a 20mL syringe.
- Change irritant drugs to an alternative (e.g. cyclizine → haloperidol).
- Give irritant drugs by alternative route (e.g. rectal).
- Add dexamethasone 1mg or hydrocortisone 25mg[1295] to syringe driver.

Precipitation

Precipitation when mixing drugs is a sign of incompatibility and means alternative drugs or means of administering the drugs must be found. Occasionally a mixture that has been used successfully, will suddenly precipitate in the middle of an infusion. It appears to start from the cannula and crystallise up the tubing. It may be related to a reaction occurring in the subcutaneous tissue, and once it has happened, it tends to recur in the same patient. Cyclizine is most frequently the problem.

- change the site and the whole giving set - not just the syringe
- consider different diluent (do not use saline for cyclizine)
- consider alternative antiemetic/drugs
- dilute drugs to a larger volume using a 20mL syringe
- keep away from direct sunlight or heat
- separate the drugs being given into two syringe drivers

PRESCRIBING STATUS
☼ Corticosteroids •

Think List

• GTN patch •• placed over site may aid drug absorption (only evidence is from prolonging life of IV infusions[1142-1146])

Drugs used for syringe drivers

HYDROCORTISONE
  Inj. 100mg/2mL
    TSD: 25mg/24h CSCI
GLYCERYL TRINITRATE (GTN)
  Patch 5mg/24h
    TSD: Apply patch daily over infusion site (approx £12/28 days)

Subcutaneous route

It is common practice in palliative care to administer injections to patients by subcutaneous rather than intramuscular route, whenever appropriate; this is in order to minimise discomfort. The product licence for many drugs does not specifically cover SC administration.

Doctors wishing to prescribe an injection by SC route that they have not previously used, should:

• Be aware that:
  – absorption may be slower than by IM route
  – bioavailability (and therefore efficacy) may be less than by IM route
  – irritant drugs may cause a greater inflammatory reaction SC than IM
• Ensure that the volume is not too great (2ml absolute maximum, preferably 1ml maximum).
• Refer to appropriate sources of evidence:
  – Palliative Care Formulary[1]
  – Local Palliative Care Centres
  – Drug Information Centres
• Do not use if the patient is 'shocked' or hypovolaemic because peripheral vasoconstriction may severely limit absorption.

Drugs not to be given by SC route

• antibiotics
• most NSAIDs (ketorolac appears to be well tolerated)
• diazepam (any preparation)
• chlorpromazine

Drugs licensed for SC injection

• diamorphine
• hyoscine hydrobromide
• octreotide
• levomepromazine (methotrimeprazine)

Drugs frequently given by sc route in palliative care

Drug - Licensed for	CSCI	SC inj.	IM inj.	IV inj.
Alfentanil	✗	✗	✗	✓
Clonazepam	✗	✗	✗	✓
Cyclizine	✗	✗	✓	✓
Dexamethasone	✗	✗	✓	✓
Diamorphine	✓	✓	✓	✓
Fentanyl	✗	✗	✓	✓
Furosemide	✗	✗	✓	✓
Glycopyrronium	✗	✗	✓	✓
Granisetron	✗	✗	✗	✓
Haloperidol	✗	✗	✓	✓
Hyoscine butylbromide	✗	✗	✓	✓
Hyoscine HBr (hydrobromide)	✗	✓	✓	✗
Ketamine	✗	✗	✓	✓
Ketorolac	✗	✗	✓	✓
Levomepromazine (methotrimeprazine)	✓	✓	✓	✓
Lorazepam	✗	✗	✓	✓
Metoclopramide	✗	✗	✓	✓
Midazolam	✗	✗	✓	✓
Octreotide	✗	✓	✗	✓
Ondansetron	✗	✗	✓	✓

COMPLEMENTARY & ALTERNATIVE MEDICINES

Cannabis & derivatives

Cannabis and derivatives (cannabinoids) such as nabilone and dronabinol (delta-9-tetrahydrocannabinol) have been used for:
- anorexia *(p.35)*
- nausea & vomiting *(p.19)*
- dyspnoea
- muscle spasm and pain in multiple sclerosis

SEE ALSO

📖 Reviews[60,476,477]

Further information on the Internet at:

http://www.druginfo.nsw.gov.au/druginfo/reports/medical_cannabis.html
http://www.kenes.com/eapcresearch/abstracts/172.htm

Cannabinoid drug preparations

Nabilone is the only (synthetic) cannabinoid licensed in the UK, for chemotherapy-induced nausea and vomiting. Dronabinol is the main psychoactive constituent of cannabis which has been used in the U.S.

NABILONE ⊖

 Caps. 250µg[†] 1mg
  TSD: 1mg b.d. **PO** (£320.32)
  250µg available on named-patient basis - Cambridge labs. 0191 296 9369

EPA - Eicosapentaenoic acid

EPA (eicosapentaenoic acid) is an omega-3 fatty acid from fish oil. Experimental work and initial trials offer promise for successful management of cancer-related cachexia. Ongoing trials are using much higher doses than are commercially available i.e. 4-8g/day. Side effects include diarrhoea and sardine-smelling burping.[1296,1297]

Alternative cancer treatments

Essiac

Essiac is a herbal mixture; the four main constituents are burdock root, Indian rhubarb, sheep sorrel, and slippery elm. It is taken orally. No adverse effects have been reported in association with its medicinal use, although allergic dermatitis and a laxative effect may be caused by the constituent herbs.

📖 Reviews[1298,1299]

The full text of the CMAJ review is available at:

http://www.cma.ca/cmaj/series/therapy.htm

Green tea

Green tea is made from unfermented, steamed or pan-fried tea leaves. It is taken orally as a cup of tea. No adverse effects have been reported in association with its medicinal use. It does contain a significant amount of caffeine (as does ordinary black tea), which can cause restlessness, insomnia or ventricular ectopics.

📖 Reviews[1298,1300]

The full text of the CMAJ review is available at:
http://www.cma.ca/cmaj/series/therapy.htm

Mistletoe (Iscador)

Iscador is prepared by fermenting the mistletoe plant with the bacterium Lactobacillus plantarum. The preparation is filtered and prepared in ampoules for injection. Local inflammation at the injection site is common, together with fever, headache and chills. No other toxic effects have been identified. However, ingestion of the plant or injection of some constituents can cause seizures or bradycardia.

📖 Reviews[1298,1301]

The full text of the CMAJ review is available at:
http://www.cma.ca/cmaj/series/therapy.htm

Vitamins A, C and E

Supplementary vitamins A, C and E are claimed to potentiate the immune system. Vitamin A can cause headache, irritability, pruritus and perioral dermatitis; megadoses can cause liver damage. High doses of vitamin C can cause gastritis, heartburn, nausea & vomiting, headaches and rash, but is usually well tolerated. Vitamin E has little associated toxicity.

📖 Reviews[1298,1302]

The full text of the CMAJ review is available at:
http://www.cma.ca/cmaj/series/therapy.htm

714-X

714-X is a camphor compound, chemically combined with nitrogen, ammonium salts, sodium chloride and ethanol. It is claimed to decrease tumour size and increase appetite and well-being. It is based on a bizarre (nutty) theory whereby this chemical inhibits the 'somatidian macrocycle'. It is prepared as a sterile solution and administered by injecting it into the groin, or nasally.

It appears to cause few side effects, although local erythema and tenderness at the injection site are common.

📖 Reviews[1298,1302]

The full text of the CMAJ review is available at:
http://www.cma.ca/cmaj/series/therapy.htm

Shark cartilage

Shark cartilage extract is said to inhibit angiogenesis and thus tumour growth. It is classified as a food supplement by the American FDA, and there is no convincing evidence of benefit in clinical trials.[1303]

Further information can be found at:
http://www.realife.com/cancer.html
http://cancer.med.upenn.edu/support/tips/tip22.html

Hydrazine sulphate

Hydrazine sulphate is an industrial chemical used in the manufacture of rocket-fuel, insecticides and rust-prevention treatments. Hydrazine sulphate interferes with gluconeogenesis in vitro. Claims that it inhibits tumour growth are unproven, however there is some evidence that it may affect cancer-induced anorexia and cachexia, and there is a reasonable body of published literature in the journals.[1304-1310]

The US Cancer Institute has declared that it should not be recommended as a routine treatment, as there is no convincing evidence of its effectiveness. Its case continues to be championed by Dr Joseph Gold at the Syracuse Cancer Institute USA, claiming that the negative results of studies were because other medicines were taken concurrently by patients in these studies which counteracted the effects of the hydrazine; these included all tranquillisers, alcohol, phenothiazine antiemetics, and antidepressants.

The drug is unlicensed and unavailable in the UK, but supplies may be sent from the Syracuse Institute at the patient's request, following contact by the patient's doctor.

Nausea, pruritus, drowsiness, excitation or peripheral neuropathies may develop in up to 10% of patients. It is also an MAOI inhibitor, so precautions need to be taken against interactions with certain foods and other medication. There is no specific advice relating to hydrazine, but usual advice is to avoid specified foods or medicines for up to 2 weeks after stopping MAOIs.

Dose recommended by Syracuse Institute: (for 9 stone patient) 60mg capsule x 1 daily for 3 days; 1 capsule b.d. for 3 days; 1 capsule t.d.s. for 6 weeks

Interactions with food and medicines

The Syracuse Institute recommend: No tranquillisers, barbiturates, alcohol or anti-depressants. No cured food including bacon, burgers, and marmite. Only cottage cheese, no other cheeses.

MAOI card from Pharmaceutical Society and BMA advises: no cheese, pickled herring, or broad beans; no Bovril, Oxo, Marmite, or other meat or yeast extract; avoid Chianti wine completely; alcohol in moderation.

SEE ALSO
⇨ *Drug interactions:* MAOIs *(p.211)*
Other interactions are mentioned in the BNF.

Additional Information

Further information can be obtained from The Syracuse Cancer Research Institute, New York, USA. Internet site: *http://scri.ngen.com/*
📖 Independent reviews[1298,1311]
The full text of the CMAJ review is available at:
http://www.cma.ca/cmaj/series/therapy.htm

EMERGENCIES IN PALLIATIVE CARE

Spinal Cord Compression

Compression of the spinal cord or cauda equina by epidural disease (blood borne metastasis or extension from a vertebral metastasis) or by vertebral collapse, can lead eventually to paraplegia or quadriplegia.

- 70% thoracic spine
- 10% cervical spine
- 20% lumbar spine

Presenting signs & symptoms
- 75% have weakness - of legs (+ arms/hands if cervical)
- 90% have pain
    - tenderness over affected vertebra
    - may be radicular pain only
- 50% have sensory level on examination
- 40% have sphincter dysfunction - a late sign, except with cauda equina compression

Management
Although the overall outcome from treatment is not good, the potential difference that successful treatment can make to a patient's quality of life is enormous. **Treatment outcome is better, the earlier it is started.**[1312-1314] Corticosteroids alone may be appropriate for some patients with very advanced cancer, especially if their mobility or performance status was already poor. Nevertheless, **making an urgent appropriate management decision is the emergency.**

Discuss immediately with senior colleague or oncologist about further management, or follow local protocol for emergency management:

1) Urgent investigation is usually appropriate if further treatment considered:
    - MRI is the investigation of choice
2) An urgent multidisciplinary management decision is ideally needed to decide appropriate treatment option:
    - radiotherapy (occasionally chemotherapy)
    - surgical decompression
3) If this is impractical, contact the oncologist as radiotherapy is the most commonly used treatment.
4) Dexamethasone 8mg b.d. should be started immediately:
    - give first dose stat. on suspicion whilst waiting for referral arrangements
    - give by injection SC or IV if patient vomiting
    - give intravenously if symptoms have developed rapidly in last 48h
5) Treat pain and other symptoms, whilst awaiting further treatment.

PRESCRIBING STATUS
☼ Corticosteroids ®

SEE ALSO
⇨ *Corticosteroids (p.126)*
📖 Reviews[1315-1318] & Guidelines[510,1319]

Additional Information

Very high doses of steroids have been recommended[1319] (up to 96mg dexamethasone), but there is no evidence of their additional benefit, and evidence of increased adverse effects.[1320,1321]

Massive Terminal Haemorrhage

Definition (as used here): major arterial haemorrhage from a patient in whom active treatment is not appropriate or possible, and which **will inevitably cause death in minutes.** Loss of more than 1.5 litres (two pints) in 30 seconds. Usually associated with tumour erosion of aorta or pulmonary artery (causing haematemesis or haemoptysis), carotid or femoral artery (external bleeding). If the haemorrhage is so massive then the only appropriate management may be to stay with the patient attempting to comfort any distress.

Massive haemorrhage is often heralded by smaller bleeds. If a major haemorrhage is anticipated, an IV cannula should be inserted. Green or blue towels should be available to help control the spread of blood, and appropriate drugs (drawn up in syringe) may be kept available by the bedside.

Management of massive haemorrhage

By definition, this will be a terminal event. The aim of treatment is to sedate as quickly as possible to relieve patient distress. Speed (of access to the drug, and administration) is paramount. Give drugs by IV route if at all possible; if not, give by deep IM injection.

The drug doses given below deliberately err on the large side to ensure rapid onset, and predictable effect. If haemorrhage is brisk, but not inevitably and rapidly fatal, use lower doses appropriate for managing distress i.e. midazolam 5-10mg IM.

Midazolam

- Some patients on regular benzodiazepines are very tolerant to their sedative effects.
- Midazolam 10mg will sedate most patients, but occasional patients (often heavy alcohol drinkers) may have little effect from several times this dose.
- If the IV route is not accessible, the large volumes needed may not be practical.
- Midazolam 50mg/10mL[‡] ampoule is available as a special order.

Opioid analgesics

- Haemorrhage is not painful and the analgesic effect is not needed.
- Strong opioids are usually locked in 'controlled drug' cupboards, leading to a delay in administering them.
- Diamorphine needs to be dissolved, leading to delay.
- A variable dose may be needed: patients on regular opioids for pain will need an appropriate dose e.g. diamorphine 10mg if opioid naïve, or twice the 4-hourly equivalent dose e.g. 60mg if on diamorphine 180mg/24h CSCI.

Ketamine

- The effect of a standard dose of ketamine is more predictable than opioids or benzodiazepines.
- As a guide, the anaesthetic dose is approx 150mg IV or 500mg IM.

If a specific plan has not been made for an individual patient, the following can be used for rapid terminal sedation:

1) Ketamine 250mg by IV injection, or
2) Midazolam 30-50mg IV, or
3) Ketamine 500mg IM (2.5mL in each of two IM sites), or
4) Midazolam 20-30mg IM (2-2.5mL in each of two IM sites)

PRESCRIBING STATUS

☼ Ketamine ●● - *Palliative care units only where policy approved*

SEE ALSO

⇨ *Bleeding & haemorrhage (p.147)*

Drugs for massive haemorrhage

KETAMINE
   Inj. 500mg/10mL, 1000mg/10mL
MIDAZOLAM
   Inj. 10mg/2mL, 50mg/10mL‡
   50mg/10ml available as special order

REFERENCE

PRACTICE NOTES

Referral Criteria

Palliative Care is defined as:
"The active total care of patients whose disease is not responsive to curative treatment, where the control of pain, of other symptoms and of psychological, social and spiritual problems is paramount, and where the goal is the best quality of life for the patient and their family."

Who to refer
Referral to a Palliative Care Team is appropriate for any patients with an incurable, progressive, and fatal illness (usually, but not always, cancer). It is particularly recommended for:
- young patients, or patients with young children in the family
- patients with rapidly progressive disease
- patients with disease presenting unexpected, difficult to control, or rapidly progressing symptoms
- distressing symptoms, when no relief has been achieved within 48h
- psycho-social distress in patient or family relating to the diagnosis or in facing death
- where reassurance of a second opinion is sought - by patient, family or other health care professional

Diagnosis
Most patients referred to a palliative care team have cancer that is beyond the stage of being curable. Many will still be receiving treatment from an oncologist or surgeon, but this treatment will be palliative in intention, and referral to a palliative care team need not wait until the oncologist or surgeon has finished their treatment.
Patients with other progressive, incurable diseases (such as motor neuron disease, Parkinson's, multiple sclerosis, and end-stage respiratory or cardiac disease) may benefit from referral if control of symptoms is difficult, or there is distress relating to the terminal nature of their illness.

Early referral
Early referral is helpful where problems are anticipated:
- symptoms that have been difficult to control, even if now controlled
- numerous symptoms
- complex problems (social, psychological, and physical)
- strong psychological reaction to the diagnosis
- young patients, or patients with young children in the family

How to refer
Referral letters with background information on the patient and illness, together with a reason for referral, are very helpful. To avoid delay, consider faxing a referral letter, or telephoning. Telephone referral may be beneficial, allowing initial advice to be given before the patient is seen, and to discuss the urgency of the referral or issues that are difficult to write in a letter.

Who to refer to

Most palliative care teams work as a multi-professional team of doctors, nurses and allied professionals. A patient referred to any member of the team, will be assessed and seen by other members of the team if appropriate. However, direct referral to a specific team member may avoid delay.

Refer to doctors patients with:

* symptoms difficult to control
* anxiety or depressive symptoms
* complex symptom problems (with psycho-social elements)
* unexpected symptoms or disease progression (e.g. unexplained confusion)

Refer to nurses patients or families for:

* on-going emotional support for patient and family
* monitoring of symptom control and guidance for patients (e.g. patient starting on morphine)

Physiotherapists, occupational therapists, and social workers may also take direct referrals.

Breaking Bad News

These are short guidance notes developed for a junior doctors' handbook.

Find the time and as private a place as possible (Can you leave your bleep?)

Try to see the patient with a relative or with a nurse who can go over information later.

Try to find out what the patient knows e.g. "What have you been told about your illness?"

Try to find out how much they want to know: e.g. "Are you the sort of person who likes to know everything about your illness or just some of the details?"

Give a warning shot that there is bad news coming e.g. "I'm afraid the test results were not very good".

Slowly and simply give the news, checking they understand and gauge their response as you go along, to know how far to go - you may need to stop half way.

Never say "there is nothing that can be done", do not lie, but offer realistic hope e.g. controlling symptoms, getting you home, treating pain etc.

Summarise at the end, give an opportunity for questions and leave patients with a definite plan for the future and check back that plan is understood.

Arrange to go back and discuss further, later or the next day as the patient will only take in about 20% of what was said.

Always tell the nurse looking after the patient of the conversation and write in notes.

Resuscitation Guidelines (DNAR's)

The issue of resuscitation guidelines is a very sensitive one, not least in palliative care.[1322-1324] Developing Unit or Trust policies need to take account of the fact that:

- most patients admitted to palliative care units have a terminal illness,
- many patients are admitted in distressing circumstances,
- for many patients, discussion of resuscitation at this time would cause unnecessary additional distress.

Notes: Terminal illness has been defined for these purposes as active, progressive, incurable disease, from which death can reasonably be expected within twelve months.[1324]

BMA and RCN joint guidelines

Recent BMA and RCN joint guidelines[1325] have been issued. They state that CPR must be initiated in the event of a cardiac or respiratory arrest in the absence of a DNAR (do not attempt resuscitation) order, or when the expressed wishes of the patient are unknown.

National Hospice Council statement[1324]

"There is evidence to suggest that, for terminally ill patients, the harms of CPR are likely to outweigh the possible benefits.

Evidence indicates that, almost invariably, CPR either fails to re-establish cardiopulmonary function, or succeeds only to result in further cardiopulmonary arrest with no intervening hospital discharge.

- CPR is inappropriate if:
    - there is virtually no chance of CPR re-establishing cardiopulmonary function; **or**
    - successful resuscitation would probably result in a quality of life unacceptable to the patient; **or**
    - it is contrary to the competent patient's expressed wishes.
- CPR may be appropriate if:
    - there is a reasonable chance of CPR re-establishing cardiopulmonary function; **and**
    - successful resuscitation would probably result in a quality of life acceptable to the patient; **and**
    - it is the competent patient's expressed wish.

There is no **ethical** obligation to discuss CPR with the majority of palliative care patients, for whom such treatment, following assessment, is judged to be futile. In the context of open and honest discussion, the raising of such issues may be redundant and potentially distressing.

If the likely outcome of CPR is uncertain, anticipatory decisions either to implement or withhold CPR should be sensitively explored with the patient. Both the likelihood of success and the resulting quality of life will be appropriate issues for discussion. Review of any such decision may be appropriate with change in the patient's clinical situation.

Should a patient be likely to benefit from CPR and would wish for it, the extent of CPR facilities and expertise available in any admitting unit ought to be discussed with the patient, ideally prior to admission. Limited availability of such facilities in specialist palliative care units need not undermine appropriateness of admission in early disease, as patients may accept such admission on the understanding that initial resuscitative measures will be instituted and transfer to a unit equipped to undertake CPR will be arranged in the event of a cardiac arrest actually occurring.

Consideration should be given to CPR policy early in the involvement of the clinical team. In the absence of an anticipatory decision or a valid advance refusal, at the time of cardiopulmonary arrest, the patient is by definition incompetent to make a decision regarding CPR and therefore it is the doctor's legal responsibility to act in the patient's best interests."

Living Wills

A 'Living Will' is also known as an Advance Directive or Advance Statement.[1326-1328]

BMA Code of Practice on Advance Statements[1329] - Summary

- Although not binding on health professionals, advance statements deserve thorough consideration and respect.
- Where valid and applicable, advance directives (refusals) must be followed.
- Health professionals consulted by people wishing to formulate an advance statement or directive should take all reasonable steps to provide accurate factual information about the treatment options and their implications.
- Where an unknown and incapacitated patient presents for treatment some checks should be made concerning the validity of any directive refusing life-prolonging treatment. In all cases, it is vital to check that the statement or refusal presented is that of the patient being treated and has not been withdrawn.
- If the situation is not identical to that described in the advance statement or refusal, treatment providers may still be guided by the general spirit of the statement if this is evident. It is advisable to contact any person nominated by the patient as well as the GP to clarify the patient's wishes. If there is doubt as to what the patient intended, the law requires the exercise of a best interests judgement.
- If an incapacitated person is known to have had sustained and informed objections to all or some treatment, even though these have not been formally recorded, health professionals may not be justified in proceeding. This applies even in an emergency.
  If witnessed and made at a time when the patient was competent and informed, such objections may constitute an oral advance directive. Health professionals will need to consider how much evidence is available about the patient's decisions and how convincing it seems. All members of the health care team can make a useful contribution to this process.
  In the absence of any indication of the patient's wishes, there is a common law duty to give appropriate treatment to incapacitated patients when the treatment is clearly in their best interests.

What to Do After Death

These are short guidance notes developed for a junior doctors' handbook.
Sit down in a quiet room with the relatives and explain to them what has happened. Allow relatives time to absorb the information and check back with them they have understood. If the death has been unexpected, they will be in a state of shock and initially will not take in anything you say. Give them time to ask questions and, if appropriate, arrange a time to see them again to answer further questions they will have. Let the family know you care.
If they wish to view the body, ensure they are accompanied by a competent member of staff. Give them time to be with the body. Some relatives may wish to hold the body, particularly if a child has died, or wish to help with laying out the body.
Hospital switchboards usually have a list of different ministers of religion who may need to be contacted
Other patients on the ward will be aware a death has occurred. The medical and nursing staff together should decide who is going to speak to the other patients and what they are going to be told. These other patients will also feel grief; the hospital chaplain may be helpful at this time.
Consider whether referral to the Coroner is necessary.

Funeral arrangements
Can all be done through the undertaker of the family's choice, who will advise them. If there is no next of kin, the social work department will arrange a funeral

Organ donation
Should be requested from suitable patients. Some relatives find it a great comfort to donate organs, others do not wish to. Their response cannot be predicted, so gentle tactful asking is required.

Doctor's administrative checklist
- Record the certification of death in medical case-notes, together with the cause of death, and stated time of death.
- Check whether organ donation has been requested.
- Check whether referral to the coroner is required. *(p. 193)*
- Write the medical 'death certificate' i.e. notification of death.
- Complete part 1 of the cremation form, if required; arrange for a second doctor to complete part 2.
- Ensure other professionals involved in the care of the patient are informed as soon as possible, including:
  - members of the primary care team - GP and district nurse
  - members of the palliative care team - community 'Macmillan' nurses etc.
  - social services and social worker
  - oncologist and other medical/surgical doctors
  - specialist nurses e.g. stoma, diabetic nurses
- Ensure arrangements are made for bereavement follow-up, depending on need, and on local resources.

Certification Of Death

These are short guidance notes developed for a junior doctors' handbook.
If you attended the patient during his/her last illness, you have a statutory
duty to issue a medical certificate of the cause of death, unless you have
reported the death to the coroner and he/she advises you that you do not
need to issue a certificate.

You must not issue a death certificate if you did not attend the deceased
during his/her last illness.

In cases of doubt the Coroner or his Officer are available for you to discuss
any matter relating to the above with them.

**NB: It is not always necessary that a Post Mortem is required in deaths that
are reported to the Coroner.**

Sometimes when patients die within 24h of admission but the diagnosis is
known and the patient known to the team, the coroner will allow you to sign
part A on the death certificate and issue it to the relatives **after** notifying and
discussing the death.

Referral To The Coroner

Cases that are notifiable to the coroner
- Cause of death is unknown.
- Deaths within 24h of admission to hospital, or person brought in dead.
- When the doctor attending the patient did not see him/her within preceding
  14 days prior to death.
- Death related to injury however remotely or, if accident cause is alleged by
  relatives or friends.
- Deaths due to industrial diseases, even if only a contributory factor,
  including asbestosis, pneumoconiosis, Farmers Lung etc.
- Patients dying in receipt of Industrial Injuries pensions or disability pensions
  if related to the cause of death.
- Death not thought to be of natural cause.
- Suspected suicide.
- Death related to suspicious or criminal action.
- Deaths within 24h of operation or administration of an anaesthetic, or any
  time subsequently, if cause of death is thought to be related to either.
- Deaths of persons in Hospital in legal custody (e.g.: under the Mental
  Health Act).
- Deaths where there is a question of self neglect or neglect by others.
- Deaths from hypothermia.
- Deaths from food poisoning.
- Deaths related to alcoholism acute or chronic.
- Deaths related to abuse of drugs or to drug addiction.
- Deaths related to medical mishap or where the relatives have criticised
  Hospital medical or nursing Management, if related to the cause of death.
- Patients that are potential organ donors if their death would be reportable
  to the Coroner.
- In parts of Wales, ALL ex-miners must be routinely reported to the Coroner.

Clinical Genetics

Referral Criteria devised for the Cancer Genetics Service in Wales[1330]

Breast Cancer
- 1 first degree relative diagnosed at 40 years or less
- 2 first degree relatives at 60 years or less (on the same side of the family)
- 3 first or second degree relatives any age (on the same side of the family)
- 1 first degree male breast cancer
- A first degree relative with bilateral breast cancer

N.B. breast cancer can also be inherited through the paternal side of the family

Breast/Ovarian Cancer
- Minimum: 1 of each cancer in first degree relatives
(If only one of each cancer, the breast cancer diagnosed under 50 years)
- A first degree relative who has both breast and ovarian cancer

Ovarian Cancer
- 2 or more ovarian cancers, at least one first degree relative affected (on the same side of the family)

Colon Cancer
- 1 first degree relative diagnosed at age 40 or less
- 2 first degree relatives at 60 years or less (on the same side of the family)
- 3 relatives, all on the same side of the family, (at least 1 should be a first degree relative)
- Familial Adenomatous Polyposis
- Hereditary non polyposis colorectal cancer (revised Amsterdam criteria)

Other Cancer Syndromes
- Patient from a family with a known single gene cancer syndrome: von Hippel-Lindau disease, multiple endocrine neoplasm, retinoblastoma
- "Related Cancers": There are some rare cancer syndromes (e.g. Li Fraumeni syndrome and Cowden syndromes) where a variety of different cancers occur within a family. Where there is a high index of suspicion, the possibility of referral should be discussed on an individual basis

Travel Abroad & Holiday Insurance

Patients planning to go away on holiday, especially if flying abroad, need to consider the following issues:[1331-1333]
• travel abroad with controlled drugs
• travel insurance
• medical clearance for air travel

Taking controlled drugs abroad

When a patient who has been prescribed controlled drug medication by their doctor wishes to either:
• take a holiday outside the UK, or
• return abroad to their own country,

then a number of steps need to be taken to ensure that they have no problems with customs and excise.

1) The Home Office Licensing Department should be telephoned to check particular restrictions 020 7273 3126 or 020 7273 3806. They will then advise whether or not a licence is required for export.
   – If the quantity of drugs concerned falls below levels pre-determined by the Home Office, then export is allowed under the *Open General Licence* system.
   – If above these levels, then a *Personal Export Licence* will be required and at least ten days should be allowed for processing the application.
   – These documents do not have any legal status outside the UK and are only issued to comply with the Misuse of Drugs Act and facilitate passage through UK customs control.
2) An application needs to be supported by a doctor's letter* which must include:
   – patient's name and address
   – quantities (total) of drugs to be carried
   – strength and form drugs will be dispensed
   – dates of travel to and from UK
3) The Home Office Licensing Department will then request details of the country or countries to be visited and they will then supply the telephone numbers for the appropriate embassies involved.
4) The individual embassies will then need to be contacted for each country to check any import restrictions that may apply.
5) Medication should always be taken in its original packaging, labelled with the patient's name, drug, dose and quantity.

Quantities of drugs allowed abroad under *Open General Licence*:
• morphine 1.2 g
• diamorphine HCl injection 1350mg
• oxycodone 900mg
• hydromorphone 360mg
• fentanyl 45mg (9 x 50µg/h patches)
• methadone 500mg
  benzodiazepines 900mg

The Home Office try to keep these formalities to a minimum. Note that diamorphine can be a problem in some countries (e.g. diamorphine is illegal to import into the USA) and therefore it is important to follow these guidelines to ensure that the patient does not experience any difficulties.

* As for any planned holiday, a signed letter from a doctor on headed notepaper giving details of the patient's diagnosis, medical condition, and professionals' telephone numbers, as well as detailing medication, can avoid a lot of potential problems.

Travel Insurance for Patients with Cancer

Patients with cancer or serious illness can find it difficult to obtain travel insurance for holidays abroad. Some companies will refuse to arrange any insurance at all; others will provide insurance, but will exclude any claim made for cancellation, illness etc. that is a result of a previously known illness. There are some insurance companies that will provide full travel and medical insurance for holidays abroad. They will almost always require a medical report, and will take into account the age, condition, and destination of the patient. The following companies may be able to help; inclusion does not imply that they are recommended.

Companies change their policies over time. If you know of any other sources of travel insurance for such patients, or find that those listed below no longer provide suitable insurance, please e-mail the details to *travel@pallmed.net*

Insurance companies	
OurWay Travel	020 8313 3900 Maximum age 60 yrs. All accompanying friends & family must take out insurance under same policy. Worldwide travel.
P J Hayman & Co.	02392 419000 "Solutions" policy. No medical certificate required. Maximum age 79 yrs. Worldwide travel.
M J Fish & Co.	01772 724442 No upper age limit. Cover not given for 'terminally ill' patients. All patients require medical screening. Worldwide travel.
Medicover	0870 35 3028 In association with CancerBACUP. Patients with expected prognosis more than 4 months from return date of holiday.
AllClear Plus	01277 267584 No upper age limit. No specific exclusions. Each situation individually rated and premiums can be quite high.
Citibond	020 8771 6431 Maximum age 60 yrs. All accompanying friends & family must take out insurance under same policy. Maximum duration of travel 31 days. Worldwide travel.
Brunsdon & Co.	0117 942 6877 Various exclusions. All applicants assessed over the telephone.
Perry Gamble & Co.	020 8542 1122 Various exclusions. All applicants assessed over the telephone.

Other companies that may help

Free Spirit Travel Insurance	01483 255888
J.D. Consultants	01689 859102/3/4
Leisure Care Insurance	01793 750150
Thomas Cook Retail	01733 417444
Club Direct Travel	01243 817766
Boots Travel Insurance	0845 840 2020

Insurance brokers

British Insurance & Investment Brokers	020 7623 9043
Motts Insurance Broker	029 2070 0635
Marrs Insurance Brokers	02083 662222

Air Travel

All patients should be advised to contact the carrier's Airline Medical Officer in advance to seek medical clearance to travel. Apart from ensuring appropriate arrangements are made for patients with mobility problems or general debility, the effect of reduced oxygen cabin pressure during flight must be considered.

Conditions that may preclude air travel, or need prior medical clearance, include:

- dyspnoea, especially oxygen dependency
- anaemia
- ischaemic heart disease or heart failure
- intestinal obstruction
- pneumothorax
- confusion
- mobility problems
- extreme general debility

As a rough guide, patients who can walk 50-100 metres at a steady pace without becoming unduly breathless, needing oxygen, or becoming cyanosed should cope with the reduced cabin pressure.

Driving

Drugs and Fitness to Drive

GMC guidelines state that doctors have a duty to inform patients, when prescribing medication that may impair their driving, that the patient has a legal duty to inform the DVLA of any circumstances that may render them unfit to drive. Although there is no legal obligation to do so, it is also appropriate to advise patients that motor insurance policies usually require patients to inform them of any change in their medical circumstances for the policy to remain valid.

Many drugs used in palliative care may impair cognition and motor skills. These include:

- opioid analgesics
- antidepressants - tricyclic antidepressants especially
- benzodiazepines - diazepam, lorazepam
- phenothiazines - levomepromazine, prochlorperazine
- antihistamines - cyclizine
- others - ketamine, baclofen etc.

In cases where a patient is obviously unfit to drive (through medication or any other medical cause) and refuses to comply, doctors have a clear responsibility to continue to encourage the patient to stop driving, and ultimately disclose information to the medical advisor at the DVLA if necessary.

Opioid analgesics[1331,1334-1336]

In cancer patients receiving long-term morphine with stable doses, morphine has only a slight and selective effect on functions relating to driving.[1337] When specific tests used to assess driving ability are used, long-term opioid usage has not been shown to significantly impair the perception, cognition, coordination or behaviour relevant to driving.[1338]

Patients undergoing a significant increase in opioid dose ($\geq 30\%$) do experience significant cognitive impairment, that disappears after 1 week of the increase.[1334]

- Patients should be advised not to drive for 1 week after starting an opioid analgesic, and for 1 week after any dose increase.
- There seems to be no justification in treating opioid analgesics any differently from other drugs that may impair performance.

Brain tumours

The diagnosis of a glioma (grade 3 or 4), other malignant intracranial tumour, or cerebral secondary deposits must be notified to the DVLA, and will result in a ban from driving for at least 2 years after treatment.[1339]

Exemption from Compulsory Seat Belt Wearing

Exemption from wearing seat-belts may be appropriate for some patients with hepatomegaly, or other intra-abdominal disease. Application forms for a Certificate of Exemption are available from the NHS Response Line: 0541 555455. Enquiries to 020 7944 2043

Investigations

Blood tests

- Blood tests should never be taken 'as a routine'.
- Blood tests may be taken to confirm or exclude a diagnosis e.g. anaemia or hypercalcaemia - **if** this may:
  - help with management decisions (e.g. symptom control)
- Blood tests may also help assess disease progression **if** this will in turn:
  - help with management decisions (e.g. deteriorating renal function may make plans for discharge inappropriate), or
  - help the patient understand his/her disease (e.g. demonstrating deteriorating liver function tests may help in explaining to the patient why he/she is not getting better)

The table below assumes that taking action on the test is appropriate e.g. blood transfusion would be appropriate if test shows anaemia.
(RBL = renal-bone-liver includes urea & electrolytes, liver function tests and serum calcium.)

Indication	Blood test	Rationale
Dyspnoea or fatigue - AND Appears clinically anaemic	FBC	Blood transfusion
Fatigue Hypotonia/myaesthenia Especially if risk of hypokalaemia (diuretics diarrhoea etc.)	RBL	Treat hypokalaemia
Bone pain	RBL	Treat hypercalcaemia
Nausea or vomiting	RBL	Treat hypercalcaemia Diagnosing renal failure or liver failure may guide antiemetic use
Confusion or drowsiness	RBL Glucose - if on steroids or PMH diabetes	Treat hypercalcaemia Diagnosing renal failure or liver failure may help guide management Treat diabetes/hyperglycaemia
Thirst or dry mouth Especially if taking diuretic or recent fluid loss from diarrhoea, vomiting etc.	RBL Glucose - if on steroids or PMH diabetes	Reducing diuretic if dehydrated IVI for rehydration if reversible cause of dehydration Treat diabetes/hyperglycaemia
Symptomatically hypotensive Clinically dehydrated	RBL Glucose - if on steroids or PMH diabetes	Reducing diuretic if dehydrated IVI for rehydration if reversible cause of dehydration Treat diabetes/hyperglycaemia

Indication	Blood test	Rationale
Persistent bleeding	FBC, Clotting screen	Treat clotting disorder Detect and/or treat thrombocytopenia Monitor for anaemia
Any unexplained / rapid deterioration	FBC, RBL Glucose - if on steroids or PMH diabetes	Treat hypercalcaemia Diagnosing renal failure or liver failure may help guide management Treat diabetes/hyperglycaemia
Restless legs syndrome	Iron	Treat iron deficiency
Patient on warfarin	Check INR on admission	High incidence of poorly controlled INR in palliative care patients
Secondary blood tests		
Fatigue Drowsiness Confusion Nausea AND hypocalcaemia or hypokalaemia	Magnesium	Treat hypomagnesaemia
Microcytic anaemia	Iron	Treat iron deficiency anaemia
Macrocytic anaemia	Serum B12 and folate	Treat B12 or folate deficiency

Microbiology investigations

MSU

Urinalysis checks will show a positive result to blood and/or protein in >90% of urinary tract infections (UTIs). Much of the reaction is to blood or white cells in the urine, as the body's response to infection. Special circumstances when this is not the case include: infection in an immunosuppressed patient (usually a diabetic / septicaemic patient), or a UTI in an obstructed urinary tract e.g. in a bladder tumour obstructing a ureter, infection can develop in the obstructed kidney, which is effectively isolated from the rest of the urinary tract. Generally, urinalysis should be performed first, and an MSU only sent if urinalysis is positive.

CSU

Up to 5% of healthy people (male > female) have bacteriuria (bacteria found in the urine) without symptoms of a UTI. In patients with a catheter this figure is very much higher. Attempts to sterilise the urine in patients with catheters by treating with antibiotics are only successful as long as the patient continues to take the drug. Bacteriuria always returns on stopping.

In view of this, only investigate patients with urinary catheters who have symptoms that might relate to a UTI, and that warrant treatment e.g.

- dysuria, frequency or urgency
- suprapubic pains - 'bladder spasms'
- loin pain
- toxic symptoms e.g. confusion, nausea & vomiting

Always do a urinalysis first and only send an MSU/CSU if positive. Unpleasant-smelling urine indicates infection rather than simple bacteriuria but does not by itself warrant investigation unless the patient considers it a problem.

MRI

MRI cannot be performed on patients who have:
- cardiac pacemaker (the magnetic field may interfere with function)
- any ferrous/magnetic metal in their body - including
    - aneurysm clip in the brain
    - cochlear implant
    - metal fragment in the eye
    - shrapnel

Hip replacements are made of non-ferrous metal and do not exclude an MRI

IV Contrast Studies

Radiological examinations requiring IV contrast to be given (IVP, CT san etc.) can precipitate lactic acidosis in patients taking metformin. The metformin should be stopped well in advance of the investigation.

Flu Vaccination

Annual immunisation with influenza vaccine is recommended for those of all ages with:
- immunosuppression due to disease or treatment
- chronic respiratory or heart disease
- chronic renal failure
- diabetes mellitus

and for persons who are:
- aged over 65 years
- residents of nursing and residential homes

There is evidence that is still effective in cancer patients.[1340]
The flu vaccine is a preparation of inactivated virus, and will not cause influenza in immunosuppressed patients. The main contraindication is an allergy to eggs.
⇨ *Viral infections (p.121)*

Needlestick Injury And HIV

The risk of HIV transmission following needlestick injury involving contaminated blood is about 0.4%. Zidovudine treatment reduces the transmission rate by about 80%. Ideally treatment should start within 1-2h of such exposure.[1341]

Falls

All patients who have had a fall should have:
- blood pressure lying & standing, to check for postural hypotension
- medication reviewed, especially
  - hypotensive drugs: antimuscarinics, beta-blockers, phenothiazines etc.
  - sedative drugs: benzodiazepines, opioid analgesics etc.
  - anticonvulsants (ataxia)
  - corticosteroids (proximal myopathy)
- neurological assessment for:
  - spinal cord compression
  - cerebellar dysfunction
  - Parkinson's disease or extrapyramidal symptoms
- physiotherapist assessment for:
  - balance
  - transfers
  - gait

⇨ Guidelines[1342]

Walking sticks

A physiotherapist can best give advice on the use of walking sticks. However, many patients will start using a walking stick without guidance, and the following simple advice can help ensure appropriate use:
- A walking stick should usually be used on the **opposite** side from the affected leg if painful on weight-bearing (to halve the weight carried through the affected leg).
- Use on the **same** side if neurological or muscle leg weakness, for extra support.
- To check the correct height, the handle of the walking stick should be level with the wrist joint when then arm is resting beside the body.
- A rubber cap on the end of the stick will help prevent it slipping.

PROCEDURES

Paracentesis

General
Paracentesis[1343] is a simple procedure, which can be performed as a day case (usually only removing 2-4 litres maximum), or as an in-patient. In tense, symptomatic ascites there may be up to 12 litres ascites present. Removal of 4-6 litres is usually enough to give symptomatic relief; more than 4-6 litres increases the risk of hypovolaemia and adverse effects, but may allow longer until ascites re-accumulates. For an ill patient, small volume paracentesis repeated as needed may be preferable.

Indications
For indications ⇨ *Ascites p.37*
- pain, discomfort, or tightness due to stretching of the abdominal wall
- dyspnoea, usually exacerbated by exertion, due to raising of the diaphragm
- vomiting due to the 'squashed stomach' syndrome

Patients are usually symptomatic only when the abdominal wall is tensely distended. Patients who are also bothered by ankle (or generalized) oedema, may fare better with diuretic therapy.

Complications
After a large volume paracentesis, the large fluid shifts from circulating volume into extracellular fluid can decompensate the patient's cardiovascular system leading to hypovolaemia, and in severe cases, collapse and renal failure. A low albumen or sodium level will exacerbate this effect.

The cannula site may continue to leak ascites after removal. If a limited, partial paracentesis has been performed, this may rarely become a continuing leak over days to weeks.

Bowel perforation is a risk, especially if intestinal obstruction is present.

Infection is a rare complication, providing aseptic technique is used.

Investigations
An ultrasound scan will confirm the presence of ascites, and may determine if it is 'pocketed' by tumour adhesions. A scan should be performed if:
- ascites is not easily clinically identified
- vomiting - or any indication of bowel obstruction/distension

A serum albumen and U&E should be taken if:
- more than 4-6 litres is to be removed, and the patient has oedema, or
- the patient is clinically dehydrated, or
- the patient has reacted badly to a previous paracentesis

Platelet count and clotting screen if the patient has any symptoms of bleeding or unexplained bruising.

Contraindications
- local or systemic infection
- coagulopathy - platelets < 40 or INR > 1.4

Limit paracentesis to 4-6 litres maximum if:
- hepatic or renal failure (creatinine > 250)
- albumen < 30 or sodium < 125

The procedure

- Patient should be asked to pass urine before the procedure.
- Blood pressure should be measured and recorded.
- Patient should lie in a semi-recumbent position.
- It may be helpful for them to tilt 30 degrees towards the side of the paracentesis.
- Use left iliac fossa unless local disease is present, and avoid inferior epigastric artery (see below).
- Confirm that site is dull to percussion.
- Using aseptic technique, give local anaesthetic to skin.
- A large bore IV cannula or Bonanno catheter can be used (⇨ p.236).
- Do not clamp to control rate of drainage - malignant ascites can be very proteinaceous and is likely to block the catheter if clamped off.

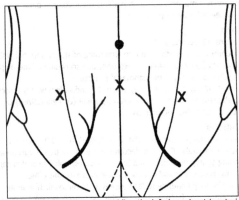

Usual sites for paracentesis, avoiding the inferior epigastric arteries.

Large volume paracentesis (> 6 litres)

If it is intended to drain to dryness, or > 6 litres:

- Stop diuretics (if used solely for ascites) 48h before procedure.
- Check blood pressure and pulse every 30 minutes during paracentesis, then hourly for 6h.
- IV dextran 70 or gelatine infusion (*Haemaccel* or *Gelofusine*) 150mL for every litre of ascites drained, given during the paracentesis or shortly afterwards will reduce hypovolaemia.[1344]

Management of complications

Hypovolaemia:

- Volume expanders (as above) should be given.

Leak from paracentesis site:

- Usually dry gauze dressings are sufficient and the leak will stop after a few hours to days.
- Enbucrilate tissue adhesive *(Histoacryl)* has been used to seal the skin on withdrawal of the cannula after paracentesis.[1345]
- Colostomy bags can be used to collect ascites if large volumes leak.
- A purse-string suture around the site may be used.

Follow-up care

Ascites will usually re-form after a paracentesis; this can vary between one and many weeks. Diuretics may reduce the rate of re-accumulation, or prevent it becoming so tense again. Repeated paracentesis on as-needed basis is appropriate management for patients with advanced cancer.

⇨ *Ascites (p.37)*

Pleural aspiration (Thoracocentesis)

General

Aspiration of a pleural effusion[1343] can give symptomatic relief from dyspnoea. A pleural effusion large enough to cause dyspnoea will be detectable clinically. Aspiration of 300-500mL fluid will usually give some symptomatic improvement, but up to 1.5 litres may be aspirated in some cases.

Complications

Haemothorax can occur, either from damage to lung or from vascular pleural tumour.

Pneumothorax can occur due to puncture of the lung; significant pneumothorax is unlikely after an uncomplicated aspiration if simple precautions are taken. A routine check X-ray after aspiration is not essential in a palliative care setting.

If a small cannula is used for aspiration (e.g. IV cannula) as opposed to a large-bore chest drain, very little air can enter through the cannula if reasonable care is taken.

Aspiration of a very large effusion that is causing the heart and mediastinum to be pushed to one side may cause cardiovascular embarrassment.

Infection is a rare complication, providing aseptic technique is used.

Investigations

Chest X-ray will show a pleural effusion, but can be difficult to differentiate from collapse/consolidation if both are present. An ultrasound scan will confirm the presence of pleural effusion, and many radiographers will mark a site for aspiration if requested.

Chest X-ray or ultrasound scan should be performed if:

• pleural effusion has not previously been confirmed radiologically
• effusion is not easily clinically identified

Platelet count and clotting screen if the patient has any symptoms of bleeding or unexplained bruising.

Contraindications

• local skin infection
• coagulopathy - platelets < 40 or INR > 1.4
• the presence of local pleural tumour is a relative contraindication, as tumour cells may be 'seeded' in the chest wall

The procedure

• Patient should sit on a chair leaning forward over a bedside table with a pillow on it, resting their head on folded arms.
• Use site marked by ultrasound scan, or
• Posterior chest wall, medial to the angle of the scapula, one intercostal space below the upper limit of dullness to percussion (mid-axillary line can also be used).

- Confirm that site is dull to percussion.
- Avoid the inferior border of the rib above; the neurovascular bundle runs in a groove inferior to the rib.
- Local anaesthetic to skin - advance the needle until pleural fluid is obtained; this will confirm the site for aspiration, and minimise risk of pneumo- or haemothorax if lung is punctured.
- Introduce a large-bore IV cannula with syringe attached until fluid is obtained, then advance a further 0.5-1 cm to ensure plastic cannula is in pleural space.
- Asking the patient to exhale against pursed lips (to increase intrathoracic pressure), remove metal trochar and immediately attach a 50/60mL syringe via a three-way tap.
- Aspirate fluid 50mL at a time, until:
  - 1 litre drained (1500mL maximum), or
  - patient starts to cough, or
  - giddiness, light-headedness or chest discomfort
- Remove the cannula and immediately seal with flexible collodion B.P., and cover with a dressing.

Management of complications

Follow-up care

All patients should be monitored and warned to report any worsening of dyspnoea which may be due to haemo- or pneumothorax. If the pleural fluid was stained with fresh blood, the patient should be observed more carefully with blood pressure and pulse recording.

A pleural effusion will often re-form after aspiration; this can vary between one and many weeks. Pleurodesis should be considered early in the disease, before loculations have formed from repeated aspirations. Indwelling pleural catheters have been used for persistent effusions[1346,1347] or pleuro-peritoneal (Denver) shunts.[284] Repeated aspiration on as-needed basis is an appropriate management for patients with advanced cancer.

⇨ *Dyspnoea (p.89)*

CLINICAL REFERENCE

Opioid Potency Ratios

Approximate equivalent morphine doses of weak opioid analgesics.

	Route	Typical dose	Total 24h dose	Equivalent morphine 24h dose	4-hourly oral morphine dose	Relative potency to oral morphine (24h)
Codeine[1]	oral	60mg q.d.s	240mg	24mg	4mg	0.1
Dihydrocodeine[1]	oral	60mg q.d.s	240mg	24mg	4mg	0.1
Buprenorphine[1]	sublingual	200µg t.d.s	0.6mg	36mg	6mg	60
Pethidine[1348]	oral	100mg q.d.s.	400mg	50mg	12.5mg	0.125
Pethidine[1348]	IM	100mg q.d.s.	400mg	150mg	25mg	0.375
Tramadol[1]	oral	50mg q.d.s.	200mg	40mg	6.6mg	0.2

Dextromoramide 5mg has approximately the same peak effect as morphine 15mg,[1] but is shorter acting

Approximate equivalent doses of strong opioid analgesics.

	Route	Period	Opioid naive	TSD	Incremental doses (mg)					Relative potency to oral morphine (24h)
Morphine	oral	4h	5mg	10mg	15	20	30	45	60	1
Morphine SR	oral	12h	15mg	30mg	45	60	90	135	180	1
Morphine	sc	4h	2.5mg	5mg	7.5	10	15	22.5 (25)	30	2
Morphine	CSCI	24h	15mg	30mg	45	60	90	135	180	2
Diamorphine	sc	4h	1.6mg (2.5mg)	3.5mg (5mg)	5	6.6 (7.5)	10	15	20	3
Diamorphine	CSCI	24h	10mg	20mg	30	40	60	90	120	3
Oxycodone	oral	4h	2.5mg	5mg	7.5	10	15	22.5 (25)	30	2
Oxycodone SR	oral	12h	7.5mg (10mg)	15mg (20mg)	22.5 (20)	30	45 (40)	67.5 (60)	90 (80)	2
Oxycodone	CSCI	24h	10mg	20mg	30	40	60	90	120	3
Fentanyl	patch	-			25µg/h		50µg/h	75µg/h	100µg/h	150
Fentanyl	CSCI	24h	0.2mg	0.4mg	0.6 (0.5)	0.8 (0.75)	1.2 (1)	1.8 (1.5)	2.4 (2)	150
Alfentanil	CSCI	24h	1mg	2mg	3	4	6	9	12	30

Important: see notes over

Hydromorphone

	Route	Period	Opioid naïve	TSD	Incremental doses (mg)					Relative potency to oral morphine (24h)
					15	20	30	45	60	
Morphine	oral	4h	5mg	10mg	15	20	30	45	60	1
Morphine SR	oral	12h	15mg	30mg	45	60	90	135	180	1
Hydromorphone	oral	4h	≤ 1.3mg	1.3-2.6mg	2.6-3.9	2.6-5.2	3.9-7.8	6.5-11.7	7.8-15.6	3.75-7.5
Hydromorphone SR	oral	12h	2-4mg	4-8mg	6-12	8-16	12-24	18-36	24-48	3.75-7.5

Hydromorphone PO 3.6-7.5:1 morphine PO[605,635,636] (7.5:1 data sheet *Palladone*)
Hydromorphone SC 3.1-8.5:1 morphine SC[605,635,637]
Hydromorphone SC 5:1 hydromorphone PO[605]
Hydromorphone SC 1:23 fentanyl SC[647]
Hydromorphone SC 2:1 oxycodone SC[626]
Hydromorphone PO 4:1 oxycodone PO[605]

Potency ratios for hydromorphone vary more than others, and probably relate to inter-individual variations in metabolism or bioavailability.

When converting between hydromorphone and morphine, use the lower equivalent dose of the range.

When converting between hydromorphone and another opioid use two methods if possible (convert first via the oral morphine equivalent using the previous table; then use a direct conversion using potency ratios given to the right); use the lowest equivalent dose.

General notes

When converting between strong opioids, considerable inter-patient variation will occur.

- Always reassess the patient carefully and anticipate the need to titrate the dose either upwards or downwards.
- If converting from a less sedating opioid (e.g. fentanyl or alfentanil) to morphine or diamorphine at doses that equate to 180mg oral morphine in 24h or greater, consider reducing the morphine/diamorphine dose by anything up to 30% (even more for very high doses), as the sedative effects may be much greater for an 'equianalgesic' dose.
- Incomplete cross-tolerance is sometimes seen between any two opioids; at doses higher than those given in the tables, consider reducing the new opioid dose by anything up to 30-50%. (⇨ *Alternative opioids p.71*)

Conversion tables

All doses in the tables are in milligrams unless otherwise specified.

Doses in *(italics)* are nearest that can be achieved from preparations available, or are closest convenient.

TSD (typical starting dose) is for patients progressing from a regular weak opioid.

Potency ratios

Note that potency ratios are quoted, not equivalence ratios i.e.

- morphine SC 2:1 morphine PO
  - morphine SC is twice as potent as orally
  - morphine SC 1mg ≈ morphine PO 2mg

Additional Information

Potency ratios reported for these drugs vary widely; the main conversion table is internally consistent with the following potency ratios:

- morphine SC 2:1 morphine PO[638]
- diamorphine SC 3:1 morphine PO[638]
- fentanyl patch 1:1 fentanyl SC[647]
- fentanyl patch 150:1 morphine PO (150:1 data sheet *Durogesic;* 100:1)[667]
- fentanyl SC 75:1 morphine SC (85:1; 68:1)[645,647]
- oxycodone SC 1.5:1 morphine SC (1.2-1.9:1)[626]
- oxycodone PO 2:1 morphine PO (2:1 data sheet *OxyContin;* 1.5:1)[624,625]
- alfentanil SC 10:1 diamorphine SC[676]
- fentanyl 5:1 alfentanil (4-10:1)[681]

SEE ALSO
⇨ *Morphine & Diamorphine (p.65), Alternative opioids (p.71)*
⇨ *Oxycodone (p.74), Hydromorphone (p.75), Fentanyl (p.76)*
⇨ *Alfentanil (p.80), Sufentanil (p.80), Remifentanil (p.80)*
⇨ *Methadone (p.81), Tramadol (p.71)*
📖 Reviews[1349-1351]

Drug Interactions

The potential for drug interactions is high in palliative care due to polypharmacy.[1352] The following are some selected drug interactions which are pertinent to palliative care prescribing.

Warfarin
The anticoagulation effect of warfarin can be affected by many drugs.[1353]
Anticoagulation may increase with:
- dextropropoxyphene (co-proxamol)
- NSAIDs *(⇨ p.61)*
- amiodarone
- erythromycin, clarithromycin
- quinolone antibiotics (e.g. ciprofloxacin)
- metronidazole
- fluconazole, itraconazole, miconazole, ketoconazole
- stanozolol

Amiodarone
A number of drugs used concomitantly with amiodarone increase the risk of ventricular arrhythmias and the advice is to avoid them:
- tricyclic antidepressants (amitriptyline etc.)
- phenothiazines, haloperidol
- flecainide
- quinine
- erythromycin (parenteral)

The low doses of haloperidol (antiemetic) and TCAs (neuropathic pain) used in palliative care probably carry a low risk, but one that cannot be dismissed.[1354]

MAOIs (antidepressants) and selegiline
There is a serious and potentially fatal interaction (serotonin syndrome[857]) between **pethidine** and MAOIs.[537,1355] A similar reaction is seen with selegiline, an MAO-B inhibitor.

No adverse interaction normally occurs in patients on MAOIs given morphine, but there are two isolated and unexplained reports of patients on MAOIs who showed hypotension, marked in one case and accompanied by unconsciousness (and rapidly and effectively reversed by naloxone). Some very limited evidence also suggests that no interaction occurs with methadone.[537]

The concurrent use of MAOIs and phenothiazines is usually safe and effective. The exception appears to be **levomepromazine** (methotrimeprazine) which has been implicated in two fatal reactions with pargyline and tranylcypromine.[537]

Anticonvulsants
Carbamazepine[858,859] levels are increased (risk of toxicity) with:
- dextropropoxyphene[487,488] (co-proxamol)
- clarithromycin, erythromycin
- fluoxetine, fluvoxamine

Phenytoin levels are increased (toxicity) by:
- clarithromycin, metronidazole, trimethoprim
- fluconazole, miconazole
- omeprazole

- fluoxetine, fluvoxamine
- aspirin
- diltiazem, nifedipine
- amiodarone

Carbamazepine and phenytoin levels are decreased (risk of fits) by corticosteroids.

Carbamazepine, phenytoin and phenobarbital can reduce the efficacy of corticosteroids. This two-way interaction[909,910] is common when managing patients with cerebral tumours.

Antifungal drugs (imidazoles)
(Fluconazole, miconazole, itraconazole, and ketoconazole).
- all enhance warfarin anticoagulation
- fluconazole, miconazole increase phenytoin levels
- fluconazole, miconazole increase sulphonylureas e.g. gliclazide, glibenclamide (risk of hypoglycaemia)
- fluconazole increases celecoxib levels[349] – halve celecoxib dose
- itraconazole, ketoconazole and possibly fluconazole increase sedation with midazolam

PPIs (proton pump inhibitors)
- omeprazole increases blood diazepam levels (increase sedation)
- omeprazole enhances anticoagulation effect of warfarin

Metronidazole
- disulfiram-like reaction with alcohol
- enhances anticoagulation with warfarin
- increases phenytoin blood levels (toxicity)
- increases blood levels of fluorouracil (5-FU) increasing toxicity

SSRI antidepressants
- fluoxetine, fluvoxamine increase carbamazepine or phenytoin blood levels (toxicity)
- fluoxetine increases plasma levels of flecainide
- serious reaction with MAOIs, selegiline (serotonin syndrome)[857]
- increased serotonergic effects with St John's wort (avoid)

St John's wort
- increased serotonergic effects with SSRIs (avoid)
- reduced anticoagulant effect of warfarin
- reduced plasma levels of carbamazepine, phenytoin, phenobarbital (risk of fits)
- reduced plasma levels of digoxin

Dextropropoxyphene (in co-proxamol)
- increases blood levels of carbamazepine up to 6-fold[487,488] (toxicity)
- enhanced anticoagulation effect of warfarin

Regular paracetamol may also affect warfarin anticoagulation.[529-535]

Torsades de pointes
An increasing number of drugs have been recognised to prolong the QT interval and potentially cause torsades de pointes, a serious cardiac arrhythmia.[1356] A register of drugs that cause QT prolongation is available on the internet at http://www.torsades.org

Paediatric Prescribing

The following information is given as a rough guide for quick reference only. Further advice should be sought when prescribing for children in palliative care.[3,1357,1358]

Many of the following drugs, doses or indications are unlicensed in children.

Analgesics

Drug	Route	2-12 yr	12-18 yr	Notes
Morphine	PO/PR	0.15mg/kg	10mg	4-hourly starting doses
Diamorphine	CSCI	0.3mg/kg/24h	20mg	24h starting dose
	SC/IM	0.05mg/kg	5mg	4-hourly as needed
Naproxen	PO/PR	5-10mg/kg		b.d. Maximum 1g/day

Antiemetics

Drug	Route	2-12 yr	12-18 yr	Notes
Cyclizine	PO/IM	>5 years 25mg	25-50mg	Up to t.d.s. as needed
Haloperidol	PO		0.5-2mg	1-3 times daily. Increased risk of extra-pyramidal side-effects in children.
Chlorpromazine	PO	5-15mg	10-25mg	Repeat up to q.d.s.
Metoclopramide	PO/IM	0.1mg/kg	<60kg 5mg >60kg 10mg	2-3 times daily. Increased risk of extra-pyramidal side-effects in children.

Sedatives

Drug	Route	2-12 yr	12-18 yr	Notes
Diazepam	PO/PR	0.25-0.5mg/kg	5-10mg	Repeated as needed
Promethazine (*Phenergan*)	PO	10-25mg	25-50mg	Repeated every 6h as needed. Also antiemetic (antihistamine.
Midazolam	CSCI	0.3mg/kg/24h		
	SC	0.7mg/kg		

Antisialogogue (for death rattle)

Drug	Route	2-18 yr	Notes
Hyoscine hydrobromide	SC	0.01-0.02mg/kg	Repeat every 4h as needed
Glycopyrronium	SC	4µg/kg	Repeat every 6-8h as needed. Doses for drooling much lower.

Average weights

Average weights for **healthy** children:

Age	Mean weight Kg	% Adult dose
Newborn	3.5	12.5
6 months	8	22
1 year	10	25
3 years	15	33
5 years	20	40
7 years	25	50
12 years	40	75
Adult male	70	100
Adult female	60	100

NB Wt. in stones x 6 ≈ wt. in Kg.
The percentage adult dose should only be used as a rough guide when paediatric doses in mg/kg are not available.

Blood Results

Normal ranges vary depending on patient characteristics and between different laboratories. The following are given as a rough guide for quick reference.

Haematology

	Male	Female
Haemoglobin	13.0-16.7 g/dl	11.8-15.0 g/dl
Haematocrit (PCV)	38.5-50.1%	36.0-44.5%
MCV	83.6-97.6 fl	77.1-97.6 fl
MCHC	32.7-34.6 g/dl	32.7-33.2 g/dl
MCH	28.0-34.6 pg	27.8-33.2 pg
Red Cell Count	$4.27\text{-}5.63 \times 10^{12}/L$	$3.85\text{-}4.68 \times 10^{12}/L$
Platelets	$150\text{-}450 \times 10^9/L$	$150\text{-}400 \times 10^9/L$
Total WCC	$4.1\text{-}10.1 \times 10^9/L$	$4.2\text{-}11.9 \times 10^9/L$

White cell differential

Neutrophils	$2.0\text{-}8.3 \times 10^9/L$	40-75%
Lymphocytes	$1.2\text{-}3.5 \times 10^9/L$	20-45%
Monocytes	$0.2\text{-}0.8 \times 10^9/L$	2-10%

Haematinics

Serum Iron	13-32 µmol/L
TIBC	36-72 µmol/L
Serum B12	200-450 pg/mL
Serum Folate	3.2-15.0 ng/mL
Red Cell Folate	180-300 ng/mL
ESR	0-20 mm/hr

Coagulation

Prothrombin time	12-17 sec (INR 0.8-1.2)
APTT (KCCT)	28-40 sec (APTT ratio 0.8-1.2)
Fibrinogen	150-400mg/dl
FDP's	< 5µgFE/mL
Protein C	70-120%
Protein S	60-120%
Antithrombin III	80-130%

Biochemistry
Urea and Electrolytes
Sodium	133-148 mmol/L
Potassium	3.5-5.2 mmol/L
Chloride	95-110 mmol/L
Urea	3.4-7.2 mmol/L
Creatinine	50-115 mmol/L
Magnesium	0.7-1.0 mmol/L

Glucose & Diabetes
RBS	>11.0 mmol/L	Diabetic
Fasting glucose	3.3-6.0 mmol/L	Normal
	6.0-7.0 mmol/L	Needs tolerance test
	>7.0 mmol/L	Diabetic
Glycosylated HbA$_1$	5-8%	Non-diabetic
	<10%	Good control
	10-12%	Moderate control
	15% +	Poor control

Liver Function Tests
Total Protein	63-82 g/L
Bilirubin	<17 mmol/L
Globulin	18-32 g/L
Albumen	35-50 g/L
Ca^{++} corrected	2.1-2.6 mmol/L*
PO4$^-$	0.8-1.45 mmol/L
Amylase	70-300 IU/L
Alkaline phosphatase	20-130 IU/L
AST (SGOT)	<40 IU/L
ALT (SGPT)	<50 IU/L
Gamma GT	12-43 IU/L

*To correct calcium for low albumen, add 0.02 for every gram of albumen below 40 g/L.

Cardiac enzymes
Creatinine kinase	25-195 iu/L
Lactate dehydrogenase (LDH)	70-250 iu/L

Urine
Sodium	100-250 mmol/24h
Potassium	14-120 mmol/24h
Osmolality	350-1000 mosmol/kg
Cortisol (free)	<280 nmol/24h

Anticonvulsants - therapeutic range
Carbamazepine	6-12 mg/L	(25-50 µmol/L)
Clonazepam	0.025-0.075 mg/L	(0.08-0.24 µmol/L)
Phenytoin	10-20 mg/L	(40-80 µmol/L)
Phenobarbital	10-30 mg/L	(45-130 µmol/L)

Values quoted are for 'trough' levels i.e. taken just before next dose is due.
Therapeutic ranges are given as a very rough guide only, as there is poor correlation between clinical effect and blood levels.

Anticoagulation Target INRs

Target INR[1092]	Indication
2.0-2.5	DVT prophylaxis
2.5	Treatment of DVT and PE (or recurrence in patients not on warfarin)
3.5	Recurrent DVT and PE in patients receiving warfarin, Mechanical prosthetic heart valves

INR should be within 0.5 of the target INR.

⇨ *Anticoagulation (p.145)*

Emergency Medicine Reference

Emergency drug doses

	Route	Adult	Child
Anaphylaxis/asthma			
Adrenaline 1:1,000 (epinephrine)	IM	0.5mL	0.1mL/yr
Aminophylline	IV 20mins	250-500mg	5mg/kg
	infusion	0.5mg/kg/hr	1mg/kg/hr
Chlorphenamine (chlorpheniramine)	IV	10mg	200µgm/kg
Salbutamol	IV slow	0.25mg	4µgm/kg
	SC, IM	0.5mg	
	neb.	5mg	2.5mg
Hydrocortisone	IV	100-300mg	
Fits/sedation			
Diazepam	IV, PR	10mg	0.25-0.5mg/kg
Diabetes - hypoglycaemia			
Glucagon	IM	1mg >12yrs	0.5mg <12yrs

Mask & Airway sizes

Airway Size		Mask Size	
1	Child	1 - 2	Child
2	Adult female	3	Teenage
3	Adult male	4	Female
4	Large	5	Male
		6	Large

Endotracheal Intubation

Age	ET Tube	Oral Length
0 -3 months	3.5mm	11cms
3 - 6 months	4.0	12
6 months -1yr	4.5	12.5
2	5.0	13
4	5.5	14
6	6.0	15
8	6.5	16
10	7.0	17
12	7.5	18
14	8.0	21
Adult		
Male	9.0	23
Female	8.0	21.5

Tracheostomy tube sizes

Age	Inside Diam.	F.G. Ch	Suction catheter F.G. Ch
0 - 3 months	3.5mm	14	8
3 - 6 months	4.0	16	8
6 months - 1yr	4.5	18	8
2	5.0	20	10
4	5.5	22	10
6	6.0	24	10
8	6.5	26	10
10	7.0	28	10
12	7.5	30	10
14	8.0	33	12
Adult			
Male	9.0mm	36	14
Female	8.0mm	33	12

Fluids

Approximate daily maintenance fluid requirements

Age	Maintenance mL/day
0 yr.	525
3 months	720
6 months	900
1yr	1000
2	1300
4	1500
6	2000
8	2250
10	2400
12	2800
14	3000
16	3000
Adult	3000

Pain Terminology

All definitions (except those with asterisks) are from the International Association for the Study of Pain.[1359]

GENERAL TERMS

Pain - An unpleasant sensory and emotional experience associated with actual or potential tissue damage, or described in terms of such damage.

Nociception - pain produced by the stimulation of specific peripheral receptors (nociceptors) and conveyed by neurones dedicated to transmitting pain.

Nociceptor - A receptor preferentially sensitive to a noxious stimulus or to a stimulus which would become noxious if prolonged.

Noxious stimulus - A noxious stimulus is one which is damaging to normal tissues.

Neuropathic pain - Pain initiated or caused by a primary lesion or dysfunction in the nervous system.

Neuropathy - A disturbance of function or pathological change in a nerve.

Neuralgia - Pain in the distribution of a nerve or nerves.

Neurogenic pain - Pain initiated or caused by a primary lesion, dysfunction, or transitory perturbation in the peripheral or central nervous system.

Peripheral neurogenic pain - Pain initiated or caused by a primary lesion or dysfunction or transitory perturbation in the peripheral nervous system.

Peripheral neuropathic pain - Pain initiated or caused by a primary lesion or dysfunction in the peripheral nervous system.

Nerve compression pain * - Pain from functional and reversible dysfunction of the nervous system. Also sometimes called nociceptive neurogenic pain.

Neuritis - Inflammation of a nerve or nerves.

Central pain - Pain initiated or caused by a primary lesion or dysfunction in the central nervous system.

Sympathetic dependent pain * (Also called sympathetic maintained pain) - A type of neuropathic pain dependent on the sympathetic nervous system, and associated with dysfunction of the sympathetic autonomic nervous system.

Causalgia - A syndrome of sustained burning pain, allodynia, and hyperpathia after a traumatic nerve lesion, often combined with vasomotor and pseudomotor dysfunction and later trophic changes.

CLINICAL DESCRIPTIONS

Allodynia - Pain due to a stimulus which does not normally provoke pain (lowered threshold: stimulus and response mode differ).

Dysaesthesia - An unpleasant abnormal sensation, whether spontaneous or evoked.

Hyperalgesia - An increased response to a stimulus which is normally painful (increased response: stimulus and response mode are the same).

Hyperaesthesia - Increased sensitivity to stimulation, excluding the special senses.

Hyperpathia - A painful syndrome characterized by an abnormally painful reaction to a stimulus, especially a repetitive stimulus, as well as an increased threshold (raised threshold: stimulus and response mode may be the same or different, increased response). Results in a pain of delayed onset that outlasts the stimulus.

Hypoalgesia - Diminished pain in response to a normally painful stimulus (raised threshold: stimulus and response mode are the same, lowered response).

Hypoaesthesia - Decreased sensitivity to stimulation, excluding the special senses.

Paraesthesia - An abnormal sensation, whether spontaneous or evoked.

Anaesthesia dolorosa - Pain in an area or region which is anaesthetic.

Deafferentation pain * - Pain in an area of deficient sensation. A term best avoided.

Opioid resistant pain * (Opioid insensitive pain) - A clinical description of a pain that cannot be fully controlled by opioid analgesia.

OTHER

Pain threshold - The least experience of pain which a subject can recognize. This level usually remains remarkable constant.

Pain tolerance level - The greatest level of pain which a subject is prepared to tolerate. This can vary enormously.

Psychological factors * - The psychological state of the patient will modulate the perception of pain whatever its underlying mechanism. If pain is exaggerated above what might normally be expected from a particular stimulus this 'exaggeration' is sometimes loosely termed the *psychological component* of the pain.

Psychosomatic pain * - Nociceptive pain with an underlying psychological cause e.g. anxiety causing increased muscle tension leading in turn to headache due to the muscle pain.

Psychogenic pain * - Pain experienced when there is no proven or suspected physiological cause or pathology.

General Assessment Questions

Twelve core assessment questions. Adapted from Emanuel, 1998.[1360]

Area of patient's experience	Suggested assessment question
Physical symptoms	What symptom bothers you most?
Pain	How much pain have you had in the last week?
Depression	Are you feeling depressed?
Financial	Is your illness causing much financial hardship to you or your family?
Carers	How much help do you need with your personal care? How much help have you needed from someone in your family?
Social support	Is there someone you can confide in and talk to about yourself or your problems? How often is there someone to have a good time with?
Spirituality	Do you have a faith? Since your illness have you become more or less spiritual or religious?
Hopes & expectations	Is there a something special, like an event, that would add a great deal of meaning to your life?
Advance care planning	Have you talked to your family, or anyone, about your preferences for medical care in case of a life-threatening situation?

Mental state assessment

COASTMAP is a useful mnemonic for factors to evaluate in a mental state examination:

Consciousness	Alertness Attention Concentration
Orientation	To person, place, and time
Activity	Agitated or retarded
Speech	Rate (pressure of speech) Content Dysphasia
Thought	Cognitive function Insight Reasoning
Memory	Long-term and short-term
Affect & mood	Depression Irritability Angry
Perceptions	Misinterpretation Hallucinations

Criteria for diagnosing Depression

Criteria for Major Depressive Episode - DSM IV[1361]

- Five (or more) of the following symptoms have been present during the same 2-week period and represent a change from previous functioning; at least one of the symptoms is either (1) depressed mood or (2) loss of interest or pleasure.

  Note: - Do not include symptoms that are clearly due to a general medical condition, or mood-incongruent delusions or hallucinations.

  - depressed mood most of the day, nearly every day, as indicated by either subjective report (e.g., feels sad or empty) or observation made by others (e.g., appears tearful).
  - markedly diminished interest or pleasure in all, or almost all, activities most of the day, nearly every day (as indicated by either subjective account or observation made by others)
  - significant weight loss when not dieting or weight gain (e.g., a change of more than 5% of body weight in a month), or decrease or increase in appetite nearly every day.
  - insomnia or hypersomnia nearly every day
  - psychomotor agitation or retardation nearly every day (observable by others, not merely subjective feelings of restlessness or being slowed down)
  - fatigue or loss of energy nearly every day
  - feelings of worthlessness or excessive or inappropriate guilt (which may be delusional) nearly every day (not merely self-reproach or guilt about being sick)
  - diminished ability to think or concentrate, or indecisiveness, nearly every day (either by subjective account or as observed by others)
  - recurrent thoughts of death (not just fear of dying), recurrent suicidal ideation without a specific plan, or a suicide attempt or a specific plan for committing suicide
- The symptoms do not meet criteria for a Mixed Episode.
- The symptoms cause clinically significant distress or impairment in social, occupational, or other important areas of functioning.
- The symptoms are not due to the direct physiological effects of a substance (e.g., a drug of abuse, a medication) or a general medical condition (e.g., hypothyroidism).
- The symptoms are not better accounted for by Bereavement, i.e., after the loss of a loved one, the symptoms persist for longer than 2 months or are characterized by marked functional impairment, morbid preoccupation with worthlessness, suicidal ideation, psychotic symptoms, or psychomotor retardation.

Endicott's criteria

Endicott (1984) has published useful ways of modifying the usual screening and diagnostic procedures for depressive disorders in cancer patients.[1362]

- fearful or depressed appearance
- social withdrawal or reduced talkativeness
- psychomotor agitation or retardation
- depressed and non-reactive mood
- pessimism/brooding self-pity
- diminished pleasure or interest
- worthlessness or excessive guilt
- suicidal thoughts/recurrent thoughts of death

Mini-Mental Score

A test devised for the serial testing of cognitive mental state on a neurogeriatric ward. A score of 20 or less was found essentially in patients with dementia, delirium, schizophrenia, or affective disorder, and not in normal elderly people or in patients with a primary diagnosis of neurosis or personality disorder.[1363,1364]

Instructions for administration	Maximum Score
Orientation	
What is the date (year) (season) (date) (day) (month)? Ask for the date. Then ask specifically for parts omitted, e.g., "Can you also tell me what season it is?" One point for each correct.	5
Where are we: (state) (county) (town) (hospital) (floor) Ask in turn "Can you tell me the name of this hospital?" (town, county, etc.). One point for each correct.	5
Registration	
Ask the patient if you may test his memory. Then say the names of 3 unrelated objects, clearly and slowly, about one second for each. After you have said all 3, ask him to repeat them. This first repetition determines his score (0-3; give 1 point for each correct answer), but keep saying them until he can repeat all 3, up to 6 trials. If he does not eventually learn all 3, recall cannot be meaningfully tested. Count trials and record.	3
Attention and calculation	
Serial 7's. Ask the patient to begin with 100 and count backwards by 7. Stop after 5 subtractions (93, 86, 79, 72, 65). Score the total number of correct answers. 1 point for each correct. If the patient cannot or will not perform this task, ask him to spell the word "world" backwards. Score the number of letters in correct order e.g. dlrow = 5, dlorw = 3.	5

Recall
Ask the patient if he can recall the 3 words you previously   3
asked him to remember. Score 0-3. Give 1 point for each
correct.

Language
Naming: Name a pencil, and watch.   2
Show the patient a wrist watch and ask him what it is.
Repeat for pencil. Score 0-2.

Repetition: Ask the patient to repeat the sentence after   1
you: "No ifs, ands or buts." Allow only one trial. Score 0
or 1.

3-Stage command: "Take a paper in your right hand, fold it   3
in half, and put it on the floor".
Give the patient a piece of plain blank paper and repeat the
command. Score 1 point for each part correctly executed.

Reading: Read and obey the following: "CLOSE YOUR   1
EYES"
On a blank piece of paper print the sentence "Close your
eyes", in letters large enough for the patient to see clearly.
Ask him to read it and do what it says. Score 1 point only if
he actually closes his eyes.

Writing: Give the patient a blank piece of paper and ask   1
him to write a sentence for you. Do not dictate a sentence,
it is to be written spontaneously. It must contain a subject
and verb and be sensible. Correct grammar and punctuation
are not necessary.

Copying: On a clean piece of paper, draw intersecting   1
pentagons, each side about 1 in., and ask him to copy it
exactly as it is. All 10 angles must be present and 2 must
intersect to score 1 point. Tremor and rotation are ignored.

TOTAL SCORE   (Max. 30)

Assess the patient's level of consciousness along a continuum, from alert
on the left to coma on the right:

_____

Alert   Drowsy   Stupor   Coma

Neurology

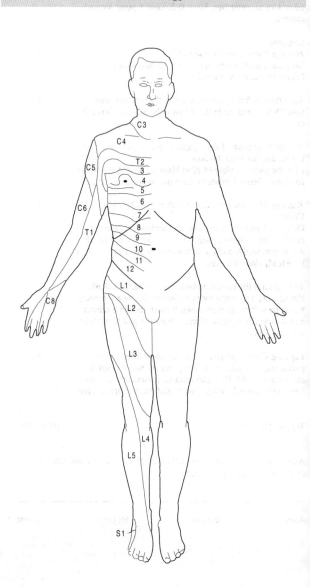

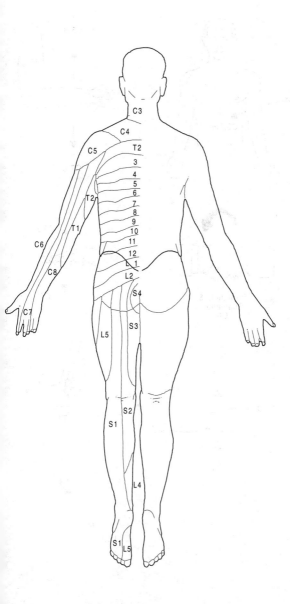

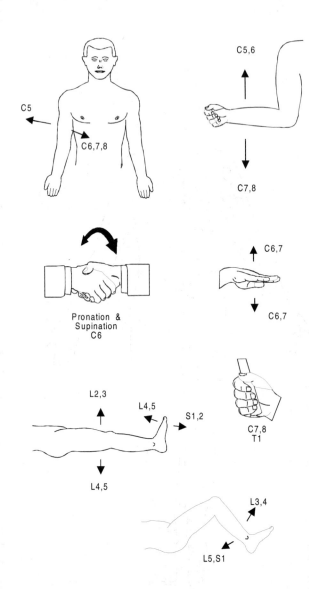

C5

C6,7,8

C5,6

C7,8

Pronation &
Supination
C6

C6,7

C6,7

C7,8
T1

L2,3

L4,5

S1,2

L4,5

L3,4

L5,S1

Family Tree

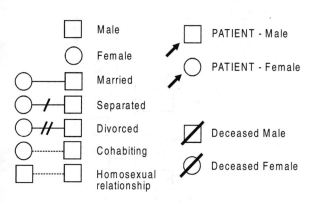

2nd AND 3rd MARRIAGES

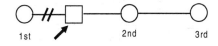

PARENTS

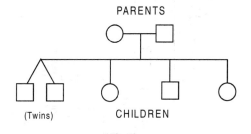

NB Alternative system: ⊗ for the Patient and ● for Deceased

Example of Family Tree

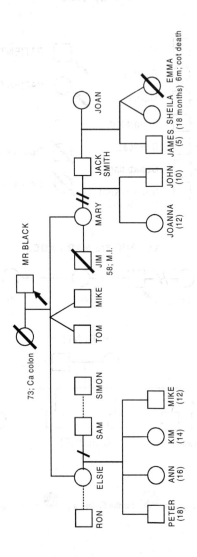

Peak Expiratory Flow Rate

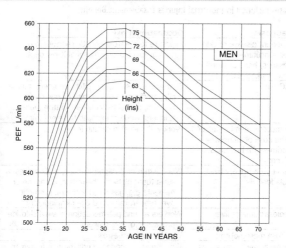

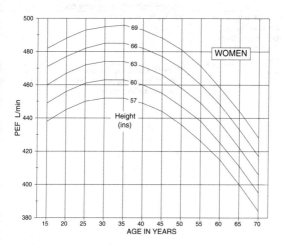

Occupational Causes Of Cancer

Diseases included in Industrial Injuries Disablement Benefit:

Diagnosis	Occupational risk
Malignant disease of skin or subcutaneous tissues, bone or blood e.g. leukaemia.	Exposure to electro-magnetic radiation e.g. nuclear fuel industry, hospital X-ray dept.
SCC skin.	Exposure to arsenic, tar, pitch, bitumen, mineral oil, paraffin or soot e.g. bituminous shale workers, optical lens makers, cotton mule spinners, workers exposed to tarry fumes.
Ca mucous membranes of the nose or sinuses or primary Ca bronchus or lung.	Work with nickel in certain forms
Primary Ca urinary tract, bladder.	Work with α or β-naphthylamine, aniline dyes, a substituted diphenyl, benzidine, auramine or magenta e.g. gas retort workers, synthetic dye, rubber, cable and chemical industry.
Angiosarcoma of liver	Workers around polymerisation of vinyl chloride process, e.g. PVC makers
Diffuse mesothelioma	Working with asbestos
Ca nasal cavity or sinuses	Working with wooden goods, or with footwear made from leather or fibre board
Primary Ca lung when there is evidence of asbestosis or bilateral diffuse pleural thickening	Work with asbestos
Lung Ca	Work in a tin mine. Exposure to bis(chloromethyl)ether, zinc-, calcium- or strontium- chromate

Help & Advice For Patients

UK National Resources
Macmillan Cancer Relief
Funds Macmillan nurses: referral via GP or hospital. Information line; financial help through patient grants. Applications for patient grants through hospital and hospice nurses, social workers and other health care professionals. (London)
☎ 0845 601 6161
🖥 http://www.macmillan.org.uk/
@ information_line@macmillan.org.uk

Marie Curie Cancer Care
Hands-on palliative nursing care, available through the local district nursing service. Also runs in-patient centres: admission by referral from GP or consultant. Both the services are free of charge. (London)
☎ 020 7235 3325
🖥 http://www.mariecurie.org.uk/

Tenovus Cancer Information Centre (Wales)
Information and support for patients, their families, carer. Helpline staffed by experienced cancer trained nurses, counsellors and social workers. Individual counselling service; free literature.
Velindre Hospital, Whitchurch, Cardiff CF14 2TL
☎ 0808 808 1010
🖥 http://www.tenovus.org.uk/

CancerBACUP
Helps people with cancer, their families and friends live with cancer. Cancer nurses provide information, emotional support and practical advice by telephone or letter. Booklets, factsheets, a newsletter, website and CD-ROM provide information. (London)
☎ 0808 800 1234
🖥 http://www.cancerbacup.org.uk/

Cancerlink
Provides emotional support and information. Register of over 600 cancer support and self-help groups nationwide. Free training and consultancy in setting up and running groups. (London)
Freephone Information Helpline: 0800 132905 (textphone available for deaf and hard of hearing)
Freephone Helpline for young people affected by cancer: 0800 591028
Freephone Asian Cancer Information Helpline in Bengali, Hindi, Punjabi, and Urdu: 0800 590415
@ Cancerlink@canlink.demon.co.uk

Bereavement
Asian Family Counselling Service
Includes bereavement counselling.
☎ 020 8997 5749

CancerBACUP Counselling
☎ 020 7833 2451

CRUSE
Bereavement counselling
☎ 020 8940 4818

Gay Bereavement Counselling Services
☎ 020 8455 8894

National Association of Bereavement Services
☎ 020 7247 1080

The Compassionate Friends
A self-help group of parents whose son or daughter (of any age, including adults) has died from any cause.
☎ 0117 953 9639

Samaritans / Age Concern / Citizens Advice Bureaux
☎ from local directory

Carers
Carers National Association
Information and support to people caring for relatives and friends. Free leaflets and information sheets.
☎ 0345 573369 (Mon-Fri 10am-midday, 2pm-4pm)
☎ 029 2088 0176 (Cardiff)

Crossroads - Caring for Carers
Provide a range of services for carers, including care in the home to enable the carer to have a break.
☎ 01788 573653

Children
ACT - Association for Children with Life-Threatening or Terminal Conditions and their Families.
☎ 0117 922 1556 (Bristol)

Complementary Therapies
Bristol Cancer Help Centre
☎ 0117 980 9500

British Acupuncture Council
☎ 020 8 964 0222

British Homoeopathic Association
☎ 020 7 935 2163

National Federation of Spiritual Healers
☎ 01932 783 164

Institute for Complementary Medicine
☎ 020 7 237 5165
🖳 *http://www.members.aol.com/ICMedicine*
@ *ICMedicine@aol.com*

Conditions other than cancer
Parkinson's Disease Society
☎ 020 7388 3513

Stroke Association
☎ 020 7490 7999

British Brain and Spine Foundation
Helpline provides information and support about neurological disorders for
patients, carers and health professionals.
☎ 0808 808 1000
@ *info@bbsf.org.uk*
🖳 *http://www.bbsf.org.uk/*

Alzheimer's Disease Society
☎ 020 7306 0606

Motor Neurone Disease Association
Professional and general enquiries: 0604 250505
Helpline: 0345 626262

Counselling
British Association for Counselling
☎ 01788 578328

Specific Cancers
Brain Tumour Foundation
☎ 020 8336 2020
@ *btf.uk@virgin.net*

Breast Cancer Care
☎ 0500 245 345
@ *information@breastcancercare.org.uk*
🖳 *http://www.breastcancercare.org.uk/*

Lymphoma Association
☎ 01844 291500 (Mon-Fri 10am-8pm)
🖳 *http://www.lymphoma.org.uk/*

Oesophageal Patients' Association
☎ 0121 704 9860

Ovacome
A support organisation for women with ovarian cancer.
☎ 07071 781861
@ *ovacome@ovacome.org.uk*
🖳 *http://www.ovacome.org.uk/ovacome*

Prostate Cancer Charity
☎ (Mon-Fri 10am-4pm) 020 8 383 1948
🖳 *http://www.prostate-cancer.org.uk/*
@ *info@prstate-cancer.org.uk*

Prostate Cancer Support Association (PSA)
☎ 020 8 446 3896 (10am-8pm)

Prostate Help Association
🖳 *http://www.pha.u-net.co.uk/*
@ *phillip@pha.u-net.com*

The Roy Castle Lung Cancer Foundation
☎ 0800 358 7200
🖳 *http://www.roycastle.org/*

Specific health problems

Changing Faces
Offers information, social skills training and counselling for people with facial disfigurements.
☎ 020 7 706 4232
🖥 http://www.changingfaces.co.uk/

British Colostomy Association
☎ 0118 939 1537
Freephone: 0800 32842

Impotence Association
☎ 020 8 767 7791
🖥 http://www.impotence.org.uk/

Let's Face It
A contact point for people of any age coping with facial disfigurement.
☎ 01252 879 630
Tel/Fax: 020 8 931 2829

Lymphoedema Support Network
☎ 020 7 351 4480
🖥 http://www.lymphoedema.org/
@ ADMINLSN@lymphoedema.freeserve.co.uk

National Association of Laryngectomee Clubs
☎ 020 7 381 9993

SPOD
Association to aid sexual and personal relationships of people with a disability.
☎ 020 7 607 8851

Urostomy Association
☎ 01245 224294

Specific patient groups

Chai
Lifeline Cancer Support and Centre for Health
Emotional, physical, practical and spiritual support to Jewish cancer patients, their families and friends.
☎ 020 8 202 4567
🖥 http://chai-lifeline.org.uk
@ info@chai-lifeline.org.uk

Gayscan
Offers completely confidential help and support to gay men living with cancer, their partners and carers.
Helpline: 020 8 446 3896

National Network for Palliative Care of People with Learning Disability
☎ 020 8846 1629
(See references[1365-1368])

Benefits And Social Services

The rules regarding financial benefits from Social Security are complicated, but the following is a short summary of the many benefits available. Further information is available from the local Social Security or Benefits Agency office; the reference number for leaflets with further information are given below:

Attendance Allowance

For disabled people aged 65 or over who need help with personal care because of their illness or disability. Normally the help must have been needed for at least six months, but under certain circumstances there are special rules so that they can get their benefit quickly and easily. (DS702; HB5)

Disability Living Allowance

For people under 65 who need help with personal care, getting around or both, because they are ill or disabled. Normally help must have been needed for at least three months, but under certain circumstances there are special rules so that they can get their benefit quickly and easily. (DS704; HB5)

Disability Working Allowance

For people who are able to work at least 16 hours a week, but have an illness or disability that limits their earning capacity. To claim a person must be aged 16 or over and have a qualifying benefit. DWA does not depend on National Insurance contributions. (Claim pack DWA1; DWA Helpline 01722 883311; leaflets DS703; HB4)

Invalid Care Allowance

For people aged 16-65 who are spending at least 35 hours a week caring for a severely disabled person who is in receipt of the middle or highest rate of Disability Living Allowance care component or Attendance Allowance. They must not earn more then £50 a week or be in full-time education. (Claim pack DS700; leaflets SD4; HB5)

Incapacity Benefit

People who are incapable of work and are employed, but who cannot get Statutory Sick Pay from their employer, or who are self-employed, or unemployed may get Incapacity Benefit if they have paid enough NI contributions. (Changeover pack SSP1 from employer, or SC1 for self-employed and unemployed; leaflet DS1)

Severe Disablement Allowance

For people between 16 and 65 who have not been able to work for at least 28 consecutive weeks because of illness or severe disablement and cannot get Incapacity Benefit because they have not paid enough NI contributions. (Claim pack from Social Security; leaflets SD1; HB5)

Statutory Sick Pay

Employed people who are sick for four or more days in a row may qualify for SSP from their employers for a maximum of 28 weeks. (Leaflet SD1)

Industrial Injuries Disablement Benefit

For those who are disabled as a result of an accident at work or as a result of a prescribed industrial disease. They may also be entitled to *Constant Attendance Allowance* and *Exceptionally Severe Disablement Allowance*. *Reduced Earnings Allowance* can also be paid if the accident happened or the disease started before 1ˢᵗ October 1990 and as a result the person cannot return to the same job or do work of the same standard. (Claim form from Social Security; leaflet NI6)

Income Support
For people aged 16 or over whose income is below a certain level, and who are not required to be available for work because they are sick, disabled, a lone parent, aged 60 or over, or getting Invalid Care Allowance. (Claim pack from Social Security; leaflet IS20)

Council Tax Discount Scheme
Disabled people and carers may receive discounts on Council Tax. (Contact Local Authority; leaflet *Council Tax: a guide to your bill,* available from 020 7890 4203)

Council Tax Benefit
People on a low income may receive help to pay council tax. (Claim forms from local Council; leaflets GL17; RR2)

Housing Benefit
Paid by local councils for people who need help with rent. The person must not have over £16,000 in savings. (claim forms from local Council; leaflets GL16; RR2)

Help with health costs
Help may be available for: free NHS prescriptions, free NHS dental treatment, free NHS sight test, maximum value of a voucher towards the cost of glasses or contact lenses, free NHS wigs and fabric supports, repayment of travel costs to hospital and back for NHS treatment (HC11; HC12; HC13)

Widow's Benefits
Widow's payment, widowed mother's allowance, widow's pension. Claim form BW1: Social Security Office issues this when they receive the certificate of registration of death the Registrar gives you. The certificate should be sent to the Social Security office as soon as possible. (D49; D49S; NP45)

Funeral Payments
If a person or their partner has to arrange a funeral and receives certain benefits or allowances, they may get some help with the costs. (Form SF200; leaflets D49; D49S)

Special Equipment

Plastic (paediatric) cannulae to use with syringe driver infusions
Ohmeda Neoflon IV cannula 24G Code 1350-8
Abbocath IV cannula 26G

Heimlich valve for continuous pleural effusion drainage
Vygon Heimlich valve Code 669.10

Drainage catheter for paracentesis
Modified Bonanno suprapubic bladder drainage catheter - Becton Dickenson & Co. Code 408289 Approx. £30 each
Available from: Hospital Management and Supplies, Brook House, 4 The Lakes, Bedford Road, Northampton, NN4 7YD

International Non-Proprietary Drug Names (INN's)

Below are listed some of the International drug names (rINN) which are taking over from British Approved Names (BAN). The list is not exhaustive. Further details in the BNF.

British approved name (BAN)	International non-proprietary name (INN)[843]
Acyclovir	Aciclovir
Adrenaline	Epinephrine
Amoxycillin	Amoxicillin
Amphetamine	Amfetamine
Bendrofluazide	Bendroflumethiazide
Benzhexol	Trihexyphenidyl
Benztropine	Benzatropine
Cephalexin	Cefalexin
Cephradine	Cefradine
Chlormethiazole	Clomethiazole
Chlorpheniramine	Chlorphenamine
Cholestyramine	Colestyramine
Colistin sulphomethate	Colistimethate
Cyclosporin	Ciclosporin
Danthron	Dantron
Dexamphetamine	Dexamfetamine
Dimethicone	Dimeticone
Dothiepin	Dosulepin
Frusemide	Furosemide
Hydroxyurea	Hydroxycarbamide
Indomethacin	Indometacin
Lignocaine	Lidocaine
Methotrimeprazine	Levomepromazine
Mitozantrone	Mitoxantrone
Phenobarbitone	Phenobarbital
Salcatonin	Calcitonin (salmon)
Sodium picosulphate	Sodium picosulfate
Stilboestrol	Diethylstilbestrol

BIBLIOGRAPHY

1   Twycross R, Wilcock A, Thorp S. *Palliative Care Formulary*. Abingdon: Radcliffe Medical Press, 1998.
2   Palliative Care Formulary (on-line edition). 2001. (http://www.palliativedrugs.com)
3   Doyle D, Hanks GWC, MacDonald N, eds. *Oxford textbook of palliative medicine*. 2nd ed. Oxford: Oxford University Press, 1997.
4   Twycross R. *Symptom management in advanced cancer*. 3rd ed. Oxford: Radcliffe Medical Press, 2001.
5   Atkinson CV, Kirkham SR. Unlicensed uses for medication in a palliative care unit. *Palliat Med* 1999;13:145-52.[A]
6   Todd J, Davies A. Use of unlicensed medication in palliative medicine (letter). *Palliat Med* 1999;13:446
7   National Institute for Clinical Excellence. *Guidance on the use of proton pump inhibitors (PPI) in the treatment of dyspepsia*, 2000. (http://www.nice.org.uk, accessed Feb 2001)
8   Nelson KA, Walsh TD. Metoclopramide in anorexia caused by cancer-associated dyspepsia syndrome (CADS). *J Palliat Care* 1993;9:14-18.[A]
9   Bruera E, et al. A double-blind, crossover study of controlled-release metoclopramide and placebo for the chronic nausea and dyspepsia of advanced cancer. *J Pain Symptom Manage* 2000;19:427-35.[A]
10 Welling LR, Watson WA. The emergency department treatment of dyspepsia with antacids and oral lidocaine. *Ann Emerg Med* 1990;19:785-8.[A]
11 Byrne MF, Murray FE. Formulary management of proton pump inhibitors. *Pharmacoeconomics* 1999;16:225-46.[A]
12 Horn J. The proton-pump inhibitors: similarities and differences. *Clin Ther* 2000;22:266-80.[A]
13 Brummer RJM, Geerling BJ, Stockbrugger RW. Acute and chronic effect of lansoprazole and omeprazole in relation to food intake (abstract). *Gut* 1995;37:T127
14 Moules I, et al. Gastric acid inhibition by the proton pump inhibitor lansoprazole is unaffected by food. *Br J Clin Res* 1993;4:153-61
15 Kromer W, Horbach S, Luhmann R. Relative efficacies of gastric proton pump inhibitors: their clinical and pharmacological basis. *Pharmacology* 1999;59:57-77.[A]
16 Stedman CA, Barclay ML. Review article: comparison of the pharmacokinetics, acid suppression and efficacy of proton pump inhibitors. *Aliment Pharmacol Ther* 2000;14:963-78.[A]
17 Hookman P, Siegel CI, Hendrix TR. Failure of oxethazaine to alter acid-induced esophageal pain. *Am J Dig Dis* 1966;11:811-3
18 Piper JM, et al. Corticosteroid use and peptic ulcer disease: role of nonsteroidal anti-inflammatory drugs. *Ann Intern Med* 1991;114:735-40.[A]
19 Hawkins C, Hanks GW. The gastroduodenal toxicity of nonsteroidal anti-inflammatory drugs. A review of the literature. *J Pain Symptom Manage* 2000;20:140-51
20 Ellershaw JE, Kelly MJ. Corticosteroids and peptic ulceration. *Palliat Med* 1994;8:313-9.[A]
21 De Abajo FJ, Rodriguez LA, Montero D. Association between selective serotonin reuptake inhibitors and upper gastrointestinal bleeding: population based case-control study. *Br Med J* 1999;319:1106-9.[A]
22 Dickinson T, et al. Association between SSRIs and upper gastrointestinal bleeding. Self treatment with non-steroidal drugs may be confounding factor (letter). *Br Med J* 2000;320:1406
23 Dunn NR, Pearce GL, Shakir SA. Association between SSRIs and upper gastrointestinal bleeding. SSRIs are no more likely than other drugs to cause such bleeding (letter). *Br Med J* 2000;320:1405-6
24 Po AL. Antidepressants and upper gastrointestinal bleeding (editorial). *Br Med J* 1999;319:1081-2
25 Williams D, Kelly A, Feely J. Association between SSRIs and upper gastrointestinal bleeding. Coprescription of antiulcer drugs with SSRIs is fairly common (letter). *Br Med J* 2000;320:1405; discussion 06

26 Eisenchlas JH, et al. Efficacy of levomepromazine for refractory emesis in 45 advanced cancer patients (abstract). *J Pain Symptom Manage* 2000;20:S63

27 Twycross RG, Barkby GD, Hallwood PM. The use of low dose levomepromazine (methotrimeprazine) in the management of nausea and vomiting. *Prog Palliat Care* 1997;5:49-53.^{A}

28 Higi M, et al. Pronounced antiemetic activity of the antipsychotic drug levomepromazine in patients receiving cancer therapy. *J Cancer Res Clin Oncol* 1980;97:81-86

29 O'Donnell V. Levomepromazine use for the treatment of nausea and vomiting (letter). *Prog Palliat Care* 1999;7:121

30 Ferris FD, et al. Transdermal scopolamine use in the control of narcotic-induced nausea. *J Pain Symptom Manage* 1991;6:389-93.^{A}

31 Chung F, et al. Ondansetron is more effective than metoclopramide for the treatment of opioid-induced emesis in post-surgical adult patients. Ondansetron OIE Post-Surgical Study Group. *European Journal of Anaesthesiology* 1999;16:669-77.^{A}

32 Alexander R, et al. Comparison of ondansetron and droperidol in reducing postoperative nausea and vomiting associated with patient-controlled analgesia. *Anaesthesia* 1995;50:1086-8.^{A}

33 Wynn RL, Essien E, Thut PD. The effects of different antiemetic agents on morphine-induced emesis in ferrets. *Eur J Pharmacol* 1993;241:47-54.^{A}

34 Sussman G, et al. Intravenous ondansetron for the control of opioid-induced nausea and vomiting. International S3AA3013 Study Group. *Clin Ther* 1999;21:1216-27.^{A}

35 Altomare DF, et al. Oral erythromycin improves gastrointestinal motility and transit after subtotal but not total gastrectomy for cancer. *Br J Surg* 1997;84:1017-21.^{A}

36 Annese V, et al. Erythromycin accelerates gastric emptying by inducing antral contractions and improved gastroduodenal coordination. *Gastroenterology* 1992;102:823-8.^{A}

37 Annese V, et al. Cisapride and erythromycin prokinetic effects in gastroparesis due to type 1 (insulin-dependent) diabetes mellitus. *Aliment Pharmacol Ther* 1997;11:599-603.^{A}

38 Burt M, et al. Erythromycin stimulates gastric emptying after esophagectomy with gastric replacement: a randomized clinical trial. *J Thorac Cardiovasc Surg* 1996;111:649-54.^{A}

39 Chen JD, et al. Effects of octreotide and erythromycin on gastric myoelectrical and motor activities in patients with gastroparesis. *Dig Dis Sci* 1998;43:80-9.^{A}

40 Collard JM, et al. Erythromycin enhances early postoperative contractility of the denervated whole stomach as an esophageal substitute. *Ann Surg* 1999;229:337-43.^{A}

41 Delatour F, et al. Effect of a single oral dose of two erythromycin ethylsuccinate formulations on gastric emptying in healthy volunteers: a scintigraphic study. *Fundam Clin Pharmacol* 1998;12:292-7.^{A}

42 Desautels G, et al. Gastric emptying response to variable oral erythromycin dosing in diabetic gastroparesis. *Dig Dis Sci* 1995;40:141-6.^{A}

43 DiBaise JK, Quigley EM. Efficacy of prolonged administration of intravenous erythromycin in an ambulatory setting as treatment of severe gastroparesis: one center's experience. *J Clin Gastroenterol* 1999;28:131-4.^{A}

44 Erbas T, et al. Comparison of metoclopramide and erythromycin in the treatment of diabetic gastroparesis. *Diabetes Care* 1993;16:1511-4.^{A}

45 Jones KL, et al. The effect of erythromycin on gastric emptying is modified by physiological changes in the blood glucose concentration. *Am J Gastroenterol* 1999;94:2074-9.^{A}

46 Jones KL, et al. Hyperglycemia attenuates the gastrokinetic effect of erythromycin and affects the perception of postprandial hunger in normal subjects. *Diabetes Care* 1999;22:339-44.^{A}

47 Petrakis J, et al. Enhancement of gastric emptying of solids by erythromycin in patients with Roux-en-Y gastrojejunostomy. *Archives Of Surgery* 1998;133:709-14.^{A}

48 Ueberschaer B, et al. Effect of 4 x 250 mg erythromycin on human gastrointestinal transit. *Zeitschrift Fur Gastroenterologie* 1995;33:340-4.^{A}

49 Ehrenpreis ED, Zaitman D, Nellans H. Which form of erythromycin should be used to treat gastroparesis? A pharmacokinetic analysis. *Aliment Pharmacol Ther* 1998;12:373-6.^{A}

50 Bertolucci LE, DiDario B. Efficacy of a portable acustimulation device in controlling seasickness. *Aviat Space Environ Med* 1995;66:1155-8.^{A}

51 Hu S, et al. P6 acupressure reduces symptoms of vection-induced motion sickness. *Aviat Space Environ Med* 1995;66:631-4.[A]

52 Dibble SL, et al. Acupressure for nausea: results of a pilot study. *Oncol Nurs Forum* 2000;27:41-7.[A]

53 Vickers AJ. Can acupuncture have specific effects on health? A systematic review of acupuncture antiemesis trials. *J R Soc Med* 1996;89:303-11.[A]

54 Lao L, et al. Electroacupuncture reduces morphine-induced emesis in ferrets: a pilot study. *J Altern Complement Med* 1995;1:257-61.[A]

55 Brown S, et al. Acupressure wrist bands to relieve nausea and vomiting in hospice patients: do they work? *Am J Hosp Palliat Care* 1992;9:26-9.[A]

56 Pan CX, et al. Complementary and alternative medicine in the management of pain, dyspnea, and nausea and vomiting near the end of life: a systematic review. *J Pain Symptom Manage* 2000;20:374-87

57 Watson JP, Mannix KA, Matthewson K. Percutaneous endoscopic gastroenterostomy and jejunal extension for gastric stasis in pancreatic carcinoma. *Palliat Med* 1997;11:407-10.[A]

58 Pirl WF, Roth AJ. Remission of chemotherapy-induced emesis with concurrent olanzapine treatment: a case report. *Psychooncology* 2000;9:84-7

59 Lundberg JC, et al. Initial results of an investigation of the efficacy of olanzapine for the relief of opioid-induced nausea in cancer pain patients (abstract). *Blood* 1999;94(S1):424b.[A]

60 Tramer MR, et al. Cannabinoids for control of chemotherapy induced nausea and vomiting: quantitative systematic review. *Br Med J* 2001;323:16-21

61 Gonzalez-Rosales F, Walsh D. Intractable nausea and vomiting due to gastrointestinal mucosal metastases relieved by tetrahydrocannabinol (dronabinol). *J Pain Symptom Manage* 1997;14:311-4.[A]

62 Flynn J, Hanif N. Nabilone for the management of intractable nausea and vomiting in terminally staged AIDS. *J Palliat Care* 1992;8:46-7

63 Smyth JF. The problem of emesis induced by cancer chemotherapy. *Clinician* 1988;6:2-12

64 Marley JE, Joy MD. Alleviation of motion sickness by nifedipine (letter). *Lancet* 1987;ii:1265

65 Davis MP, Walsh D. Treatment of nausea and vomiting in advanced cancer. *Support Care Cancer* 2000;8:444-52.[A]

66 Tyler LS, Lipman AG. Nausea and vomiting in palliative care. *J Pharm Care Pain Symptom Control* 2000;8:163-81.[A]

67 *Nausea and vomiting.* In: National Cancer Institute CancerNet PDQ database, 2000. (http://cancernet.nci.nih.gov/pdq/, accessed 9 Dec 2000)

68 Twycross R, Back I. Clinical management. Nausea and vomiting in advanced cancer. *Eur J Palliat Care* 1998;5:39-45

69 Bentley A, Boyd K. Use of clinical pictures in the management of nausea and vomiting: a prospective audit. *Palliat Med* 2001;15:247-53

70 Clissold SP, Heel RC. Transdermal hyoscine (Scopolamine). A preliminary review of its pharmacodynamic properties and therapeutic efficacy. *Drugs* 1985;29:189-207.[A]

71 Gordon C, et al. Transdermal scopolamine: human performance and side effects. *Aviat Space Environ Med* 1986;57:236-40.[A]

72 Williams PI, Smith M. An assessment of prochlorperazine buccal for the prevention of nausea and vomiting during intravenous patient-controlled analgesia with morphine following abdominal hysterectomy. *European Journal of Anaesthesiology* 1999;16:638-45.[A]

73 Tramer MR, et al. Efficacy of 5-HT3 receptor antagonists in radiotherapy-induced nausea and vomiting: a quantitative systematic review. *Eur J Cancer* 1998;34:1836-44.[A]

74 Del Giglio A, et al. Granisetron is equivalent to ondansetron for prophylaxis of chemotherapy-induced nausea and vomiting: results of a meta-analysis of randomized controlled trials. *Cancer* 2000;89:2301-8.[A]

75 Blackwell CP, Harding SM. The clinical pharmacology of ondansetron. *Eur J Cancer Clin Oncol* 1989;25:S21-S24

76 Cole RM, et al. Successful control of intractable nausea and vomiting requiring combined ondansetron and haloperidol in a patient with advanced cancer. *J Pain Symptom Manage* 1994;9:48-50.[A]

77 Pereira J, Bruera E. Successful management of intractable nausea with ondansetron: a case study. *J Palliat Care* 1996;12:47-50

78 Mystakidou K, et al. Comparison of tropisetron and chlorpromazine combinations in the control of nausea and vomiting of patients with advanced cancer. *J Pain*

Symptom Manage 1998;15:176-84.[A]

79   Yamakuni H, et al. Probable involvement of the 5-hydroxytryptamine(4) receptor in methotrexate-induced delayed emesis in dogs. *J Pharmacol Exp Ther* 2000;292:1002-7.[A]

80   Barrajon E, De las Penas R. Randomised double blind crossover study comparing ondansetron, granisetron and tropisetron. A cost-benefit analysis. *Support Care Cancer* 2000;8:323-33.[A]

81   Currow DC, et al. Use of ondansetron in palliative medicine. *J Pain Symptom Manage* 1997;13:302-7.[A]

82   Tyers MB, Bunce KT, Humphrey PPA. Pharmacological and anti-emetic properties of ondansetron. *Eur J Cancer Clin Oncol* 1989;25:S15-S19

83   Bymaster FP, et al. In vitro and in vivo biochemistry of olanzapine: a novel, atypical antipsychotic drug. *J Clin Psychiatry* 1997;58(S10):28-36.[A]

84   Richelson E. Receptor pharmacology of neuroleptics: relation to clinical effects. *J Clin Psychiatry* 1999;60:5-14.[A]

85   McCallum RW, et al. Gastric pacing improves emptying and symptoms in patients with gastroparesis. *Gastroenterology* 1998;114:456-61;598-601.[A]

86   Rabine JC, Barnett JL. Management of the patient with gastroparesis. *J Clin Gastroenterol* 2001;32:11-8.[A]

87   Isbister WH, Elder P, Symons L. Non-operative management of malignant intestinal obstruction. *J R Coll Surg Edinb* 1990;35:369-72

88   Davis MP, Furste A. Glycopyrrolate: a useful drug in the palliation of mechanical bowel obstruction (letter). *J Pain Symptom Manage* 1999;18:153-4

89   Mercadante S, et al. Comparison of octreotide and hyoscine butylbromide in controlling gastrointestinal symptoms due to malignant inoperable bowel obstruction. *Support Care Cancer* 2000;8:188-91.[A]

90   Ripamonti C, et al. Role of octreotide, scopolamine butylbromide, and hydration in symptom control of patients with inoperable bowel obstruction and nasogastric tubes: a prospective randomized trial. *J Pain Symptom Manage* 2000;19:23-34.[A]

91   Mercadante S, et al. Octreotide in relieving gastrointestinal symptoms due to bowel obstruction. *Palliat Med* 1993;7:295-9.[A]

92   Riley J, Fallon MT. Octreotide in terminal malignant obstruction of the gastrointestinal tract. *Eur J Palliat Care* 1994;1:23-5

93   Mercadante S. Bowel obstruction in home-care cancer patients: 4 years experience. *Support Care Cancer* 1995;3:190-3.[A]

94   Binkert CA, et al. Benign and malignant stenoses of the stomach and duodenum: treatment with self-expanding metallic endoprostheses. *Radiology* 1996;199:335-8.[A]

95   Baere de, et al. Self-expanding metallic stents as palliative treatment of malignant gastroduodenal stenosis. *Am J Roentgenol* 1997;169:1079-83.[A]

96   Hyodo T, Yoshida Y, Imawari M. A new endoscopic metallic stenting method for duodenal stenosis: a preliminary report. *J Gastroenterol* 1999;34:577-81.[A]

97   Venu RP, et al. Self-expandable metal stents for malignant gastric outlet obstruction: a modified technique. *Endoscopy* 1998;30:553-8.[A]

98   Soetikno RM, et al. Palliation of malignant gastric outlet obstruction using an endoscopically placed Wallstent. *Gastrointest Endosc* 1998;47:267-70.[A]

99   Singer SB, Asch M. Metallic stents in the treatment of duodenal obstruction: technical issues and results. *Can Assoc Radiol J* 2000;51:121-9.[A]

100   Park HS, et al. Upper gastrointestinal tract malignant obstruction: initial results of palliation with a flexible covered stent. *Radiology* 1999;210:865-70.[A]

101   Nevitt AW, et al. Expandable metallic prostheses for malignant obstructions of gastric outlet and proximal small bowel. *Gastrointest Endosc* 1998;47:271-6.[A]

102   Dresner SM, et al. Percutaneous endoscopic duodenostomy: the relief of obstruction in advanced gastric carcinoma. *Palliat Med* 1999;13:165-7.[A]

103   Ward J, Johnson M, Renwick I. Palliation of gastric outlet obstruction by a self-expanding metallic stent. *CME Bulletin Palliat Med* 2000;2:49-50.[A]

104   Ashby MA, et al. Percutaneous gastrostomy as a venting procedure in palliative care. *Palliat Med* 1991;5:147-50

105   Gemlo B, et al. Home support of patients with end-stage malignant bowel obstruction using hydration and venting gastrostomy. *Am J Surg* 1986;152:100-04

106   Arnell T, et al. Colonic stents in colorectal obstruction. *American Surgeon* 1998;64:986-8.[A]

107   Baron TH, et al. Expandable metal stents for the treatment of colonic obstruction: techniques and outcomes. *Gastrointest Endosc* 1998;47:277-86.[A]

108   Canon CL, et al. Treatment of colonic obstruction with expandable metal stents: radiologic features. *Am J Roentgenol* 1997;168:199-205.[A]

109 Choo IW, et al. Malignant colorectal obstruction: treatment with a flexible covered stent. *Radiology* 1998;206:415-21.[A]

110 Dohmoto M, Hünerbein M, Schlag PM. Application of rectal stents for palliation of obstructing rectosigmoid cancer. *Surg Endosc* 1997;11:758-61.[A]

111 Mainar A, et al. Acute colorectal obstruction: treatment with self-expandable metallic stents before scheduled surgery--results of a multicenter study. *Radiology* 1999;210:65-9.[A]

112 Mishima K, et al. Expandable metallic stent treatment for malignant colorectal strictures. *Cardiovasc Intervent Radiol* 1999;22:155-8.[A]

113 Paúl Díaz L, et al. Palliative treatment of malignant colorectal strictures with metallic stents. *Cardiovasc Intervent Radiol* 1999;22:29-36.[A]

114 Kaye SB. Intestinal obstruction: how best to manage, and when is palliative chemotherapy the right option? (editorial). *Palliat Care Today* 1995;4:2

115 Ripamonti C, et al. Clinical-practice recommendations for the management of bowel obstruction in patients with end-stage cancer. *Support Care Cancer* 2001;9:223-33

116 *Constipation, impaction, and bowel obstruction.* In: National Cancer Institute CancerNet PDQ database, 2000. (http://cancernet.nci.nih.gov/pdq/, accessed 9 Dec 2000)

117 Beattie GJ, Leonard RCF, Smyth JF. Bowel obstruction in ovarian carcinoma: a retrospective study and review of the literature. *Palliat Med* 1989;3:275-80

118 Baines M. Intestinal obstruction in patients with advanced cancer. *Palliat Care Today* 1995;4:4-6

119 Baines M, Oliver DJ, Carter RL. Medical management of intestinal obstruction in patients with advanced malignant disease. *Lancet* 1985;ii:990-93

120 Feuer D. Management of intestinal obstruction. *CME Bulletin Palliat Med* 1999;1:35-40

121 Rubin J, et al. Octreotide acetate long-acting formulation versus open-label subcutaneous octreotide acetate in malignant carcinoid syndrome. *J Clin Oncol* 1999;17:600-6.[A]

122 Feuer DJ, Broadley KE. Systematic review and meta-analysis of corticosteroids for the resolution of malignant bowel obstruction in advanced gynaecological and gastrointestinal cancers. Systematic Review Steering Committee. *Ann Oncol* 1999;10:1035-41.[A]

123 Feuer DJ, Broadley KE. *Corticosteroids for the resolution of malignant bowel obstruction in advanced gynaecological and gastrointestinal cancer (Cochrane Review).* In: The Cochrane Library, Issue 3, 2000. (http://hiru.mcmaster.ca/cochrane, accessed 5 Dec 2000)

124 Laval G, et al. The use of steroids in the management of inoperable intestinal obstruction in terminal cancer patients: do they remove the obstruction? *Palliat Med* 2000;14:3-10.[A]

125 De Conno F, et al. Continuous subcutaneous infusion of hyoscine butylbromide reduces secretions in patients with gastrointestinal obstruction. *J Pain Symptom Manage* 1991;6:484-6.[A]

126 Mercadante S. Scopolamine butylbromide plus octreotide in unresponsive bowel obstruction (letter). *J Pain Symptom Manage* 1998;16:278-80

127 Cremer SA, Gelfand DW. Esophageal bezoar resulting from enteral feedings. *Jpen Journal of Parenteral and Enteral Nutrition* 1996;20:371-3.[A]

128 Escamilla C, et al. Intestinal obstruction and bezoars. *J Am Coll Surg* 1994;179:285-8.[A]

129 Krupp KB, Johns P, Troncoso V. Esophageal bezoar formation in a tube-fed patient receiving sucralfate and antacid therapy: a case report. *Gastroenterol Nurs* 1995;18:46-8.[A]

130 Stack PE, Thomas E. Pharmacobezoar: an evolving new entity. *Dig Dis Sci* 1995;13:356-64.[A]

131 Dickman A, Littlewood C. *The syringe driver in palliative care.* 5th ed: ARD Publications: St Helens and Knowsley Hospitals, 1998.

132 Hassel B. Treatment of biliary colic with nitroglycerin (letter). *Lancet* 1993;342:1305

133 Attar A, et al. Comparison of a low dose polyethylene glycol electrolyte solution with lactulose for treatment of chronic constipation. *Gut* 1999;44:226-30.[A]

134 Ungar A. Movicol in treatment of constipation and faecal impaction. 2000;61:37-40.[A]

135 Culbert P, Gillett H, Ferguson A. Highly effective new oral therapy for faecal impaction. *Br J Gen Pract* 1998;48:1599-600

136 Culbert P, Gillett H, Ferguson A. Highly effective oral therapy (polyethylene

glycol/electrolyte solution) for faecal impaction and severe constipation. *Clin Drug Invest* 1998;16:355-60.^

137 Sykes NP. A volunteer model for the comparison of laxatives in opioid-related constipation. *J Pain Symptom Manage* 1996;11:363-9.^

138 Culpepper-Morgan JA, et al. Treatment of opioid-induced constipation with oral naloxone: a pilot study. *Clin Pharmacol Ther* 1992;52:90-5.^

139 Robinson BA, Johansson L, Shaw J. Oral naloxone in opioid-associated constipation (letter). *Lancet* 1991;338:581-2

140 Sykes NP. Oral naloxone in opioid-associated constipation (letter). *Lancet* 1991;337:1475

141 Sykes NP. An investigation of the ability of oral naloxone to correct opioid-related constipation in patients with advanced cancer. *Palliat Med* 1996;10:135-44

142 Sykes N. Clinical management. The treatment of morphine-induced constipation. *Eur J Palliat Care* 1998;5:12-5

143 Meissner W, et al. Oral naloxone reverses opioid-associated constipation. *Pain* 2000;84:105-9.^

144 Fallon MT. Constipation in cancer patients: Prevalence, pathogenesis, and cost-related issues. *Eur J Pain* 1999;3:3-7.^

145 Sykes N. Constipation in palliative care. *Palliat Care Today* 1997;5:55

146 Campbell T, et al. The management of constipation in people with cancer. *Int J Palliat Nurs* 2001;7:110-19

147 Beckwith MC. Constipation in palliative care patients. *J Pharm Care Pain Symptom Control* 1999;7:47-57

148 Sykes NP. A clinical comparison of laxatives in a hospice. *Palliat Med* 1991;5:307-14

149 Ippen H. Red skin and Dorbanex. *Br Med J* 1974;4:345

150 Bunney MH, Noble IM. Red skin and Dorbanex (letter). *Br Med J* 1974;2:731

151 Barth JH, et al. A cutaneous complication of Dorbanex therapy. *Clinical And Experimental Dermatology* 1984;9:95-96

152 Donowitz M. Magnesium-induced diarrhea and new insights into the pathobiology of diarrhea (editorial). *N Engl J Med* 1991;324:1059-60

153 Henriksson R, et al. The effect of ondansetron on radiation-induced emesis and diarrhoea. *Acta Oncol* 1992;31:767-69.^

154 Schworer H, et al. Treatment of diarrhea in carcinoid syndrome with ondansetron, tropisetron, and clonidine. *Am J Gastroenterol* 1995;90:645-8.^

155 Gupta TP, Ehrinpreis MN. Candida-associated diarrhea in hospitalized patients. *Gastroenterology* 1990;98:780-5.^

156 Baillie-Johnson HR. Octreotide in the management of treatment-related diarrhoea. *Anticancer Drugs* 1996;7(S1):11-5.^

157 Romeu J, et al. Efficacy of octreotide in the management of chronic diarrhoea in AIDS. *AIDS* 1991;5:1495-99

158 Oberg K. The use of octreotide in the management of carcinoid syndrome. *Somatostatin Analogues and the Gastrointestinal Tract* 1993;1:1-2

159 Mercadante S. Octreotide in the treatment of diarrhoea induced by coeliac plexus block. *Pain* 1995;61:345-46

160 Kornblau S, et al. Management of cancer treatment-related diarrhea. Issues and therapeutic strategies. *J Pain Symptom Manage* 2000;19:118-29.^

161 Farthing MJ. The role of somatostatin analogues in the treatment of refractory diarrhoea. *Digestion* 1996;57(S1):107-13.^

162 Beckwith MC, Lipman AG. Diarrhea in palliative care patients. *J Pharm Care Pain Symptom Control* 1999;7:91-108.^

163 Fontaine O, Gore SM, Pierce NF. Rice-based oral rehydration solution for treating diarrhoea. *Cochrane Database Syst Rev* 2000:CD001264.^

164 Gore SM, Fontaine O, Pierce NF. Impact of rice based oral rehydration solution on stool output and duration of diarrhoea: meta-analysis of 13 clinical trials. *Br Med J* 1992;304:287-91.^

165 Ramakrishna BS, et al. Amylase-resistant starch plus oral rehydration solution for cholera. *N Engl J Med* 2000;342:308-13.^

166 Rovera G, et al. The use of clonidine for the treatment of high intestinal output following small bowel transplantation. *Transplantation Proceedings* 1997;29:1853-4

167 Mercadante S. Diarrhea in terminally ill patients: pathophysiology and treatment. *J Pain Symptom Manage* 1995;10:298-309.^

168 *Radiation enteritis.* In: National Cancer Institute CancerNet PDQ database, 2000. (http://cancernet.nci.nih.gov/pdq/, accessed 9 Dec 2000)

169 Ooms LA, Degryse AD, Janssen PA. Mechanisms of action of loperamide. *Scand*

J Gastroenterol Suppl 1984;96:145-55.[A]

170 Shee CD, Pounder RE. Loperamide, diphenoxylate, and codeine phosphate in chronic diarrhoea. *Br Med J* 1980;280:524

171 Schuermans V, et al. Loperamide (R 18 553), a novel type of antidiarrheal agent. Part 6: Clinical pharmacology. Placebo-controlled comparison of the constipating activity and safety of loperamide, diphenoxylate and codeine in normal volunteers. *Arzneimittel-Forschung* 1974;24:1653-7

172 Palmer KR, Corbett CL, Holdsworth CD. Double-blind cross-over study comparing loperamide, codeine and diphenoxylate in the treatment of chronic diarrhea. *Gastroenterology* 1980;79:1272-75

173 Mercadante S. The role of octreotide in palliative care. *J Pain Symptom Manage* 1994;9:406-11.[A]

174 Mercadante S. Treatment of diarrhoea due to enterocolic fistula with octreotide in a terminal cancer patient. *Palliat Med* 1992;6:257-9

175 Williams C. 3M Cavilon No Sting Barrier Film in the protection of vulnerable skin. *Br J Nurs* 1998;7:613-5.[A]

176 Jeyarajah AR, et al. Effective palliation of a colovaginal fistula using a self-expanding metal stent. *Gastoint End* 1997;46:367-9

177 Green DE, Phillips GL Jr. Vaginal prosthesis for control of vesicovaginal fistula. *Gynecol Oncol* 1986;23:119-23.[A]

178 Goh PM, Kum CK, Toh EH. Endoscopic patch closure of malignant esophagotracheal fistula using Histoacryl glue. *Surg Endosc* 1994;8:1434-5.[A]

179 Walls AW, Regnard CF, Mannix KA. The closure of an abdominal fistula using self-polymerizing silicone rubbers - case study. *Palliat Med* 1994;8:59-62.[A]

180 Shand A, et al. Palliation of a malignant gastrocolic fistula by endoscopic human fibrin sealant injection. *Eur J Gastroenterol Hepatol* 1997;9:1009-11.[A]

181 Oneschuk D, Bruera E. Successful management of multiple enterocutaneous fistulas in a patient with metastatic colon cancer. *J Pain Symptom Manage* 1997;14:121-4.[A]

182 Moertel CG, et al. Corticosteroid therapy of preterminal gastrointestinal cancer. *Cancer* 1974;33:1607-09

183 Willox J, et al. Prednisolone as an appetite stimulant in patients with cancer. *Br Med J* 1984;288:27

184 Bruera E, et al. Action of oral methylprednisolone in terminal cancer patients: a prospective randomized double-blind trial. *Cancer Treat Rep* 1985;69:751-54

185 Popiela T, Lucchi R, Giongo F. Methylprednisolone as palliative therapy for female terminal cancer patients. The Methylprednisolone Female Preterminal Cancer Study Group. *Eur J Cancer Clin Oncol* 1989;25:1823-9.[A]

186 Nelson KA, et al. Assessment of upper gastrointestinal motility in the cancer-associated dyspepsia syndrome. *J Palliat Care* 1993;9:27-31.[A]

187 Beal JE, et al. Long-term efficacy and safety of dronabinol for acquired immunodeficiency syndrome-associated anorexia. *J Pain Symptom Manage* 1997;14:7-14.[A]

188 Beal JE, et al. Dronabinol as a treatment for anorexia associated with weight loss in patients with AIDS. *J Pain Symptom Manage* 1995;10:89-97.[A]

189 Rimmer T. Clinical management. Treating the anorexia of cancer. *Eur J Palliat Care* 1998;5:179-81

190 Nelson K, et al. A phase II study of delta-9-tetrahydrocannabinol for appetite stimulation in cancer-associated anorexia. *J Palliat Care* 1994;10:14-8.[A]

191 Bruera E, et al. Thalidomide in patients with cachexia due to terminal cancer: preliminary report. *Ann Oncol* 1999;10:857-9

192 Peuckmann V, Fisch M, Bruera E. Potential novel uses of thalidomide: focus on palliative care. *Drugs* 2000;60:273-92.[A]

193 Calabrese L, Fleischer AB. Thalidomide: current and potential clinical applications. *Am J Med* 2000;108:487-95.[A]

194 Carey I. Cancer cachexia. *Palliat Care Today* 2000;9:20-22

195 Mantovani G, et al. Managing cancer-related anorexia/cachexia. *Drugs* 2001;61:499-514.[A]

196 Rimmer T. Anorexia and malignancy. *CME Bulletin Palliat Med* 1999;1:69-72

197 Davis MP, Dickerson D. Cachexia and anorexia: cancer's covert killer. *Support Care Cancer* 2000;8:180-7.[A]

198 Lovel T, Dunlop R. OICPC Therapeutic Highlights: Cachexia. *Prog Palliat Care* 2000;8:133-34

199 Bruera E. Pharmacological treatment of cachexia: any progress? *Support Care Cancer* 1998;6:109-13.[A]

200 Tyler LS, Lipman AG. Anorexia and cachexia in palliative care patients. *J Pharm*

Care Pain Symptom Control 1999;7:11-22.^

201 *Nutrition.* In: National Cancer Institute CancerNet PDQ database, 2000. (http://cancernet.nci.nih.gov/pdq/, accessed 9 Dec 2000)

202 Gluck M, Pope CE, 2nd. Chronic hiccups and gastroesophageal reflux disease: the acid perfusion test as a provocative maneuver. *Ann Intern Med* 1986;105:219-20

203 Traube M. The spectrum of the symptoms and presentations of gastroesophageal reflux disease. *Gastroenterol Clin North Am* 1990;19:609-16.^

204 De Conno F, Polastri D. Clinical features and symptomatic treatment of liver metastasis in the terminally ill patient. *Ann Ital Chir* 1996;67:819-26.^

205 Burcharth F, Agger P. Singultus: a case of hiccup with diaphragmatic tumour. *Acta Chir Scand* 1974;140:340-41

206 Al Deeb SM, et al. Intractable hiccup induced by brainstem lesion. *J Neurol Sci* 1991;103:144-50.^

207 Fischer AQ, McLean WT, Jr. Intractable hiccups as presenting symptom of brainstem tumor in children. *Childs Brain* 1982;9:60-63

208 Kozik M, Owsianowska T. Persistent hiccoughs as the predominant symptom with a tumour of the medulla oblongata. *J Neurol* 1976;212:91-93

209 Stotka VL, et al. Intractable hiccough as the primary manifestation of brain stem tumor. *Am J Med* 1962;32:313-15

210 LeWitt PA, Barton NW, Posner JB. Hiccup with dexamethasone therapy (letter). *Ann Neurol* 1982;12:405-06

211 Baethge BA, Lidsky MD. Intractable hiccups associated with high dose intravenous methylprednisolone therapy. *Ann Intern Med* 1986;104:58-59

212 Hardo PG. Intractable hiccups: an early feature of Addison's disease. *Postgrad Med J* 1989;65:918-19.^

213 Jones JS, Lloyd T, Cannon L. Persistent hiccups as an unusual manifestation of hyponatremia. *J Emerg Med* 1987;5:283-87.^

214 Salem MR. Hiccups and pharyngeal stimulation. *JAMA* 1968;204:551

215 Madanagopolan N. Metoclopramide in hiccup. *Curr Med Res Opin* 1975;3:371-74.^

216 Williamson BW, MacIntyre IM. Management of intractable hiccup. *Br Med J* 1977;2:501-03.^

217 Friedgood C, Ripstein C. Chlorpromazine in the treatment of intractable hiccups. *JAMA* 1955;157:309

218 Intractable hiccup: baclofen and nifedipine are worth trying. *Drug Ther Bull* 1990;28:36

219 Bhalotra R. Baclofen therapy for intractable hiccoughs (letter). *J Clin Endocrinol Metab* 1990;12:122

220 Burke AM, White AB, Brill N. Baclofen for intractable hiccups (letter). *N Engl J Med* 1988;319:1353-62

221 Catalano F. Centrally acting skeletal muscle relaxants in persistent hiccups. *Acta Neurol (Napoli)* 1973;28:466-70

222 Lance JW, Bassil GT. Familial intractable hiccup relieved by baclofen (letter). *Lancet* 1989;ii:276-77

223 Oneschuk D. The use of baclofen for treatment of chronic hiccups (letter). *J Pain Symptom Manage* 1999;18:4-5

224 Walker P, Watanabe S, Bruera E. Baclofen, a treatment for chronic hiccup. *J Pain Symptom Manage* 1998;16:125-32.^

225 Yaqoob M, Prabhu P, Ahmad R. Baclofen for intractable hiccups (letter). *Lancet* 1989;ii:562-63

226 Brigham B, Bolin T. High dose nifedipine and fludrocortisone for intractable hiccups (letter). *Med J Aust* 1992;157:70

227 Lipps DC, et al. Nifedipine for intractable hiccups. *Neurology* 1990;40:531-32

228 Mukhopadhyay P, et al. Nifedipine for intractable hiccups. *N Engl J Med* 1986;314:1256

229 Quigley C. Nifedipine for hiccups (letter). *J Pain Symptom Manage* 1997;13:313

230 McKeogh M. Dexamethasone for intractable hiccoughs in a patient with AIDS and PML (letter). *Palliat Med* 1994;8:337-8

231 De Ruysscher D, Spaas P, Specenier P. Treatment of intractable hiccup in a terminal cancer patient with nebulized saline (letter). *Palliat Med* 1996;10:166-67

232 Ives TJ, et al. Treatment of intractable hiccups with intramuscular haloperidol. *Am J Psychiatry* 1985;142:1368-69.^

233 Wilcock A, Twycross R. Midazolam for intractable hiccup. *J Pain Symptom Manage* 1996;12:59-61.^

234 Jacobson PL, Messenheimer JA, Farmer TW. Treatment of intractable hiccups

with valproic acid. *Neurology* 1981;31:1458-60

235 McFarling DA, Susac JO. Letter: Carbamazepine for hiccoughs. *JAMA* 1974;230:962

236 Davis JN. Diphenylhydantoin for hiccups (letter). *Lancet* 1974;1:985-87

237 Petroski D, Patel AN. Diphenylhydantoin for intractable hiccups (letter). *Lancet* 1974;1:724-28

238 Kissel P, Royer R, Vicari F. (Amitriptyline in the therapy of hiccup). *Bull Mem Soc Med Hop Paris* 1967;118:849-54

239 Parvin R, et al. Amitriptyline for intractable hiccup (letter). *Am J Gastroenterol* 1988;83:1007-08

240 Peabody CA, et al. Intractable hiccups treated with amitriptyline (letter). *Am J Psychiatry* 1988;145:1036-37

241 Stalnikowicz R, Fich A, Troudart T. Amitriptyline for intractable hiccups. *N Engl J Med* 1986;315:64-65

242 Teodorowicz J, Zimny M. The effect of ketamine in patients with refractory hiccup in the postoperative period. Preliminary report. *Anaesth Resusc Intensive Ther* 1975;3:271-72.[A]

243 Shantha TR. Ketamine for the treatment of hiccups during and following anesthesia: a preliminary report. *Anesth Analg* 1973;52:822-24

244 Tavakoli M, Corssen G. Control of hiccups by ketamine: a preliminary report. *Ala J Med Sci* 1974;11:229-30

245 Finch JW. Rapid control of persistent hiccups by orphenadrine citrate. *Med Times* 1966;94:485-88

246 Askenasy JJ, Boiangiu M, Davidovitch S. Persistent hiccup cured by amantadine (letter). *N Engl J Med* 1988;318:71-76

247 Duffy MC, et al. Hiccough relief with cisapride (letter). *Lancet* 1992;340:121-24

248 Gregory GA, Way WL. Methylphenidate for the treatment of hiccups during anesthesia. *Anesthesiology* 1969;31:89-90

249 Macris SG, Gregory GA, Way WL. Methylphenidate for hiccups. *Anesthesiology* 1971;34:200-01

250 Nathan MD, Leshner RT, Keller AP. Intractable hiccups. *Laryngoscope* 1980;90:1612-18.[A]

251 Gardner AMN. Glucagon stops hiccups. *Br Med J* 1985;290:822

252 Gilston A. Nikethamide for hiccough (letter). *Anaesthesia* 1979;34:1059-62

253 Li X, Yi J, Qi B. Treatment of hiccough with auriculo-acupuncture and auriculo-pressure: a report of 85 cases. *J Tradit Chin Med* 1990;10:257-59

254 Li F, Wang D, Ma X. Treatment of hiccoughs with auriculoacupuncture. *J Tradit Chin Med* 1991;11:14-16

255 Wong SK. Treatment of hiccough by acupuncture (letter). *Med J Malaysia* 1983;38:80-81

256 Yan LS. Treatment of persistent hiccupping with electro-acupuncture at "hiccup-relieving" point. *J Tradit Chin Med* 1988;8:29-30

257 Zhao CX. Acupuncture and moxibustion treatment of hiccup. *J Tradit Chin Med* 1989;9:182-83

258 Fesmire FM. Termination of intractable hiccups with digital rectal massage (letter). *Ann Emerg Med* 1988;17:868-73

259 Odeh M, Bassan H, Oliven A. Termination of intractable hiccups with digital rectal massage. *J Intern Med* 1990;227:145-46.[A]

260 Fodstad H, Blom S. Phrenic nerve stimulation (diaphragm pacing) in chronic singultus. *Neurochirurgia (Stuttg)* 1984;27:115-16.[A]

261 Fodstad H. The Swedish experience in phrenic nerve stimulation. *PACE* 1987;10:246-51.[A]

262 Kolodzik PW, Eilers MA. Hiccups (singultus): review and approach to management. *Ann Emerg Med* 1991;20:565-73.[A]

263 Rousseau P. Hiccups in terminal disease. *Am J Hosp Palliat Care* 1994;11:7-10

264 Bobele M. Nonmedical management of intractible hiccups: a brief review of the literature. *Psychol Rep* 1987;61:225-26

265 Souadjian JV, Cain JC. Intractable hiccup: etiologic factors in 220 cases. *Postgrad Med J* 1968;43:72-77

266 Bhargava RP, Datta S, Badgaiya R. A simple technique to stop hiccups (letter). *Indian J Physiol Pharmacol* 1985;29:57-58

267 Engleman EG, Lankton J, Lankton B. Granulated sugar as treatment for hiccups in conscious patients. *N Engl J Med* 1971;285:1467-70

268 Faught W, et al. Peritoneovenous shunt for palliation of gynecologic malignant ascites. *J Am Coll Surg* 1995;180:472-4.[A]

269 Schumacher DL, Saclarides TJ, Staren ED. Peritoneovenous shunts for palliation

of the patient with malignant ascites. *Ann Surg Oncol* 1994;1:378-81.^

270 Soderlund C. Denver peritoneovenous shunting for malignant or cirrhotic ascites. A prospective consecutive series. *Scand J Gastroenterol* 1986;21:1161-72.^

271 Greenway B, Johnson PJ, Williams R. Control of malignant ascites with spironolactone. *Br J Surg* 1982;69:441-42

272 Arroyo V, Gines P, Planas R. Treatment of ascites in cirrhosis. Diuretics, peritoneovenous shunt, and large-volume paracentesis. *Gastroenterol Clin North Am* 1992;21:237-56.^

273 De Simone GG. Treatment of malignant ascites. *Prog Paliat Care* 1999;7:10-16

274 Fogel MR, et al. Diuresis in the ascitic patient: a randomized controlled trial of three regimens. *J Clin Gastroenterol* 1981;3(S1):73-80.^

275 Amiel SA, Blackburn AM, Rubens RD. Intravenous infusion of frusemide as treatment for ascites in malignant disease. *Br Med J* 1984;288:1041

276 Lee A, Lau TN, Yeong KY. Indwelling catheters for the management of malignant ascites. *Support Care Cancer* 2000;8:493-99.^

277 Sabatelli FW, et al. Permanent indwelling peritoneal access device for the management of malignant ascites. *Cardiovasc Intervent Radiol* 1994;17:292-4.^

278 Mackey JR, et al. A phase II trial of triamcinolone hexacetanide for symptomatic recurrent malignant ascites. *J Pain Symptom Manage* 2000;19:193-9.^

279 Cairns W, Malone R. Octreotide as an agent for the relief of malignant ascites in palliative care patients. *Palliat Med* 1999;13:429-30

280 Mahler F, Rapin CH, MacGee W. Corynebacterium Parvum as palliative treatment in malignant ascites. *J Palliat Care* 1988;4:58-62

281 Currie JL, et al. Intracavitary Corynebacterium parvum for treatment of malignant effusions. *Gynecol Oncol* 1983;16:6-14

282 Webb HE, Oaten SW, Pike CP. Treatment of malignant ascitic and pleural effusions with Corynebacterium parvum. *Br Med J* 1978;1:338-40

283 Twycross RG, Lack S. *Control of alimentary symptoms in far advanced cancer.* London: Churchill Livingstone, 1986.

284 Lee KA, et al. Management of malignant pleural effusions with pleuroperitoneal shunting. *J Am Coll Surg* 1994;178:586-8.^

285 McNamara P. Paracentesis - an effective method of symptom control in the palliative care setting? *Palliat Med* 2000;14:62-4

286 Sharma S, Walsh D. Management of symptomatic malignant ascites with diuretics: two case reports and a review of the literature (Review). *J Pain Symptom Manage* 1995;10:237-42.^

287 Henry DA, O'Connell DL. Effects of fibrinolytic inhibitors on mortality from upper gastrointestinal haemorrhage. *Br Med J* 1989;298:1142-6.^

288 Von Holstein CC, Eriksson SB, Kallen R. Tranexamic acid as an aid to reducing blood transfusion requirements in gastric and duodenal bleeding. *Br Med J* 1987;294:7-10.^

289 Biggs JC, Hugh TB, Dodds AJ. Tranexamic acid and upper gastrointestinal haemorrhage: a double blind trial. *Gut* 1976;17:729-34

290 Barer D, et al. Cimetidine and tranexamic acid in the treatment of acute upper gastrointestinal tract bleeding. *N Engl J Med* 1983;308:1571-75

291 Brown C, Rees WDW. Drug treatment for acute upper gastrointestinal bleeding. *Br Med J* 1992;304:135-36

292 McCormick PA, Ooi H, Crosbie O. Tranexamic acid for severe bleeding gastric antral vascular ectasia in cirrhosis. *Gut* 1998;42:750-2.^

293 Gonzales-Rosales F, et al. Chronic bleeding secondary to an unresectable duodenal adenocarcinoma controlled with sucralfate and famotidine (letter). *Palliat Med* 1998;12:205-6

294 Grover N, Johnson A. Aminocaproic acid used to control upper gastrointestinal bleeding in radiation gastritis. *Dig Dis Sci* 1997;42:982-4

295 Dean A, Tuffin P. Fibrinolytic inhibitors for cancer-associated bleeding problems. *J Pain Symptom Manage* 1997;13:20-4.^

296 Broadley KE, et al. The role of embolization in palliative care. *Palliat Med* 1995;9:331-5.^

297 Riley J. The role of embolization in palliative care (letter). *Palliat Med* 1996;10:168

298 McQuillan RE, et al. Use of embolization in palliative care (letter; comment). *Palliat Med* 1996;10:167-8

299 Phillips-Hughes J. The role of embolisation in the treatment of bleeding tumours. *Palliat Care Today* 1997;5:50-52

300 Reuter SR, Chuang VP, Bree RL. Selective arterial embolization for control of massive upper gastrointestinal bleeding. *Am J Roentgenol* 1975;125:119-26.^

301 Khoursheed M, Crotch-Harvey MA, Gould DA. Embolization in the palliation of

complications of inoperable primary pancreatic neoplasms. *Clin Radiol* 1994;49:784-6.[A]

302 Regnard CFB. Palliation of gastric carcinoma haemorrhage with sucralfate (letter). *Palliat Med* 1990;4:329-30

303 Tryba M, May B. Acute treatment of severe haemorrhagic gastritis with high dose sucralfate (letter). *Lancet* 1988;ii:1304

304 Avgerinos A, Armonis A, Raptis S. Somatostatin and octreotide in the management of acute variceal hemorrhage. *Hepato-Gastroenterology* 1995;42:145-50.[A]

305 Chakravarty BJ, Riley JW. Control of colonic variceal haemorrhage with a somatostatin analogue. *J Gastroenterol Hepatol* 1996;11:305-6.[A]

306 Davis WC, Kelly DM. Home infusion of vasopressin for gastrointestinal bleeding. *Am J Health Syst Pharm* 1997;54:2230-1

307 Hanisch E, Doertenbach J, Usadel KH. Somatostatin in acute bleeding oesophageal varices. Pharmacology and rationale for use. *Drugs* 1992;44(S2):24-35;70-2.[A]

308 Christiansen J, Ottenjann R, Von Arx F. Placebo-controlled trial with the somatostatin analogue SMS 201-995 in peptic ulcer bleeding. *Gastroenterology* 1989;97:568-74.[A]

309 Gagnon B, et al. Palliative management of bleeding events in advanced cancer patients. *J Palliat Care* 1998;14:50-4

310 Gurzo M, et al. (Therapeutic possibilities in the management of gastrointestinal bleeding in thrombocytopenic patients). *Orvosi Hetilap* 1994;135:805-8.[A]

311 Bjarnason I, et al. Side effects of nonsteroidal anti-inflammatory drugs on the small and large intestine in humans. *Gastroenterology* 1993;104:1832-47

312 Davies NM. Toxicity of nonsteroidal anti-inflammatory drugs in the large intestine. *Dis Colon Rectum* 1995;38:1311-21

313 Wells I. Internal iliac artery embolization in the management of pelvic bleeding (editorial; comment). *Clin Radiol* 1996;51:825-7

314 Sasai T, et al. Treatment of chronic post-radiation proctitis with oral administration of sucralfate. *Am J Gastroenterol* 1998;93:1593-5.[A]

315 Kawagoe K, Kawana T. (Intravesical or intrarectal instillation of maalox for the treatment of radiation cystitis or proctitis). *Nippon Gan Chiryo Gakkai Shi* 1989;24:1545-50.[A]

316 McElligott E, Quigley C, Hanks GW. Tranexamic acid and rectal bleeding (letter). *Lancet* 1991;337:431-32

317 Kochhar R, et al. Natural history of late radiation proctosigmoiditis treated with topical sucralfate suspension. *Dig Dis Sci* 1999;44:973-8.[A]

318 Paes TRF, et al. Alum solution in the control of intractable haemorrhage from advanced rectal carcinoma. *Br J Surg* 1986;73:192

319 Mercadante S, et al. Gastrointestinal bleeding in advanced cancer patients (letter). *J Pain Symptom Manage* 2000;19:160-2

320 Brunner G, et al. Optimizing the intragastric pH as a supportive therapy in upper GI bleeding. *Yale J Biol Med* 1996;69:225-31.[A]

321 Lau JY, et al. Effect of intravenous omeprazole on recurrent bleeding after endoscopic treatment of bleeding peptic ulcers. *N Engl J Med* 2000;343:310-6.[A]

322 Barkun AN, et al. Review article: acid suppression in non-variceal acute upper gastrointestinal bleeding. *Aliment Pharmacol Ther* 1999;13:1565-84.[A]

323 Schonhofer PS, Werner B, Troger U. Ocular damage associated with proton pump inhibitors. *Br Med J* 1997;314:1805

324 Riordan-Eva P, Sanders MD. Omeprazole and ocular damage. Facts of cases are unclear (letter). *Br Med J* 1998;316:67,68

325 Lund JN, Scholefield JH. A randomised, prospective, double-blind, placebo-controlled trial of glyceryl trinitrate ointment in treatment of anal fissure (published erratum appears in Lancet 1997 Mar 1;349(9052):656). *Lancet* 1997;349:11-4.[A]

326 Coperchini ML, Kreeger LC. Postural hypotension from topical glyceryl trinitrate ointment for anal pain (letter). *J Pain Symptom Manage* 1997;14:263-4

327 Glyceryl trinitrate for anal fissure? *DTB* 1998;36:55-56

328 Hagen NA. Sharp, shooting neuropathic pain in the rectum or genitals: pudendal neuralgia (editorial). *J Pain Symptom Manage* 1993;8:496

329 Hanks GW. Opioid-responsive and opioid-non-responsive pain in cancer. *British Medical Bulletin* 1991;47:718-31.[A]

330 McLoughlin R, McQuillan R. Using nifedipine to treat tenesmus (letter). *Palliat Med* 1997;11:419-20

331 Bristow A, Foster JMG. Lumbar sympathectomy in the management of rectal tenesmoid pain. *Ann R Coll Surg Engl* 1988;70:38-39.[A]

332 Hunt RW. The palliation of tenesmus. *Palliat Med* 1991;5:352-53

333 Mercadante S, Fulfaro F, Dabbene M. Methadone in treatment of tenesmus not responding to morphine escalation. *Support Care Cancer* 2001;9:129-30

334 Gevers AM, et al. Endoscopic laser therapy for palliation of patients with distal colorectal carcinoma: analysis of factors influencing long-term outcome. *Gastrointest Endosc* 2000;51:580-5.^

335 Birnbaum PL, Mercer CD. Laser fulguration for palliation of rectal tumours. *Can J Surg* 1990;33:299-301.^

336 Krajnik M, et al. Potential uses of topical opioids in palliative care - report of 6 cases. *Pain* 1999;80:121-5.^

337 Rich A, Ellershaw E. Tenesmus / rectal pain - how is it best managed? *CME Bulletin Palliat Med* 2000;2:41-44

338 Ozcan M, et al. Sucralfate for posttonsillectomy analgesia. *Otolaryngol Head Neck Surg* 1998;119:700-4.^

339 Jacobson JM, et al. Thalidomide in low intermittent doses does not prevent recurrence of human immunodeficiency virus-associated aphthous ulcers. *J Infect Dis* 2001;183:343-46.^

340 Henriquet F, et al. Thalidomide in oral aphthous ulceration in patients with HIV infection (letter). *Palliat Med* 1994;8:255-6

341 Jackson IK, Chambers MS, Lipman AG. Oral mucosal problems in palliative care patients. *J Pharm Care Pain Symptom Control* 2000;8:143-61.^

342 Oneschuk D, Hanson J, Bruera E. A survey of mouth pain and dryness in patients with advanced cancer. *Support Care Cancer* 2000;8:372-76.^

343 Turhal NS, Erdal S, Karacay S. Efficacy of treatment to relieve mucositis-induced discomfort. *Support Care Cancer* 2000;8:55-8.^

344 Regnard C. Single dose fluconazole versus five-day ketoconazole in oral candidosis (abstract). *Palliat Med* 1994;8:72-73

345 Finlay IG. Oral symptoms and candida in the terminally ill. *Br Med J* 1986;292:592-93

346 Finlay I. Oral fungal infections. *Eur J Palliat Care* 1995;2:4-7

347 OICPC therapeutic highlights: Mouth care. *Prog Palliat Care* 2000;8:276-77

348 Clarkson JE, Worthington HV, Eden OB. *Interventions for preventing oral mucositis or oral candidiasis for patients with cancer receiving chemotherapy (excluding head and neck cancer) (Cochrane Review).* In: The Cochrane Library, Issue 3, 2000. (http://hiru.mcmaster.ca/cochrane, accessed 5 Dec 2000)

349 Davies NM, et al. Clinical pharmacokinetics and pharmacodynamics of celecoxib: a selective cyclo-oxygenase-2 inhibitor. *Clin Pharmacokinet* 2000;38:225-42.^

350 Ball K, et al. Fluconazole sensitivities of Candida species isolated from the mouths of terminally ill cancer patients. *Am J Hosp Palliat Care* 1998;15:315-9.^

351 Johnson EM, et al. Itraconazole susceptibilities of fluconazole susceptible and resistant isolates of five Candida species. *J Antimicrob Chemother* 1995;36:787-93

352 White ID, et al. Morphine and dryness of the mouth. *Br Med J* 1989;298:1222-3

353 Mercadante S, et al. The use of pilocarpine in opioid-induced xerostomia. *Palliat Med* 2000;14:529-31

354 Wiseman LR, Faulds D. Oral pilocarpine: a review of its pharmacological properties and clinical potential in xerostomia. *Drugs* 1995;49:143-55.^

355 Blom M, Dawidson I, Angmar-Mansson B. The effect of acupuncture on salivary flow rates in patients with xerostomia. *Oral Surg Oral Med Oral Pathol* 1992;73:293-8.^

356 Rydholm M, Strang P. Acupuncture for patients in hospital-based home care suffering from xerostomia. *J Palliat Care* 1999;15:20-3.^

357 Cooke C, Ahmedzai S, Mayberry J. Xerostomia - a review. *Palliat Med* 1996;10:284-92.^

358 Holmes S. Xerostomia: aetiology and management in cancer patients. *Support Care Cancer* 1998;6:348-55.^

359 Sweeney MP, et al. Clinical trial of a mucin-containing oral spray for treatment of xerostomia in hospice patients. *Palliat Med* 1997;11:225-32.^

360 Davies AN. A comparison of artificial saliva and chewing gum in the management of xerostomia in patients with advanced cancer. *Palliat Med* 2000;14:197-203.^

361 Davies AN, et al. A comparison of artificial saliva and pilocarpine in the management of xerostomia in patients with advanced cancer. *Palliat Med* 1998;12:105-11.^

362 Stone P, A'Hern R. Artificial saliva versus pilocarpine for xerostomia (letter). *Palliat Med* 1999;13:81-3

363 Mandel L, Tamari K. Sialorrhea and gastroesophageal reflux. *JADA*

1995;126:1537-41

364 Rashid H, Long JD, Wadleigh RG. Management of secretions in esophageal cancer patients with glycopyrrolate. *Ann Oncol* 1997;8:198-9.[A]

365 Brodtkorb E, et al. Transdermal scopolamine in drooling. *Journal Of Mental Deficiency Research* 1988;32 (Pt 3):233-7.[A]

366 Talmi YP, et al. Reduction of salivary flow with Scopoderm TTS. *Ann Otol Rhinol Laryngol* 1988;97:128-30.[A]

367 Dreyfuss P, Vogel D, Walsh N. The use of transdermal scopolamine to control drooling. A case report. *Am J Phys Med Rehabil* 1991;70:220-2.[A]

368 Blasco PA, Stansbury JC. Glycopyrrolate treatment of chronic drooling. *Arch Pediatr Adolesc Med* 1996;150:932-5.[A]

369 Lucas V, Amass C. Use of enteral glycopyrrolate in the management of drooling (letter). *Palliat Med* 1998;12:207-8

370 Palliative Care Formulary bulletin-board (communication). 2001. (http://www.palliativedrugs.com)

371 Newall AR, Orser R, Hunt M. The control of oral secretions in bulbar ALS/MND. *J Neurol Sci* 1996;139S:43-4.[A]

372 Zeppetella G. Nebulized scopolamine in the management of oral dribbling: three case reports. *J Pain Symptom Manage* 1999;17:293-5.[A]

373 Doyle J, Walker P, Bruera E. Nebulized scopolamine (letter). *J Pain Symptom Manage* 2000;19:327-8

374 Lucas V, Schofield L. Clinical management. Treatment of drooling. *Eur J Palliat Care* 2000;7:5-7

375 Mirakhur RK, Dundee JW, Jones CJ. Evaluation of the anticholinergic actions of glycopyrronium bromide. *Br J Clin Pharmacol* 1978;5:77-84

376 Spiegel D, Sands S, Koopman C. Pain and depression in patients with cancer. *Cancer* 1994;74:2570-8.[A]

377 *Control of pain in patients with cancer*, No. 44. Edinburgh: Scottish Intercollegiate Guidelines Network (SIGN), 2000. (http://www.sign.ac.uk/guidelines)

378 Hanks GW, et al. Morphine and alternative opioids in cancer pain: the EAPC recommendations. *Br J Cancer* 2001;84:587-93.[A]

379 Caraceni A, Portenoy RK. Pain management in patients with pancreatic carcinoma. *Cancer* 1996;78:639-53.[A]

380 Hanna M, et al. The use of coeliac plexus blockade in patients with chronic pain. *Palliat Med* 1990;4:11-16

381 Prasanna A. Unilateral celiac plexus block. *J Pain Symptom Manage* 1996;11:154-7.[A]

382 Khojasteh A, et al. Roles of steroidal and nonsteroidal coanalgesics in management of cancer pain (Meeting abstract). *Proc Annu Meet Am Soc Clin Oncol* 1993;12.[A]

383 McDonnell F, Walsh D. Treatment of odynophagia and dysphagia in advanced cancer with sublingual glyceryl trinitrate. *Palliat Med* 1999;13:251-2

384 Rainer TH, et al. Cost effectiveness analysis of intravenous ketorolac and morphine for treating pain after limb injury: double blind randomised controlled trial. *Br Med J* 2000;321:1247-51.[A]

385 Clark AJ, Simpsom KH, Ellis FR. Continuous brachial plexus blockade in the management of intractable cancer pain in the arm. *Palliat Med* 1990;4:123-26

386 Amesbury B, O'Riordan J, Dolin S. The use of interpleural analgesia using bupivacaine for pain relief in advanced cancer. *Palliat Med* 1999;13:153-8.[A]

387 Irick N, Hostetter MB. Interpleural analgesia for analgesia due to metastatic lung cancer. *J Pharm Care Pain Symptom Control* 2000;8:61-67.[A]

388 Myers DP, et al. Interpleural analgesia for the treatment of severe cancer pain in terminally ill patients. *J Pain Symptom Manage* 1993;8:505-10.[A]

389 De Conno F, et al. Subcutaneous octreotide in the treatment of pain in advanced cancer patients. *J Pain Symptom Manage* 1994;9:34-8.[A]

390 Murakami R, et al. Short communication: the value of embolization therapy in painful osseous metastases from hepatocellular carcinomas; comparative study with radiation therapy. *Br J Radiol* 1996;69:1042-4.[A]

391 Lonroth H, Hyltander A, Lundell L. Unilateral left-sided thoracoscopic sympathectomy for visceral pain control: a pilot study. *Eur J Surg* 1997;163:97-100.[A]

392 Hidderley M, Weinel E. Effects of TENS applied to acupuncture points distal to a pain site. *Int J Palliat Nurs* 1997;3:185-91.[A]

393 Filshie J. Clinical management. Acupuncture in palliative care. *Eur J Palliat Care* 2000;7:41-4

394 Principles of pain control in palliative care for adults. *J R Coll Physicians Lond*

2000;34:350-52

395 *Guidelines for managing cancer pain in adults*: National Council for Hospice and Specialist Palliative Care, 1994.

396 World Health Organisation. *Cancer pain relief*. Geneva: WHO, 1986.

397 *Pain*. In: National Cancer Institute CancerNet PDQ database, 2000. (http://cancernet.nci.nih.gov/pdq/, accessed 9 Dec 2000)

398 Williams J. Clinical management. Critical appraisal of invasive therapies used to treat chronic pain and cancer pain. *Eur J Palliat Care* 2000;7:121-5

399 Caraceni A, Portenoy RK. An international survey of cancer pain characteristics and syndromes. IASP Task Force on Cancer Pain. International Association for the Study of Pain. *Pain* 1999;82:263-74.[A]

400 Cohen KL, Harris S. Efficacy and safety of nonsteroidal anti-inflammatory drugs in the therapy of diabetic neuropathy. *Arch Intern Med* 1987;147:1442-4.[A]

401 Dellemijn P. Are opioids effective in relieving neuropathic pain? *Pain* 1999;80:453-62.[A]

402 Cherny NI, et al. Opioid responsiveness of cancer pain syndromes caused by neuropathic or nociceptive mechanisms: a combined analysis of controlled, single-dose studies. *Neurology* 1994;44:857-61.[A]

403 Rowbotham MC, Reisner-Keller LA, Fields HL. Both intravenous lidocaine and morphine reduce the pain of postherpetic neuralgia. *Neurology* 1991;41:1024-8.[A]

404 Sindrup SH, Jensen TS. Efficacy of pharmacological treatments of neuropathic pain: an update and effect related to mechanism of drug action. *Pain* 1999;83:389-400.[A]

405 Sindrup SH, et al. Tramadol relieves pain and allodynia in polyneuropathy: a randomised, double-blind, controlled trial. *Pain* 1999;83:85-90.[A]

406 Harati Y, et al. Double-blind randomized trial of tramadol for the treatment of the pain of diabetic neuropathy. *Neurology* 1998;50:1842-6.[A]

407 Dellemijn PL, Vanneste JA. Randomised double-blind active-placebo-controlled crossover trial of intravenous fentanyl in neuropathic pain. *Lancet* 1997;349:753-8.[A]

408 Dellemijn PL, van Duijn H, Vanneste JA. Prolonged treatment with transdermal fentanyl in neuropathic pain. *J Pain Symptom Manage* 1998;16:220-9.[A]

409 Watson CP, Babul N. Efficacy of oxycodone in neuropathic pain: a randomized trial in postherpetic neuralgia. *Neurology* 1998;50:1837-41.[A]

410 McQuay HJ, et al. Opioid sensitivity of chronic pain: a patient-controlled analgesia method. *Anaesthesia* 1992;47:757-67.[A]

411 Ripamonti C, et al. Continuous subcutaneous infusion of ketorolac in cancer neuropathic pain unresponsive to opioid and adjuvant drugs. A case report. *Tumori* 1996;82:413-5.[A]

412 Dellemijn PL, et al. Medical therapy of malignant nerve pain. A randomised double-blind explanatory trial with naproxen versus slow-release morphine. *Eur J Cancer* 1994;30A:1244-50.[A]

413 McQuay HJ, et al. A systematic review of antidepressants in neuropathic pain. *Pain* 1996;68:217-27.[A]

414 McQuay HJ, Carroll D, Glynn CJ. Dose-response for analgesic effect of amitriptyline in chronic pain. *Anaesthesia* 1993;48:281-85

415 Drug treatment of neuropathic pain. *Drug Ther Bull* 2000;38:89-93

416 Pernia A, et al. Venlafaxine for the treatment of neuropathic pain (letter). *J Pain Symptom Manage* 2000;19:408-10

417 De Boer T. The pharmacologic profile of mirtazepine. *J Clin Psychiatry* 1996;57(S4):19-25

418 Kent JM. SNaRIs, NaSSAs, and NaRIs: new agents for the treatment of depression. *Lancet* 2000;355:911-8.[A]

419 Ritzenthaler BME, Pearson DJ. Efficacy and tolerability of mirtazepine in neuropathic pain (abstract). *Palliat Med* 2000;14:346

420 Brannon GE, Stone KD. The use of mirtazapine in a patient with chronic pain. *J Pain Symptom Manage* 1999;18:382-5.[A]

421 Ventafridda V, et al. Antidepressants increase the bioavailability of morphine in cancer patients (letter). *Lancet* 1987;i:1204

422 Ventafridda V, et al. Studies on the effects of antidepressant drugs on the antinociceptive action of morphine and on plasma morphine in rat and man. *Pain* 1990;43:155-62

423 Eija K, Tiina T, Pertti NJ. Amitriptyline effectively relieves neuropathic pain following treatment of breast cancer. *Pain* 1996;64:293-302.[A]

424 McQuay H, et al. Anticonvulsant drugs for management of pain: a systematic review. *Br Med J* 1995;311:1047-52.[A]

425 Collins SL, et al. Antidepressants and anticonvulsants for diabetic neuropathy and postherpetic neuralgia: A quantitative systematic review. *J Pain Symptom Manage* 2000;20:449-58.[A]

426 Swerdlow M, Cundill JG. Anticonvulsant drugs used in the treatment of lancinating pain. A comparison. *Anaesthesia* 1981;36:1129-32.[A]

427 Hardy JR, et al. A Phase II study to establish the efficacy and toxicity of sodium valproate in patients with cancer-related neuropathic pain. *J Pain Symptom Manage* 2001;21:204-09.[A]

428 Sinnott C, Lord D. The use of clonazepam for pain in advanced cancer (abstract). *Palliat Med* 2000;14:326

429 Devulder J, De Laat M. Lamotrigine in the treatment of chronic refractory neuropathic pain. *J Pain Symptom Manage* 2000;19:398-403.[A]

430 McCleane G. 200 mg daily of lamotrigine has no analgesic effect in neuropathic pain: a randomised, double-blind, placebo controlled trial. *Pain* 1999;83:105-7.[A]

431 Carrieri PB, et al. Efficacy of lamotrigine on sensory symptoms and pain in peripheral neuropathies (letter). *J Pain Symptom Manage* 1999;18:154-6

432 Solaro C, et al. Topiramate relieves idiopathic and symptomatic trigeminal neuralgia. *J Pain Symptom Manage* 2001;21:367-68

433 Bajwa ZH, et al. Topiramate relieves refractory intercostal neuralgia. *Neurology* 1999;52:1917

434 Gilron I, et al. Topiramate in trigeminal neuralgia: a randomized, placebo-controlled multiple crossover pilot study. *Clin Neuropharmacol* 2001;24:109-12.[A]

435 Smith TE, Chong MS. Neuropathic pain. *Hosp Med* 2000;61:760-66

436 Rocafort J, Viguria J. Gabapentin as an analgesic. *Eur J Pall Care* 2001;8:54-57

437 Backonja M, et al. Gabapentin for the symptomatic treatment of painful neuropathy in patients with diabetes mellitus: a randomized controlled trial. *JAMA* 1998;280:1831-6.[A]

438 Rowbotham M, et al. Gabapentin for the treatment of postherpetic neuralgia: a randomized controlled trial. *JAMA* 1998;280:1837-42.[A]

439 Morello CM, et al. Randomized double-blind study comparing the efficacy of gabapentin with amitriptyline on diabetic peripheral neuropathy pain. *Arch Intern Med* 1999;159:1931-7.[A]

440 Rusy LM, Troshynski TJ, Weisman SJ. Gabapentin in phantom limb pain management in children and young adults: Report of seven cases. *J Pain Symptom Manage* 2001;21:78-82.[X]

441 Dallocchio C, et al. Gabapentin vs. amitriptyline in painful diabetic neuropathy: An open- label pilot study. *J Pain Symptom Manage* 2000;20:280-85.[A]

442 Chandler A, Williams JE. Gabapentin, an adjuvant treatment for neuropathic pain in a cancer hospital. *J Pain Symptom Manage* 2000;20:82-86

443 Caraceni A, et al. Gabapentin as an adjuvant to opioid analgesia for neuropathic cancer pain. *J Pain Symptom Manage* 1999;17:441-5.[A]

444 Lossignol DA, et al. Successful treatment of neuropathic cancer pain with gabapentin (abstract). *Support Care Cancer* 2000;8:244

445 Back IN, Finlay IG. *Caudal epidural analgesia in palliative care: a review of case notes*, 2000. (http://clinmed.netprints.org)

446 Jackson MB, et al. Percutaneous cervical cordotomy for the control of pain in patients with pleural mesothelioma. *Thorax* 1999;54:238-41.[A]

447 Stuart G, Cramond T. Role of percutaneous cervical cordotomy for pain of malignant origin. *Med J Aust* 1993;158:667-70.[A]

448 Galer BS, Harle J, Rowbotham MC. Response to intravenous lidocaine infusion predicts subsequent response to oral mexiletine: a prospective study. *J Pain Symptom Manage* 1996;12:161-7.[A]

449 Jarvis B, Coukell AJ. Mexiletine. A review of its therapeutic use in painful diabetic neuropathy. *Drugs* 1998;56:691-707.[A]

450 Wallace MS, Magnuson S, Ridgeway B. Efficacy of oral mexiletine for neuropathic pain with allodynia: a double-blind, placebo-controlled, crossover study. *Reg Anesth Pain Med* 2000;25:459-67.[A]

451 Stracke H, et al. Mexiletine in the treatment of diabetic neuropathy. *Diabetes Care* 1992;15:1550-5.[A]

452 Dunlop R, et al. Analgesic effects of oral flecainide (letter). *Lancet* 1988;i:420-21

453 Sinnott C, et al. Flecainide in cancer nerve pain (letter). *Lancet* 1991;337:1347

454 Hall E. Rectal flecainide (letter). *Palliat Med* 1991;5:352

455 Foster AVM, et al. Application of Opsite film: a new and effective treatment of painful diabetic neuropathy. *Diabetic Medicine* 1994;11:768-72

456 Anghinah R, Oliveira AS, Gabbai AA. Effect of baclofen on pain in diabetic neuropathy (letter). *Muscle & Nerve* 1994;17:958-9

457 Fromm GH, Terrence CF, Chattha AS. Baclofen in the treatment of trigeminal neuralgia: double-blind study and long-term follow-up. *Ann Neurol* 1984;15:240-4.[A]

458 Fromm GH, Terrence CF. Comparison of L-baclofen and racemic baclofen in trigeminal neuralgia. *Neurology* 1987;37:1725-8.[A]

459 Fromm GH. Baclofen as an adjuvant analgesic. *J Pain Symptom Manage* 1994;9:500-09

460 Jefferson M. The use of baclofen for the treatment of postradical neck pain syndrome (abstract). *Palliat Med* 2000;14:330-31

461 Davidsen O, Lindeneg O, Walsh M. Analgesic treatment with levomepromazine in acute myocardial infarction. A randomized clinical trial. *Acta Med Scand* 1979;205:191-4.[A]

462 Pud D, et al. The NMDA receptor antagonist amantadine reduces surgical neuropathic pain in cancer patients: a doble blind, randomized, placebo controlled trial. *Pain* 1998;75:349-54

463 Eisenberg E, Pud D. Can patients with chronic neuropathic pain be cured by acute administration of the NMDA receptor antagonist amantadine? *Pain* 1998;74:337-9.[A]

464 Medrik-Goldberg T, et al. Intravenous lidocaine, amantadine, and placebo in the treatment of sciatica: a double-blind, randomized, controlled study. *Reg Anesth Pain Med* 1999;24:534-40.[A]

465 McCleane G. Topical application of doxepin hydrochloride, capsaicin and a combination of both produces analgesia in chronic human neuropathic pain: a randomized, double-blind, placebo-controlled study. *Br J Clin Pharmacol* 2000;49:574-9.[A]

466 Glynn C. An approach to the management of the patient with deafferentation pain. *Palliat Med* 1989;3:13-21

467 Max MB, et al. Association of pain relief with drug side effects in postherpetic neuralgia: a single-dose study of clonidine, codeine, ibuprofen, and placebo. *Clin Pharmacol Ther* 1988;43:363-71.[A]

468 Dickson RJ, Russell PSB. Pain unresponsive to high dose opiate drugs. *Palliat Med* 1989;3:61-64

469 Zeigler D, et al. Transdermal clonidine versus placebo in painful diabetic neuropathy. *Pain* 1992;48:403-8.[A]

470 Davis KD, et al. Topical application of clonidine relieves hyperalgesia in patients with sympathetically maintained pain. *Pain* 1991;47:309-17.[A]

471 Bernard JM, Kick O, Bonnet F. Comparison of intravenous and epidural clonidine for postoperative patient-controlled analgesia. *Anesth Analg* 1995;81:706-12.[A]

472 Cohen KL, Lucibello FE, Chomiak M. Lack of effect of clonidine and pentoxifylline in short-term therapy of diabetic peripheral neuropathy. *Diabetes Care* 1990;13:1074-7.[A]

473 Watson CP. Topical capsaicin as an adjuvant analgesic. *J Pain Symptom Manage* 1994;9:425-33.[A]

474 McQuay HJ, et al. Dextromethorphan for the treatment of neuropathic pain: a double-blind randomised controlled crossover trial with integral n-of-1 design. *Pain* 1994;59:127-33.[A]

475 Mercadante S, Casuccio A, Genovese G. Ineffectiveness of dextromethorphan in cancer pain. *J Pain Symptom Manage* 1998;16:317-22.[A]

476 Campbell FA, et al. Are cannabinoids an effective and safe treatment option in the management of pain. *Br Med J* 2001;323:13-16

477 Aston H. Cannabis in palliative care. *CME Bulletin Palliat Med* 1999;1:73-77

478 Kopf A, Ruf W. Novel drugs for neuropathic pain. *Curr Opin Anaesthesiol* 2000;13:577-83.[A]

479 Quigley C. New approaches to the management of neuropathic pain. *CME Bulletin Palliat Med* 2000;2:35-40

480 Woolf CJ, Mannion RJ. Neuropathic pain: aetiology, symptoms, mechanisms, and management. *Lancet* 1999;353:1959-64.[A]

481 Sinnott C. Neuropathic pain. *CME Bulletin Palliat Med* 1998;1:7-9

482 Back IN. *The management of neuropathic pain: questionnaire on the treatment choices of palliative medicine physicians.* 2000. (http://clinmed.netprints.org)

483 O'Reilly M. Clinical management. The role of anticonvulsants in palliative care. *Eur J Palliat Care* 1997;4:7-11

484 Kingery WS. A critical review of controlled clinical trials for peripheral neuropathic pain and complex regional pain syndromes. *Pain* 1997;73:123-39.[A]

485 Tremont-Lukats IW, Megeff C, Backonja MM. Anticonvulsants for neuropathic pain syndromes: mechanisms of action and place in therapy. *Drugs*

2000;60:1029-52.[A]

486 Wiffen P, et al. *Anticonvulsant drugs for acute and chronic pain (Cochrane Review)*. In: The Cochrane Library, Issue 3, 2000. (http://hiru.mcmaster.ca/cochrane, accessed 5 Dec 2000)

487 Oles KS, Mirza W, Penry JK. Catastrophic neurologic signs due to drug interaction: Tegretol and Darvon. *Surg Neurol* 1989;32:144-51.[A]

488 Yu YL, et al. Interaction between carbamazepine and dextropropoxyphene. *Postgrad Med J* 1986;62:231-3.[A]

489 Sang CN. NMDA-receptor antagonists in neuropathic pain: experimental methods to clinical trials. *J Pain Symptom Manage* 2000;19:S21-5.[A]

490 Hewitt DJ. The use of NMDA-receptor antagonists in the treatment of chronic pain. *Clin J Pain* 2000;16:S73-S79.[A]

491 Crosby V, Wilcock A, Corcoran R. The safety and efficacy of a single dose (500 mg or 1 g) of intravenous magnesium sulfate in neuropathic pain poorly responsive to strong opioid analgesics in patients with cancer. *J Pain Symptom Manage* 2000;19:35-9.[A]

492 Mannix K, et al. Using bisphosphonates to control the pain of bone metastases: Evidence-based guidelines for palliative care. *Palliat Med* 2000;14:455-61.[A]

493 Groff L, et al. The role of disodium pamidronate in the management of bone pain due to malignancy. *Palliat Med* 2001;15:297-307

494 Quilty PM, et al. A comparison of the palliative effects of strontium-89 and external beam radiotherapy in metastatic prostate cancer. *Radiother Oncol* 1994;31:33-40.[A]

495 Dearnaley DP, et al. Palliation of bone metastases in prostate cancer. Hemibody irradiation or strontium-89? *Clin Oncol* 1992;4:101-7.[A]

496 Rowell NP. Intralesional methylprednisolone for rib metastases: an alternative to radiotherapy? *Palliat Med* 1988;2:153-55

497 Mystakidou K, et al. Continuous subcutaneous administration of high-dose salmon calcitonin in bone metastasis: pain control and beta-endorphin plasma levels. *J Pain Symptom Manage* 1999;18:323-30.[A]

498 Marcy PY, et al. Percutaneous cementoplasty for pelvic bone metastasis. *Support Care Cancer* 2000;8:500-03.[A]

499 Marcy PY, et al. Erratum: Percutaneous cementoplasty for pelvic bone metastasis (Support Care in Cancer (2000) 8 (500-503)). *Support Care Cancer* 2000;8:510

500 Weill A, et al. Spinal metastases: indications for and results of percutaneous injection of acrylic surgical cement. *Radiology* 1996;199:241-7.[A]

501 Mathis JM, Petri M, Naff N. Percutaneous vertebroplasty treatment of steroid-induced osteoporotic compression fractures. *Arthritis Rheum* 1998;41:171-5.[A]

502 Cotten A, et al. Percutaneous vertebroplasty for osteolytic metastases and myeloma: effects of the percentage of lesion filling and the leakage of methyl methacrylate at clinical follow-up. *Radiology* 1996;200:525-30.[A]

503 Cotten A, et al. Percutaneous vertebroplasty: state of the art. *Radiographics* 1998;18:311-20; discussion 20-3.[A]

504 Cotten A, et al. Malignant acetabular osteolyses: percutaneous injection of acrylic bone cement. *Radiology* 1995;197:307-10.[A]

505 Gangi A, et al. CT-guided interventional procedures for pain management in the lumbosacral spine. *Radiographics* 1998;18:621-33.[A]

506 Weill A, Kobaiter H, Chiras J. Acetabulum malignancies: technique and impact on pain of percutaneous injection of acrylic surgical cement. *Eur Radiol* 1998;8:123-9.[A]

507 Jensen ME, et al. Percutaneous polymethylmethacrylate vertebroplasty in the treatment of osteoporotic vertebral body compression fractures: technical aspects. *Am J Neuroradiol* 1997;18:1897-904.[A]

508 Gangi A, et al. Injection of alcohol into bone metastases under CT guidance. *Journal Of Computer Assisted Tomography* 1994;18:932-5.[A]

509 Van Veldhuizen PJ, et al. Treatment of vitamin D deficiency in patients with metastatic prostate cancer may improve bone pain and muscle strength. *J Urol* 2000;163:187-90.[A]

510 British Association of Surgical Oncology Guidelines. The management of metastatic bone disease in the United Kingdom. The Breast Specialty Group of the British Association of Surgical Oncology. *Eur J Surg Oncol* 1999;25:3-23.[A]

511 Fulfaro F, et al. The role of bisphosphonates in the treatment of painful metastatic bone disease: a review of phase III trials. *Pain* 1998;78:157-69.[A]

512 Shah S, Hardy J. Non-steroidal anti-inflammatory drugs in cancer pain: a review of the literature as relevant to palliative care. *Prog Palliat Care* 2001;9:3-7

513 Mercadante S, et al. Analgesic effects of nonsteroidal anti-inflammatory drugs in

cancer pain due to somatic or visceral mechanisms. *J Pain Symptom Manage* 1999;17:351-6.^

514 Maksymowych WP. Managing acute osteoporotic vertebral fractures with calcitonin. *Canadian Family Physician* 1998;44:2160-66

515 Ernst DS, et al. A double-blind, crossover trial of intravenous clodronate in metastatic bone pain. *J Pain Symptom Manage* 1992;7:4-11.^

516 Ernst DS, et al. A randomized, controlled trial of intravenous clodronate in patients with metastatic bone disease and pain. *J Pain Symptom Manage* 1997;13:319-26.^

517 Cascinu S, et al. Different doses of pamidronate in patients with painful osteolytic bone metastases. *Support Care Cancer* 1998;6:139-43.^

518 Aeschlimann JR, Tyler LS. Drug interactions associated with cytochrome P-450 enzymes. *J Pharm Care Pain Symptom Control* 1996;4:35-53

519 Wolf CR, Smith G, Smith RL. Science, medicine, and the future: Pharmacogenetics. *Br Med J* 2000;320:987-90

520 Sindrup SH, Brosen K. The pharmacogenetics of codeine hypoalgesia. *Pharmacogenetics* 1995;5:335-46.^

521 Dayer P, Desmeules J, Striberni R. In vitro forecasting of drugs that may interfere with codeine bioactivation. *Eur J Drug Metab Pharmacokinet* 1992;17:115-20.^

522 Tegeder I, Lotsch J, Geisslinger G. Pharmacokinetics of opioids in liver disease. *Clin Pharmacokinet* 1999;37:17-40.^

523 Li Wan Po A, Zhang WY. Systematic overview of co-proxamol to assess analgesic effects of addition of dextropropoxyphene to paracetamol. *Br Med J* 1997;315:1565-71.^

524 Hanks GW, Forbes K. Co-proxamol is effective in chronic pain (letter). *Br Med J* 1998;316:1980

525 Co-proxamol or paracetamol for acute pain? *Drug Ther Bull* 1998;36:80

526 Ebert B, et al. Dextropropoxyphene acts as a noncompetitive N-methyl-D-aspartate antagonist. *J Pain Symptom Manage* 1998;15:269-74.^

527 Twycross RG, et al. OICPC Therapeutic Highlights: Paracetamol. *Prog Palliat Care* 2000;8:198-202

528 De Craen AJM, et al. Analgesic efficacy and safety of paracetamol-codeine combinations versus paracetamol alone: a systematic review. *Br Med J* 1996;313:321-25

529 Hylek EM, et al. Acetaminophen and other risk factors for excessive warfarin anticoagulation. *JAMA* 1998;279:657-62.^

530 Amato MG, et al. Acetaminophen and risk factors for excess anticoagulation with warfarin (letter). *JAMA* 1998;280:695-6; discussion 97

531 Eliason BC, Larson W. Acetaminophen and risk factors for excess anticoagulation with warfarin (letter). *JAMA* 1998;280:696-7

532 Estrada C. Acetaminophen and risk factors for excess anticoagulation with warfarin (letter). *JAMA* 1998;280:695; discussion 97

533 Gray CD. Acetaminophen and risk factors for excess anticoagulation with warfarin (letter). *JAMA* 1998;280:695; discussion 97

534 Pedell L. Acetaminophen and risk factors for excess anticoagulation with warfarin (letter). *JAMA* 1998;280:696; discussion 97

535 Riser J. Acetaminophen and risk factors for excess anticoagulation with warfarin (letter). *JAMA* 1998;280:696; discussion 97

536 Eisenberg E, et al. Efficacy and safety of nonsteroidal antiinflammatory drugs for cancer pain: a meta-analysis. *J Clin Oncol* 1994;12:2756-65.^

537 Stockley IH. *Drug Interactions.* 4th ed. London: Pharmaceutical Press, 1996.

538 Cook ME, et al. Comparative effects of nabumetone, sulindac, and ibuprofen on renal function. *J Rheumatol* 1997;24:1137-44.^

539 Swan SK, et al. Effect of cyclooxygenase-2 inhibition on renal function in elderly persons receiving a low-salt diet. A randomized, controlled trial. *Ann Intern Med* 2000;133:1-9.^

540 Rossat J, et al. Renal effects of selective cyclooxygenase-2 inhibition in normotensive salt-depleted subjects. *Clin Pharmacol Ther* 1999;66:76-84.^

541 Whelton A, et al. Effects of celecoxib and naproxen on renal function in the elderly. *Arch Intern Med* 2000;160:1465-70.^

542 Cheng JC. Nonsteroidal anti-inflammatory drugs and aspirin: a comparison of the antiplatelet effects. *Am J Ther* 1997;4:62-5.^

543 Toscani F, et al. Sodium naproxen: continuous subcutaneous infusion in neoplastic pain control. *Palliat Med* 1989;3:207-11

544 Toscani F. Sodium naproxen: continuous subcutaneous infusion in neoplastic pain control (letter). *Palliat Med* 1990;4:147

545 Hall E. Subcutaneous diclofenac: an effective alternative? (letter). *Palliat Med* 1993;7:339-40

546 Myers KG, Trotman IF. Use of ketorolac by continuous subcutaneous infusion for the control of cancer-related pain. *Postgrad Med J* 1994;70:359-62.[A]

547 Blackwell N, et al. Subcutaneous ketorolac - a new development in pain control. *Palliat Med* 1993;7:63-5.[A]

548 Burns JW, et al. Double-blind comparison of the morphine sparing effect of continuous and intermittent I.M. administration of ketorolac. *Br J Anaesth* 1991;67:235-38

549 Carretta A, et al. Efficacy of ketorolac tromethamine and extrapleural intercostal nerve block on post-thoracotomy pain. A prospective, randomized study. *Int Surg* 1996;81:224-8.[A]

550 De Conno F, et al. Tolerability of ketorolac administered via continuous subcutaneous infusion for cancer pain: a preliminary report. *J Pain Symptom Manage* 1994;9:119-21.[A]

551 Duncan AR, Hardy JR, Davis CL. Subcutaneous ketorolac (letter). *Palliat Med* 1995;9:77-8

552 Gillis JC, Brogden RN. Ketorolac. A reappraisal of its pharmacodynamic and pharmacokinetic properties and therapeutic use in pain management. *Drugs* 1997;53:139-88.[A]

553 Hughes A, Wilcock A, Corcoran R. Ketorolac: continuous subcutaneous infusion for cancer pain (letter). *J Pain Symptom Manage* 1997;13:315-6

554 Joishy SK, Walsh D. The opioid-sparing effects of intravenous ketorolac as an adjuvant analgesic in cancer pain: application in bone metastases and the opioid bowel syndrome. *J Pain Symptom Manage* 1998;16:334-9.[A]

555 Kaynaroglu V, Agalar F. Efficacy of ketorolac tromethamine and extrapleural intercostal nerve block on post-thoracotomy pain (letter). *Int Surg* 1997;82:322

556 Lippmann M, Ginsburg R. Ketorolac for post-thoracotomy pain relief (letter). *Br J Anaesth* 1994;73:281

557 Middleton RK, Lyle JA, Berger DL. Ketorolac continuous infusion: a case report and review of the literature. *J Pain Symptom Manage* 1996;12:190-4.[A]

558 Ribeiro S, Chandler S, Weinstein SM. Safety of chronic use of ketorolac tromethamine for cancer pain (Meeting abstract). *Proc Annu Meet Am Soc Clin Oncol* 1994;13.[A]

559 Staquet MJ. A double-blind study with placebo control of intramuscular ketorolac tromethamine in the treatment of cancer pain. *J Clin Pharmacol* 1989;29:1031-6.[A]

560 Toscani F, et al. Ketorolac versus diclofenac sodium in cancer pain. *Arzneimittelforschung* 1994;44:550-4.[A]

561 Virdee H, et al. Is diamorphine/ketorolac stable? *Pharm Pract* 1997;February:82-83

562 Yalcin S, et al. Ketorolac tromethamine in cancer pain. *Acta Oncol* 1997;36:231-2

563 Reinhart DI. Minimising the adverse effects of ketorolac. *Drug Safety* 2000;22:487-97.[A]

564 Resman-Targoff BH. Ketorolac: a parenteral nonsteroidal antiinflammatory drug. *DICP* 1990;24:1098-104.[A]

565 Litvak KM, McEvoy GK. Ketorolac, an injectable nonnarcotic analgesic. *Clin Pharm* 1990;9:921-35.[A]

566 Moore RA, et al. Quantitative systematic review of topically applied non-steroidal anti-inflammatory drugs. *Br Med J* 1998;316:333-8.[A]

567 Jenkins CA, Bruera E. Nonsteroidal anti-inflammatory drugs as adjuvant analgesics in cancer patients. *Palliat Med* 1999;13:183-96.[A]

568 Shah S, Hardy J. A review of the Cox-2 inhibitors. *Prog Palliat Care* 2001;9:47-52

569 Henry D, et al. Variability in risk of gastrointestinal complications with individual non-steroidal anti-inflammatory drugs: results of a collaborative meta-analysis. *Br Med J* 1996;312:1563-66

570 National Institute for Clinical Excellence. *Guidance on the use of cyclo-oxygenase (Cox) II selective inhibitors, celecoxib, rofecoxib, meloxicam and etodolac for osteoarthritis and rheumatoid arthritis*, 2001. (http://www.nice.org.uk, accessed July 2001)

571 Ventafridda V, et al. Sodium naproxen versus sodium diclofenac in cancer pain control. *Arzneimittelforschung* 1990;40:1132-4.[A]

72 Silverstein FE, et al. Gastrointestinal toxicity with celecoxib vs nonsteroidal anti-inflammatory drugs for osteoarthritis and rheumatoid arthritis: the CLASS study: A randomized controlled trial. Celecoxib Long-term Arthritis Safety Study. *JAMA* 2000;284:1247-55.[A]

73 Leese PT, et al. Effects of celecoxib, a novel cyclooxygenase-2 inhibitor, on

platelet function in healthy adults: a randomized, controlled trial. *J Clin Pharmacol* 2000;40:124-32.[A]

574 Wallace JL. Distribution and expression of cyclooxygenase (COX) isoenzymes, their physiological roles, and the categorization of nonsteroidal anti-inflammatory drugs (NSAIDs). *Am J Med* 1999;107:11S-16S; discussion 16S-17S.[A]

575 Vane SJ. Aspirin and other anti-inflammatory drugs. *Thorax* 2000;55(S2):S3-9

576 Hoskin PJ, Poulain P, Hanks GW. Controlled-release morphine in cancer pain. Is a loading dose required when the formulation is changed? *Anaesthesia* 1989;44:897-901

577 Hagen NA, Elwood T, Ernst S. Cancer pain emergencies: a protocol for management. *J Pain Symptom Manage* 1997;14:45-50.[A]

578 Kumar KS, Rajagopal MR, Naseema AM. Intravenous morphine for emergency treatment of cancer pain. *Palliat Med* 2000;14:183-8.[A]

579 McMichael H. Intravenous titration of opioids in palliative care (abstract). *Palliat Med* 1999;13:506-07

580 Fromm MF, et al. Loss of analgesic effect of morphine due to coadministration of rifampin. *Pain* 1997;72:261-7.[A]

581 Manara AR. The effect of metoclopramide on the absorption of oral controlled release morphine. *Br J Clin Pharmacol* 1988;25:518-21.[A]

582 De Bernardi M, de Bernardi F, Colombo P. Randomised crossover comparison of the pharmacokinetic profiles of two sustained release morphine sulfate formulations in patients with cancer-related pain. *Clin Drug Invest* 1997;14:S28-33

583 Bruera E, et al. Twice-daily versus once-daily morphine sulphate controlled-release suppositories for the treatment of cancer pain. A randomized controlled trial. *Support Care Cancer* 1999;7:280-3.[A]

584 Davis C. A new 24-hour morphine hydrogel suppository. *Eur J Pall Care* 2000;7:165-67

585 Mercadante S, Portenoy RK. Opioid poorly-responsive cancer pain. Part 2. Basic mechanisms that could shift dose response for analgesia. *J Pain Symptom Manage* 2001;21:255-64.[A]

586 Mercadante S, Portenoy RK. Opioid poorly-responsive cancer pain. Part 1: Clinical considerations. *J Pain Symptom Manage* 2001;21:144-50.[A]

587 Fallon MT, O'Neill B. Substitution of another opioid for morphine. Opioid toxicity should be managed initially by decreasing the opioid dose (letter). *Br Med J* 1998;317:81

588 Quevedo F, Walsh D. Morphine-induced ventilatory failure after spinal cord compression. *J Pain Symptom Manage* 1999;18:140-2.[A]

589 Pereira J, Bruera E. Emerging neuropsychiatric toxicities of opioids. *J Pharm-Care Pain Symptom Control* 1997;5:3-29.[A]

590 Potter JM, et al. Myoclonus associated with treatment with high doses of morphine: the role of supplemental drugs. *Br Med J* 1989;299:150-3.[A]

591 Mercadante S. Pathophysiology and treatment of opioid-related myoclonus in cancer patients. *Pain* 1998;74:5-9.[A]

592 Obeso JA. Therapy of myoclonus. *Clin Neurosci* 1995;3:253-7.[A]

593 Eisele JH, Jr., Grigsby EJ, Dea G. Clonazepam treatment of myoclonic contractions associated with high- dose opioids: case report. *Pain* 1992;49:231-2.[A]

594 Mercadante S, Villari P, Fulfaro F. Gabapentin for opioid-related myoclonus in cancer patients. *Support Care Cancer* 2001;9:205-06

595 Heger S, et al. Morphine induced allodynia in a child with brain tumour. *Br Med J* 1999;319:627-9

596 Sjogren P, Jensen NH, Jensen TS. Disappearance of morphine-induced hyperalgesia after discontinuing or substituting morphine with other opioid agonists. *Pain* 1994;59:313-6.[A]

597 Sjogren P, et al. Hyperalgesia and myoclonus in terminal cancer patients treated with continuous intravenous morphine. *Pain* 1993;55:93-7.[A]

598 Bowsher D. Paradoxical pain. When the metabolites of morphine are in the wrong ratio (letter). *Br Med J* 1993;306:473

599 Morley JS, et al. Paradoxical pain. *Lancet* 1992;340:1045

600 Devulder J. Hyperalgesia induced by high-dose intrathecal sufentanil in neuropathic pain. *J Neurosurg Anesthesiol* 1997;9:146-8.[A]

601 Manfredi PL, et al. Inappropriate use of naloxone in cancer patients with pain. *J Pain Symptom Manage* 1996;11:131-4.[A]

602 Slatkin NE, Rhiner M, Bolton TM. Donepezil in the treatment of opioid-induced sedation. *J Pain Symptom Manage* 2001;21:425-38

603 De Stoutz ND, Bruera E, Suarez-Almazor M. Opioid rotation for toxicity reduction

in terminal cancer patients. *J Pain Symptom Manage* 1995;10:378-84.[A]

604 Hawley P, Forbes K, Hanks GW. Opioids, confusion and opioid rotation (letter). *Palliat Med* 1998;12:63-4

605 Sarhill N, Walsh D, Nelson KA. Hydromorphone: pharmacology and clinical applications in cancer patients. *Support Care Cancer* 2001;9:84-96

606 Katcher J, Walsh D. Opioid-induced itching: morphine sulfate and hydromorphone hydrochloride. *J Pain Symptom Manage* 1999;17:70-2.[A]

607 Farrell A, Rich A. Analgesic use in patients with renal failure. *Eur J Pall Care* 2000;7:201-05

608 Fainsinger R, Toro R. Opioids, confusion and opioid rotation. *Palliat Med* 1998;12:463

609 Fallon M. Opioid rotation: does it have a role? (editorial). *Palliat Med* 1997;11:177-8

610 Fallon MT. Rationale for using alternative drugs to morphine. *Palliat Care Today* 2000;9:10,14

611 Morley JS. Opioid rotation: does it have a role? *Palliat Med* 1998;12:464-65

612 Scholes C. The theoretical basis of opioid rotation. *CME Bulletin Palliat Med* 1998;1:13-15

613 Twycross R. Opioid rotation: does it have a role? (letter). *Palliat Med* 1998;12:60-3

614 Mercadante S. Opioid rotation for cancer pain: rationale and clinical aspects. *Cancer* 1999;86:1856-66.[A]

615 Kloke M, et al. Toxicity and/or insufficient analgesia by opioid therapy: Risk factors and the impact of changing the opioid. A retrospective analysis of 273 patients observed at a single center. *Support Care Cancer* 2000;8:479-86.[A]

616 Ashby MA, Martin P, Jackson KA. Opioid substitution to reduce adverse effects in cancer pain management. *Med J Aust* 1999;170:68-71.[A]

617 Murray P. Substitution of another opioid for morphine may be useful for pain control (letter). *Br Med J* 1998;316:702-3

618 Wilder-Smith CH. Opioids in cancer pain - which one is best? *Support Care Cancer* 2001;9:71-72

619 Grond S, et al. High-dose tramadol in comparison to low-dose morphine for cancer pain relief. *J Pain Symptom Manage* 1999;18:174-9.[A]

620 Wilder-Smith CH, et al. Oral tramadol, a mu-opioid agonist and monoamine reuptake-blocker, and morphine for strong cancer-related pain. *Ann Oncol* 1994;5:141-6.[A]

621 Petzke F, et al. Slow-release tramadol for treatment of chronic malignant pain - An open multicenter trial. *Support Care Cancer* 2001;9:48-54.[A]

622 Lewis KS, Han NH. Tramadol: a new centrally acting analgesic. *Am J Health Syst Pharm* 1997;54:643-52.[A]

623 Shah S, Hardy J. Oxycodone: a review of the literature. *Eur J Pall Care* 2001;8:93-96

624 Heiskanen T, Kalso E. Controlled-release oxycodone and morphine in cancer related pain. *Pain* 1997;73:37-45.[A]

625 Bruera E, et al. Randomized, double-blind, cross-over trial comparing safety and efficacy of oral controlled-release oxycodone with controlled-release morphine in patients with cancer pain. *J Clin Oncol* 1998;16:3222-9.[A]

626 Gagnon B, et al. The use of intermittent subcutaneous injections of oxycodone for opioid rotation in patients with cancer pain. *Support Care Cancer* 1999;7:265-70.[A]

627 Maddocks I, et al. Attenuation of morphine-induced delirium in palliative care by substitution with infusion of oxycodone. *J Pain Symptom Manage* 1996;12:182-9.[A]

628 Heiskanen TE, et al. Morphine or oxycodone in cancer pain? *Acta Oncol* 2000;39:941-47.[A]

629 Heiskanen T, Olkkola KT, Kalso E. Effects of blocking CYP2D6 on the pharmacokinetics and pharmacodynamics of oxycodone. *Clin Pharmacol Ther* 1998;64:603-11.[A]

630 Cleary J, et al. The influence of pharmacogenetics on opioid analgesia: studies with codeine and oxycodone in the Sprague-Dawley/Dark Agouti rat model. *J Pharmacol Exp Ther* 1994;271:1528-34

631 Ross FB, Wallis SC, Smith MT. Co-administration of sub-antinociceptive doses of oxycodone and morphine produces marked antinociceptive synergy with reduced CNS side-effects in rats. *Pain* 2000;84:421-8.[A]

632 Lee MA, Leng MEF, Tiernan EJJ. Retrospective study of the use of hydromorphone in palliative care patients with normal and abnormal urea and creatinine. *Palliat Med* 2001;15:26-34.[A]

633 Babul N, Darke AC, Hagen N. Hydromorphone metabolite accumulation in renal

failure (letter). *J Pain Symptom Manage* 1995;10:184-6

634 Parab P, et al. Pharmacokinetics of hydromorphone after intravenous, peroral and rectal administration to human subjects. *Biopharm Drug Dispos* 1988;9:187-99.[A]

635 Lawlor P, et al. Dose ratio between morphine and hydromorphone in patients with cancer pain: a retrospective study. *Pain* 1997;72:79-85.[A]

636 Bruera E, et al. Opioid rotation in patients with cancer pain. A retrospective comparison of dose ratios between methadone, hydromorphone, and morphine. *Cancer* 1996;78:852-7.[A]

637 Dunbar PJ, et al. Clinical analgesic equivalence for morphine and hydromorphone with prolonged PCA. *Pain* 1996;68:265-70.[A]

638 Morphine in cancer pain: modes of administration. Expert Working Group of the European Association for Palliative Care. *Br Med J* 1996;312:823-6

639 Radbruch L, et al. Constipation and the use of laxatives: a comparison between transdermal fentanyl and oral morphine. *Palliat Med* 2000;14:111-9.[A]

640 Haazen L, et al. The constipation-inducing potential of morphine and transdermal fentanyl. *Eur J Pain* 1999;3:9-15.[A]

641 Ahmedzai S, Brooks D. Transdermal fentanyl versus sustained-release oral morphine in cancer pain: preference, efficacy, and quality of life. The TTS-Fentanyl Comparative Trial Group. *J Pain Symptom Manage* 1997;13:254-61.[A]

642 Donner B, et al. Long-term treatment of cancer pain with transdermal fentanyl. *J Pain Symptom Manage* 1998;15:168-75.[A]

643 Allan L, et al. Randomised crossover trial of transdermal fentanyl and sustained release oral morphine for treating chronic non-cancer pain. *Br Med J* 2001;322:1154-58

644 Mercadante S, et al. Subcutaneous fentanyl infusion in a patient with bowel obstruction and renal failure. *J Pain Symptom Manage* 1997;13:241-4.[A]

645 Paix A, et al. Subcutaneous fentanyl and sufentanil infusion substitution for morphine intolerance in cancer pain management. *Pain* 1995;63:263-9.[A]

646 Hunt R, et al. A comparison of subcutaneous morphine and fentanyl in hospice cancer patients. *J Pain Symptom Manage* 1999;18:111-9.[A]

647 Watanabe S, et al. Fentanyl by continuous subcutaneous infusion for the management of cancer pain: a retrospective study. *J Pain Symptom Manage* 1998;16:323-6.[A]

648 Higgs CM, Vella-Brincat J. Withdrawal with transdermal fentanyl (letter). *J Pain Symptom Manage* 1995;10:4-5

649 Zenz M, Donner B, Strumpf M. Withdrawal symptoms during therapy with transdermal fentanyl (fentanyl TTS)? *J Pain Symptom Manage* 1994;9:54-5

650 Davies AN, Bond C. Transdermal fentanyl and the opioid withdrawal syndrome (letter). *Palliat Med* 1996;10:348

651 Hunt R. Transdermal fentanyl and the opioid withdrawal syndrome (letter). *Palliat Med* 1996;10:347-48

652 Vielvoye-Kerkmeer AP, Mattern C, Uitendaal MP. Transdermal fentanyl in opioid-naive cancer pain patients: an open trial using transdermal fentanyl for the treatment of chronic cancer pain in opioid-naive patients and a group using codeine. *J Pain Symptom Manage* 2000;19:185-92.[A]

653 Rose PG, Macfee MS, Boswell MV. Fentanyl transdermal system overdose secondary to cutaneous hyperthermia. *Anesth Analg* 1993;77:390-1

654 Radbruch L, et al. Transdermal fentanyl for the management of cancer pain: a survey of 1005 patients. *Palliat Med* 2001;15:309-21

655 Farrar JT, et al. Oral transmucosal fentanyl citrate: randomized, double-blinded, placebo- controlled trial for treatment of breakthrough pain in cancer patients. *J Natl Cancer Inst* 1998;90:611-6.[A]

656 Payne R, et al. Long-term safety of oral transmucosal fentanyl citrate for breakthrough cancer pain. *J Pain Symptom Manage* 2001;22:575-83

657 Streisand JB, et al. Absorption and bioavailability of oral transmucosal fentanyl citrate. *Anesthesiology* 1991;75:223-9.[A]

658 Coluzzi PH, et al. Breakthrough cancer pain: a randomized trial comparing oral transmucosal fentanyl citrate (OTFC) and morphine sulfate immediate release (MSIR). *Pain* 2001;91:123-30.[A]

659 Portenoy RK, et al. Oral transmucosal fentanyl citrate (OTFC) for the treatment of breakthrough pain in cancer patients: a controlled dose titration study. *Pain* 1999;79:303-12.[A]

660 Christie JM, et al. Dose-titration, multicenter study of oral transmucosal fentanyl citrate for the treatment of breakthrough pain in cancer patients using transdermal fentanyl for persistent pain. *J Clin Oncol* 1998;16:3238-45.[A]

661 Grond S, et al. Transdermal fentanyl in the long-term treatment of cancer pain: a prospective study of 50 patients with advanced cancer of the gastrointestinal tract or the head and neck region. *Pain* 1997;69:191-8.[A]

662 Gardner-Nix J. Caregiver toxicity from transdermal fentanyl. *J Pain Symptom Manage* 2001;21:447-48

663 Zeppetella G. Sublingual fentanyl citrate for cancer-related breakthrough pain: a pilot study. *Palliat Med* 2001;15:323-28

664 Zech DF, Lehmann KA, Grond S. Transdermal (TTS) fentanyl in cancer pain management (review). *Prog Palliat Care* 1994;2:37-42

665 Hanks G. Oral transmucosal fentanyl citrate for the management of breakthrough pain. *Eur J Pall Care* 2001;8:6-9

666 Coda BA, et al. Comparative efficacy of patient-controlled administration of morphine, hydromorphone, or sufentanil for the treatment of oral mucositis pain following bone marrow transplantation. *Pain* 1997;72:333-46.[A]

667 Donner B, Zenz M. Transdermal fentanyl: a new step on the therapeutic ladder. *Anticancer Drugs* 1995;6:39-43.[A]

668 Vieira ZE, et al. Evaluation of fentanyl and sufentanil on the diameter of the common bile duct by ultrasonography in man: a double blind, placebo controlled study. *Int J Clin Pharmacol Ther* 1994;32:274-7.[A]

669 Paul JR. Analgesia of painful skin ulcers with topical gel containing fentanyl citrate - four case reports (abstract). *Palliat Med* 2000;14:335-36

670 Chen JC, et al. The opioid receptor binding of dezocine, morphine, fentanyl, butorphanol and nalbuphine. *Life Sci* 1993;52:389-96.[A]

671 Kieffer BL. Opioids: first lessons from knockout mice. *Trends Phamacol Sci* 1999;20:19-26.[A]

672 Clarke S, Kitchen I. Opioid analgesia: new information from gene knockout studies. *Curr Opin Anaesthesiol* 1999;12:609-14

673 Kitchen I. Opioid gene knockouts: new answers to old questions? *Opioid sensitivity of chronic noncancer pain.* Seattle: IASP Press, 1999:281-303.

674 Subramanian G, et al. Molecular docking reveals a novel binding site model for fentanyl at the mu-opioid receptor. *Journal of Medicinal Chemistry* 2000;43:381-91.[A]

675 Michiels M, Hendriks R, Heykants J. Radioimmunoassay of the new opiate analgesics alfentanil and sufentanil. Preliminary pharmacokinetic profile in man. *J Pharm Pharmacol* 1983;35:86-93.[A]

676 Kirkham SR, Pugh R. Opioid analgesia in uraemic patients. *Lancet* 1995;345:1185.[A]

677 Van Peer A, et al. Alfentanil kinetics in renal insufficiency. *Eur J Clin Pharmacol* 1986;30:245-7.[A]

678 Bower S, Sear JW. Disposition of alfentanil in patients receiving a renal transplant. *J Pharm Pharmacol* 1989;41:654-7.[A]

679 Stanski DR. The clinical pharmacology of alfentanil. *Eur J Anaesthesiol Suppl* 1987;1:3-11.[A]

680 Gallagher G, et al. Target-controlled alfentanil analgesia for dressing change following extensive reconstructive surgery for trauma. *J Pain Symptom Manage* 2001;21:1-2

681 Larijani GE, Goldberg ME. Alfentanil hydrochloride: a new short-acting narcotic analgesic for surgical procedures. *Clin Pharm* 1987;6:275-82.[A]

682 Scholz J, Steinfath M, Schulz M. Clinical pharmacokinetics of alfentanil, fentanyl and sufentanil. An update. *Clin Pharmacokinet* 1996;31:275-92.[A]

683 Kunz KM, Theisen JA, Schroeder ME. Severe episodic pain: management with sublingual sufentanil (letter). *J Pain Symptom Manage* 1993;8:189-90

684 Egan TD. Remifentanil pharmacokinetics and pharmacodynamics. A preliminary appraisal. *Clin Pharmacokinet* 1995;29:80-94.[A]

685 Litman RS. Conscious sedation with remifentanil during painful medical procedures. *J Pain Symptom Manage* 2000;19:468-71.[A]

686 Codd EE, et al. Serotonin and norepinephrine uptake inhibiting activity of centrally acting analgesics: structural determinants and role in antinociception. *J Pharmacol Exp Ther* 1995;274:1263-70.[A]

687 Makin MK, et al. Methadone in the management of cancer related neuropathic pain: report of five cases. *Pain Clin* 1998;10:275-79

688 Morley JS, Makin MK. The use of methadone in cancer pain poorly responsive to other opioids. *Pain Reviews* 1998;5:51-58

689 Davis MP, Walsh D. Methadone for relief of cancer pain: a review of pharmacokinetics, pharmacodynamics, drug interactions and protocols of administration. *Support Care Cancer* 2001;9:73-83

690 Sweeney C, Bruera E. New roles for old drugs: methadone. *Prog Palliat Care* 2001;9:8-10

691 Bruera E, Neumann CM. Role of methadone in the management of pain in cancer patients. *Oncology* 1999;13:1275-82.ᴬ

692 Gannon C. The use of methadone in the care of the dying. *Eur J Palliat Care* 1997;4:152-8

693 Manfredi PL, et al. Methadone analgesia in cancer pain patients on chronic methadone maintenance therapy. *J Pain Symptom Manage* 2001;21:169-74.ᴬ

694 Back IN, Finlay I. Analgesic effect of topical opioids on painful skin ulcers (letter). *J Pain Symptom Manage* 1995;10:493

695 Ramesh PR, Santhosh AR, Kumar KS. Topical morphine in Ayurveda (letter). *Palliat Med* 1998;12:64

696 Twillman RK, et al. Treatment of painful skin ulcers with topical opioids. *J Pain Symptom Manage* 1999;17:288-92.ᴬ

697 Flock P, Gibbs L, Sykes N. Diamorphine-metronidazole gel effective for treatment of painful infected leg ulcers. *J Pain Symptom Manage* 2000;20:396-97

698 Enarson MC, Hays H, Woodroffe MA. Clinical experience with oral ketamine. *J Pain Symptom Manage* 1999;17:384-6.ᴬ

699 Fisher K, Hagen NA. Analgesic effect of oral ketamine in chronic neuropathic pain of spinal origin: a case report. *J Pain Symptom Manage* 1999;18:61-6.ᴬ

700 Haines DR, Gaines SP. N of 1 randomised controlled trials of oral ketamine in patients with chronic pain. *Pain* 1999;83:283-7.ᴬ

701 Vielvoye-Kerkmeer AP, van der Weide M, Mattern C. Re: Clinical experience with oral ketamine (letter). *J Pain Symptom Manage* 2000;19:3-4

702 Broadley KE, Kurowska A, Tookman A. Ketamine injection used orally. *Palliat Med* 1996;10:247-50.ᴬ

703 Oshima E, et al. Continuous subcutaneous injection of ketamine for cancer pain (letter). *Can J Anaesth* 1990;37:385-86

704 Mercadante S, et al. Long-term ketamine subcutaneous continuous infusion in neuropathic cancer pain. *J Pain Symptom Manage* 1995;10:564-8.ᴬ

705 Mercadante S, et al. Analgesic effect of intravenous ketamine in cancer patients on morphine therapy: A randomized, controlled, double-blind, crossover, double-dose study. *J Pain Symptom Manage* 2000;20:246-52.ᴬ

706 Fine PG. Low-dose ketamine in the management of opioid nonresponsive terminal cancer pain. *J Pain Symptom Manage* 1999;17:296-300.ᴬ

707 Lloyd-Williams M. Ketamine for cancer pain [letter]. *J Pain Symptom Manage* 2000;19:79-80

708 Edmonds P. The role of ketamine in the management of chronic pain. *CME Bulletin Palliat Med* 1998;1:3-6

709 Finlay I. Ketamine and its role in cancer pain. *Pain Reviews* 1999;6:303-13

710 NMDA-Receptor Antagonists: Evolving Role in Analgesia. Proceedings of a meeting. New York City, New York, USA. May 1, 1999. *J Pain Symptom Manage* 2000;19:S1-64

711 Bennett GJ. Update on the neurophysiology of pain transmission and modulation: focus on the NMDA-receptor. *J Pain Symptom Manage* 2000;19:S2-6.ᴬ

712 Portenoy RK, et al. Enhancing opioid analgesia with NMDA-receptor antagonists: clarifying the clinical importance. A roundtable discussion. *J Pain Symptom Manage* 2000;19:S57-64

713 Price DD, et al. NMDA-receptor antagonists and opioid receptor interactions as related to analgesia and tolerance. *J Pain Symptom Manage* 2000;19:S7-11.ᴬ

714 Ferrini R. Parenteral lidocaine for severe intractable pain in six hospice patients continued at home. *J Palliat Med* 2000;3:193-200.ᴬ

715 Brose WG, Cousins MJ. Subcutaneous lidocaine for treatment of neuropathic cancer pain. *Pain* 1991;45:145-8.ᴬ

716 Linchitz RM, Raheb JC. Subcutaneous infusion of lidocaine provides effective pain relief for CRPS patients. *Clin J Pain* 1999;15:67-72.ᴬ

717 Devulder JE, et al. Neuropathic pain in a cancer patient responding to subcutaneously administered lignocaine. *Clin J Pain* 1993;9:220-3.ᴬ

718 Kalso E, et al. Systemic local-anaesthetic-type drugs in chronic pain: a systematic review. *Eur J Pain* 1998;2:3-14.ᴬ

719 Backonja MM. Local anaesthetics as adjuvant analgesics. *J Pain Symptom Manage* 1994;9:491-99

720 Rowbotham MC, et al. Lidocaine patch: double-blind controlled study of a new treatment method for post-herpetic neuralgia. *Pain* 1996;65:39-44.ᴬ

721 Devers A, Galer BS. Topical lidocaine patch relieves a variety of neuropathic pain conditions: an open-label study. *Clin J Pain* 2000;16:205-8.ᴬ

722 Argoff CE. New analgesics for neuropathic pain: the lidocaine patch. *Clin J Pain* 2000;16:S62-6.[A]

723 Sloan PA. Nitrous oxide/oxygen analgesia in palliative care. *J Palliat Care* 1986;2:43-5

724 Keating HJ, 3rd, Kundrat M. Patient-controlled analgesia with nitrous oxide in cancer pain. *J Pain Symptom Manage* 1996;11:126-30.[A]

725 Lee MA, et al. A simple method of using epidural analgesia in palliative medicine (letter). *Palliat Med* 2001;15:347-48

726 Eisenach JC, et al. Epidural clonidine analgesia for intractable cancer pain. *Pain* 1995;61:391-9.[A]

727 Becker R, et al. Continuous intrathecal baclofen infusion in the management of central deafferentation pain. *J Pain Symptom Manage* 2000;20:313-15

728 Loubser PG, Akman NM. Effects of intrathecal baclofen on chronic spinal cord injury pain. *J Pain Symptom Manage* 1996;12:241-7.[A]

729 Thompson E, Hicks F. Intrathecal baclofen and homeopathy for the treatment of painful muscle spasms associated with malignant spinal cord compression. *Palliat Med* 1998;12:119-21.[A]

730 Peat SJ, Bras P, Hanna MH. A double-blind comparison of epidural ketamine and diamorphine for postoperative analgesia. *Anaesthesia* 1989;44:555-58

731 Wulf H, Gleim M, Mignat C. The stability of mixtures of morphine hydrochloride, bupivacaine hydrochloride, and clonidine hydrochloride in portable pump reservoirs for the management of chronic pain syndromes. *J Pain Symptom Manage* 1994;9:308-11.[A]

732 Kreeger L, et al. Epidural diamorphine and bupivacaine stability study. *Palliat Med* 1995;9:315-8

733 Barnes AR, Nash S. Stability of bupivacaine hydrochloride with diamorphine hydrochloride in an epidural infusion. *Pharm World Sci* 1995;17:87-92.[A]

734 Johnson CE, et al. Compatibility of bupivacaine hydrochloride and morphine sulfate. *Am J Health Syst Pharm* 1997;54:61-4

735 Ballantyne JC, Loach AB, Carr DB. Itching after epidural and spinal opiates. *Pain* 1988;33:149-60.[A]

736 Nitescu P, et al. Bacteriology, drug stability, and exchange of percutaneous delivery systems and antibacterial filters in long-term intrathecal infusion of opioid drugs and bupivacaine in "refractory" pain. *Clin J Pain* 1992;8:324-37.[A]

737 De Cicco M, et al. Time-dependent efficacy of bacterial filters and infection risk in long-term epidural catheterization. *Anesthesiology* 1995;82:765-71.[A]

738 Bennett G, et al. Evidence-based review of the literature on intrathecal delivery of pain medication. *J Pain Symptom Manage* 2000;20:S12-S36.[A]

739 Cherry DA. The spinal administration of opioids in the treatment of acute and chronic pain: bolus doses, continuous infusion, intraventricular administration and implanted drug delivery systems. *Palliat Med* 1987;1:89-106

740 Devulder J, et al. Spinal analgesia in terminal care: risk versus benefit. *J Pain Symptom Manage* 1994;9:75-81.[A]

741 Simpson KH, Russon L. The use of intrathecal drug delivery systems in pain management. *CME Bulletin Palliat Med* 2000;2:17-20

742 Bennett G, et al. Clinical guidelines for intraspinal infusion: Report of an expert panel. *J Pain Symptom Manage* 2000;20:S37-S43.[A]

743 Du Pen SL, Williams AR. The dilemma of conversion from systemic to epidural morphine: a proposed conversion tool for treatment of cancer pain. *Pain* 1994;56:113-18.[A]

744 Kalso E, et al. Epidural and subcutaneous morphine in the management of cancer pain: a double-blind cross-over study. *Pain* 1997;67:443-9.[A]

745 Camann WR, et al. Effects of oral caffeine on postdural puncture headache. A double-blind, placebo-controlled trial. *Anesth Analg* 1990;70:181-4.[A]

746 Edmonds P. OICPC Therapeutic Highlights: Pleural effusions. *Prog Palliat Care* 2000;8:79-80

747 Chen YM, et al. Usefulness of pig-tail catheter for palliative drainage of malignant pleural effusions in cancer patients. *Support Care Cancer* 2000;8:423-26.[A]

748 Gleeson C, Spencer D. Blood transfusion and its benefits in palliative care. *Palliat Med* 1995;9:307-13

749 Simonds AK, et al. Use of expandable metal stents in the treatment of bronchial obstruction. *Thorax* 1989;44:680-81

750 Hetzel MR. Laser palliation of tracheobronchial tumours: a review. *Palliat Med* 1988;2:134-38

751 Hoskin PJ. Brachytherapy in palliative care. *CME Bulletin Palliat Med* 1999;1:45-53

752   Batchelor TT, et al. Steroid myopathy in cancer patients. *Neurology* 1997;48:1234-8.^

753   Bruera E, et al. The frequency and correlates of dyspnea in patients with advanced cancer. *J Pain Symptom Manage* 2000;19:357-62.^

754   Okuyama T, et al. Factors correlated with fatigue in disease-free breast cancer patients: application of the Cancer Fatigue Scale. *Support Care Cancer* 2000;8:215-22.^

755   Congleton J, Muers MP. The incidence of airflow obstruction in bronchial carcinoma, its relation to breathlessness, and response to bronchodilator therapy. *Resp Med* 1995;89:291-96

756   Janssens JP, de Muralt B, Titelion V. Management of dyspnea in severe chronic obstructive pulmonary disease. *J Pain Symptom Manage* 2000;19:378-92.^

757   Allard P, et al. How effective are supplementary doses of opioids for dyspnea in terminally ill cancer patients? A randomized continuous sequential clinical trial. *J Pain Symptom Manage* 1999;17:256-65.^

758   Boyd KJ, Kelly M. Oral morphine as symptomatic treatment of dyspnoea in patients with advanced cancer. *Palliat Med* 1997;11:277-81.^

759   Bruera E, et al. Subcutaneous morphine for dyspnea in cancer patients. *Ann Intern Med* 1993;119:906-7

760   Bruera E, et al. Effects of morphine on the dyspnea of terminal cancer patients. *J Pain Symptom Manage* 1990;5:341-4.^

761   Johanson GA. Should opioids or sedatives be used for dyspnea in end-stage disease. *Am J Hosp Palliat Care* 1990;July/Aug:12-13

762   Stone P, Kurowska A, Tookman A. Nebulized frusemide for dyspnoea (letter). *Palliat Med* 1994;8:258

763   Nishino T, et al. Inhaled furosemide greatly alleviates the sensation of experimentally induced dyspnea. *Am J Respir Crit Care Med* 2000;161:1963-7.^

764   Bredin M, et al. Multicentre randomised controlled trial of nursing intervention for breathlessness in patients with lung cancer. *Br Med J* 1999;318:901-4.^

765   McIver B, Walsh D, Nelson K. The use of chlorpromazine for symptom control in dying cancer patients. *J Pain Symptom Manage* 1994;9:341-5.^

766   Davis C. The role of nebulised drugs in palliating respiratory symptoms of malignant disease. *Eur J Palliat Care* 1995;2:9-15

767   Davis CL. Single dose randomised controlled trial of nebulised morphine in patients with cancer related breathlessness. *Palliat Med* 1996;10:64-65

768   Ahmedzai S, Davis C. Nebulised drugs in palliative care. *Thorax* 1997;52:575-7

769   Enck RE. The role of nebulized morphine in managing dyspnea. *Am J Hosp Palliat Care* 1999;16:373-4

770   Chandler S. Nebulized opioids to treat dyspnea. *Am J Hosp Palliat Care* 1999;16:418-22.^

771   Quelch PC, Faulkner DE, Yun JW. Nebulized opioids in the treatment of dyspnea. *J Palliat Care* 1997;13:48-52

772   Zeppetella G. Nebulized morphine in the palliation of dyspnoea. *Palliat Med* 1997;11:267-75.^

773   Stark RD, et al. Effects of small-particle aerosols of local anaesthetic on dyspnoea in patients with respiratory disease. *Clin Sci* 1985;69:29-36

774   Wilcock A, Corcoran R, Tattersfield AE. Safety and efficacy of nebulized lignocaine in patients with cancer and breathlessness. *Palliat Med* 1994;8:35-8.^

775   Filshie J, et al. Acupuncture for the relief of cancer-related breathlessness. *Palliat Med* 1996;10:145-50

776   Acupuncture, asthma and breathlessness (editorial). *Lancet* 1986;ii:1427-28

777   Curtis JL, et al. Helium-oxygen gas therapy. Use and availability for the emergency treatment of inoperable airway obstruction. *Chest* 1986;90:455-7.^

778   McGee DL, Wald DA, Hinchliffe S. Helium-oxygen therapy in the emergency department. *J Emerg Med* 1997;15:291-6.^

779   Newton-John H. Acute upper airway obstruction due to supraglottic dystonia induced by a neuroleptic. *Br Med J* 1988;297:964-65

780   Booth S. Breathlessness in advanced cance - what can we do? *Palliat Care Today* 1999;7:37-38

781   Birks C. Pathophysiology and management of dyspnoea in palliative care and the evolving role of the nurse. *Int J Palliat Nurs* 1997;3:264-5.^

782   Ripamonti C, Bruera E. Dyspnea: pathophysiology and assessment. *J Pain Symptom Manage* 1997;13:220-32.^

783   Tyler LS. Dyspnea in palliative care patients. *J Pharm Care Pain Symptom Control* 1999;7:109-27

784   Egelmeers A, et al. Palliative effectiveness of radiation therapy in the treatment of

superior vena cava syndrome. *Bull Cancer Radiother* 1996;83:153-7.[A]

785 Nicholson AA, et al. Treatment of malignant superior vena cava obstruction: metal stents or radiation therapy. *Journal Of Vascular And Interventional Radiology* 1997;8:781-8.[A]

786 Young N, Glare P. Use of a metallic stent for relief of symptoms caused by superior vena caval obstruction in a patient with advanced cancer: a case report. *J Pain Symptom Manage* 1999;18:56-60.[A]

787 Renwick I. Metallic stents in palliative care. *CME Bulletin Palliat Med* 1999;1:41-44

788 Paterson J, et al. Stenting for inferior caval obstruction (letter). *Palliat Med* 1996;10:344-5

789 O'Neill JM, et al. Stenting for superior vena caval obstruction: an effective palliative intervention. *Palliat Med* 1995;9:65

790 Morales M, et al. Treatment of catheter-induced thrombotic superior vena cava syndrome: A single institution's experience. *Support Care Cancer* 2000;8:334-38.[A]

791 *Superior vena cava syndrome*. In: National Cancer Institute CancerNet PDQ database, 2000. (http://cancernet.nci.nih.gov/pdq/, accessed 9 Dec 2000)

792 Bruera Ede, et al. Effects of oxygen on dyspnea in hypoxaemic terminal-cancer patients. *Lancet* 1993;342:13-14

793 Liss HP, Grant BJB. The effect of nasal flow on breathlessness in patients with chronic obstructive pulmonary disease. *Am Rev Respir Dis* 1988;137:1285-88

794 Booth S, et al. Does oxygen help dyspnea in patients with cancer? *Am J Respir Crit Care Med* 1996;153:1515-8.[A]

795 Royal College of Physicians. *Domiciliary oxygen therapy services: clinical guidelines and advice for prescribers*. London: RCP, 1999.

796 Campbell EJ, Baker MD, Crites-Silver P. Subjective effects of humidification of oxygen for delivery by nasal cannula. A prospective study. *Chest* 1988;93:289-93.[A]

797 Bateman NT, Leach RM. ABC of oxygen. Acute oxygen therapy. *Br Med J* 1998;317:798-801

798 Rees PJ, Dudley F. Oxygen therapy in chronic lung disease. *Br Med J* 1998;317:871-4

799 Rees PJ, Dudley F. Provision of oxygen at home. *Br Med J* 1998;317:935-8

800 Treacher DF, Leach RM. Oxygen transport-1. Basic principles. *Br Med J* 1998;317:1302-6

801 Ing AJ, Ngu MC, Breslin AB. Pathogenesis of chronic persistent cough associated with gastroesophageal reflux. *Am J Respir Crit Care Med* 1994;149:160-7.[A]

802 Glasziou P. Evidence based case report. Twenty year cough in a non-smoker. *Br Med J* 1998;316:1660-61

803 Sevelius H. Dose response to codeine in patients with chronic cough. *Clin Pharmacol Ther* 1971;12:449-55

804 Eddy NB, et al. Codeine and its alternates for pain and cough relief. 4. Potential alternates for cough relief. *Bull World Health Organ* 1969;40:639-719

805 Holmes PW, Barter CE, Pierce RJ. Chronic persistent cough: use of ipratropium bromide in undiagnosed cases following upper respiratory tract infection. *Respiratory Medicine* 1992;86:425-9.[A]

806 Lowry R, et al. Antitussive properties of inhaled bronchodilators on induced cough. *Chest* 1988;93:1186-9.[A]

807 Moroni M, et al. Inhaled sodium cromoglycate to treat cough in advanced lung cancer patients. *Br J Cancer* 1996;74:309-11.[A]

808 Poole PJ, Black PN. Oral mucolytic drugs for exacerbations of chronic obstructive pulmonary disease: systematic review. *Br Med J* 2001;322:1271-73

809 Dicpinigaitis PV, et al. Inhibition of capsaicin-induced cough by the gamma-aminobutyric acid agonist baclofen. *J Clin Pharmacol* 1998;38:364-7.[A]

810 Kamei J, Kasuya Y. Antitussive effects of Ca2+ channel antagonists. *Eur J Pharmacol* 1992;212:61-6.[A]

811 Trochtenberg S. Nebulized lidocaine in the treatment of refractory cough. *Chest* 1994;105:1592-3.[A]

812 March CR, Hardy PAJ. Interpleural infusion with bupivicaine for intractable cough. *Palliat Med* 1991;5:349-50

813 Doona M, Walsh D. Benzonatate for opioid-resistant cough in advanced cancer. *Palliat Med* 1998;12:55-8.[A]

814 Krawtz SM, et al. Palliation of massive bronchorrhoea (letter). *Chest* 1988;94:1313-14

815 Tamaoki J, et al. Inhaled indomethacin in bronchorrhea in bronchioloalveolar carcinoma: role of cyclooxygenase. *Chest* 2000;117:1213-4

816 Irwin RS, Curley FJ, Bennett FM. Appropriate use of antitussives and protussives. A practical review. *Drugs* 1993;46:80-91.[A]

817 Rawlinson F. Dyspnoea and cough. *Eur J Pall Care* 2000;7:161-64

818 Palmer LB, et al. Aerosolized antibiotics in mechanically ventilated patients: delivery and response. *Critical Care Medicine* 1998;26:31-9.[A]

819 Kamei J, et al. Involvement of haloperidol-sensitive sigma-sites in antitussive effects. *Eur J Pharmacol* 1992;224:39-43.[A]

820 Christensen V, Ladegaard_Pedersen HJ, Skovsted P. Intravenous lidocaine as a suppressant of persistent cough caused by bronchoscopy. *Acta Anaesthesiologica Scandinavica Supplementum* 1978;67:84-6.[A]

821 Yukioka H, et al. Intravenous lidocaine as a suppressant of coughing during tracheal intubation in elderly patients. *Anesth Analg* 1993;77:309-12.[A]

822 Rees GJ, et al. Palliative radiotherapy for lung cancer: two versus five fractions. *Clin Oncol* 1997;9:90-5.[A]

823 Gollins SW, et al. Long-term survival and symptom palliation in small primary bronchial carcinomas following treatment with intraluminal radiotherapy alone. *Clin Oncol* 1996;8:239-46.[A]

824 Hernandez P, et al. High dose rate brachytherapy for the local control of endobronchial carcinoma following external irradiation. *Thorax* 1996;51:354-8.[A]

825 Villanueva AG, Lo TC, Beamis JF, Jr. Endobronchial brachytherapy. *Clin Chest Med* 1995;16:445-54.[A]

826 Huber RM, et al. Palliative endobronchial brachytherapy for central lung tumors. A prospective, randomized comparison of two fractionation schedules. *Chest* 1995;107:463-70.[A]

827 Zhang JS, et al. Bronchial arteriography and transcatheter embolization in the management of hemoptysis. *Cardiovasc Intervent Radiol* 1994;17:276-9.[A]

828 Pierce RJ, et al. Endobronchial resection with the Nd-YAG laser--two years experience in an Australian unit. *Aust N Z J Med* 1990;20:120-6.[A]

829 Jones DK, Davies RJ. Massive haemoptysis. Medical management will usually arrest the bleeding. *Br Med J* 1990;300:889-90

830 Wong LT, et al. Treatment of recurrent hemoptysis in a child with cystic fibrosis by repeated bronchial artery embolizations and long-term tranexamic acid. *Pediatric Pulmonology* 1996;22:275-9.[A]

831 Chang AB, et al. Major hemoptysis in a child with cystic fibrosis from multiple aberrant bronchial arteries treated with tranexamic acid. *Pediatric Pulmonology* 1996;22:416-20

832 Back I, et al. A study comparing hyoscine hydrobromide and glycopyrrolate in the treatment of death rattle. *Palliat Med* 2001;15:329-36

833 Bennett MI. Death rattle: an audit of hyoscine (scopolamine) use and review of management. *J Pain Symptom Manage* 1996;12:229-33.[A]

834 Hughes A, et al. Audit of three antimuscarinic drugs for managing retained secretions. *Palliat Med* 2000;14:221-22

835 Lucas V. The use of glycopyrrolate by syringe driver to alleviate bronchial secretions (abstract). *Progress in Palliative Care* 1993;2:11

836 Dawson HR. The use of transdermal scopolamine in the control of death rattle. *J Palliat Care* 1989;5:31-33

837 Gallagher R. Nicotine withdrawal as an etiologic factor in delirium (letter). *J Pain Symptom Manage* 1998;16:76-7

838 Thompson SA, Duncan JS, Smith SJ. Partial seizures presenting as panic attacks. *Br Med J* 2000;321:1002-3

839 Buclin T, et al. Psychopharmacology in supportive care of cancer: a review for the clinician. IV. Other psychotropic agents. *Support Care Cancer* 2001;9:213-22

840 Jackson IK, Lipman AG. Anxiety in palliative care patients. *J Pharm Care Pain Symptom Control* 1999;7:23-35.[A]

841 Chochinov HM, et al. "Are you depressed?" Screening for depression in the terminally ill. *Am J Psychiatry* 1997;154:674-6.[A]

842 Kugaya A, et al. Successful antidepressant treatment for five terminally ill cancer patients with major depression, suicidal ideation and a desire for death. *Support Care Cancer* 1999;7:432-6.[A]

843 *British National Formulary (BNF).* 41 ed. London: BMA and Royal Pharmaceutical Society, 2001.

844 Thase ME, Entsuah AR, Rudolph RL. Remission rates during treatment with venlafaxine or selective serotonin reuptake inhibitors. *Br J Psychiatry* 2001;178:234-41.[A]

845 Andersen G, Vestergaard K, Riis JO. Citalopram for post-stroke pathological crying. *Lancet* 1993;342:837-9.[A]

846 *Depression.* In: National Cancer Institute CancerNet PDQ database, 2000. (http://cancernet.nci.nih.gov/pdq/, accessed 9 Dec 2000)

847 Pirl WF, Roth AJ. Diagnosis and treatment of depression in cancer patients. *Oncology* 1999;13:1293-301; discussion 301-2, 305-6.[A]

848 Berney A, et al. Psychopharmacology in supportive care of cancer: A review for the clinician. III. Antidepressants. *Support Cancer* 2000;8:278-86.[A]

849 Maguire P. The use of antidepressants in patients with advanced cancer. *Support Care Cancer* 2000;8:265-67

850 Martin AC, Jackson KC. Depression in palliative care patients. *J Pharm Care Pain Symptom Control* 1999;7:71-89

851 Nakano T, et al. Algorithm for the treatment of major depression in patients with advanced cancer. *Psychiatry Clin Neurosci* 1999;53:S61-5.[A]

852 Raap JW, Beckwith MC, Reimherr FW. Clinical uses and differences among the selective serotonin reuptake inhibitors. *J Pharm Care Pain Symptom Control* 2000;8:23-38.[A]

853 Edwards JG, Anderson I. Systematic review and guide to selection of selective serotonin reuptake inhibitors. *Drugs* 1999;57:507-33.[A]

854 Caley CF. Extrapyramidal reactions and the selective serotonin-reuptake inhibitors. *Ann Pharmacother* 1997;31:1481-9.[A]

855 Haddad P, Lejoyeux M, Young A. Antidepressant discontinuation reactions (editorial). *Br Med J* 1998;316:1105-6

856 Zajecka J, Tracy KA, Mitchell S. Discontinuation symptoms after treatment with serotonin reuptake inhibitors: a literature review. *J Clin Psychiatry* 1997;58:291-7.[A]

857 Sporer KA. The serotonin syndrome. Implicated drugs, pathophysiology and management. *Drug Safety* 1995;13:94-104.[A]

858 Pippenger CE. Clinically significant carbamazepine drug interactions: an overview. *Epilepsia* 1987;28(S3):S71-6.[A]

859 Spina E, Pisani F, Perucca E. Clinically significant pharmacokinetic drug interactions with carbamazepine. An update. *Clin Pharmacokinet* 1996;31:198-214.[A]

860 Linde K, Mulrow CD. *St John's wort for depression (Cochrane Review).* In: The Cochrane Library, Issue 3, 2000. (http://hiru.mcmaster.ca/cochrane, accessed 5 Dec 2000)

861 Woelk H. Comparison of St John's wort and imipramine for treating depression: randomised controlled trial. *Br Med J* 2000;321:536-9.[A]

862 Meyers CA, et al. Methylphenidate therapy improves cognition, mood, and function of brain tumor patients. *J Clin Oncol* 1998;16:2522-7.[A]

863 Stiefel F, Bruera E. Psychostimulants for hypoactive-hypoalert delirium? *J Palliat Care* 1991;7:25-6

864 Morita T, et al. Successful palliation of hypoactive delirium due to multi-organ failure by oral methylphenidate. *Support Care Cancer* 2000;8:134-7.[A]

865 Satel SL, Nelson JC. Stimulants in the treatment of depression: a critical overview. *J Clin Psychiatry* 1989;50:241-9.[A]

866 Lloyd-Williams M, Friedman T, Rudd N. A survey of antidepressant prescribing in the terminally ill. *Palliat Med* 1999;13:243-8.[A]

867 Block SD. Assessing and managing depression in the terminally ill patient. ACP-ASIM End-of-Life Care Consensus Panel. American College of Physicians - American Society of Internal Medicine. *Ann Intern Med* 2000;132:209-18.[A]

868 Frierson RL, Wey JJ, Tabler JB. Psychostimulants for depression in the medically ill. *Am Fam Physician* 1991;43:163-70.[A]

869 Woods SW, et al. Psychostimulant treatment of depressive disorders secondary to medical illness. *J Clin Psychiatry* 1986;47:12-5.[A]

870 Olin J, Masand P. Psychostimulants for depression in hospitalized cancer patients. *Psychosomatics* 1996;37:57-62.[A]

871 Gurian B, Rosowsky E. Low-dose methylphenidate in the very old. *J Geriatric Psychiatry & Neurol* 1990;3:152-4.[A]

872 Fernandez F, et al. Effects of methylphenidate in HIV-related depression: a comparative trial with desipramine. *Int J Psychiatry Med* 1995;25:53-67.[A]

873 Bruera E, et al. Methylphenidate associated with narcotics for the treatment of cancer pain. *Cancer Treat Rep* 1987;71:67-70.[A]

874 Bruera E, et al. The use of methylphenidate in patients with incident cancer pain receiving regular opiates. A preliminary report. *Pain* 1992;50:75-7.[A]

875 Bruera E, Watanabe S. Psychostimulants as adjuvant analgesics. *J Pain Symptom Manage* 1994;9:412-5.[A]

876 Kreeger L, Duncan A, Cowap J. Psychostimulants used for opioid-induced

drowsiness (letter). *J Pain Symptom Manage* 1996;11:1-2

877 Mercadante S, Serretta R, Casuccio A. Effects of caffeine as adjuvant to morphine in advanced cancer patients: a randomized, double-blind, placebo-controlled, crossover study. *J Pain Symptom Manage* 2001;21:369-72

878 Dalal S, Melzack R. Potentiation of opioid analgesia by psychostimulant drugs: a review. *J Pain Symptom Manage* 1998;16:245-53.^A

879 Wilwerding MB, et al. A randomized, crossover evaluation of methylphenidate in cancer patients receiving strong narcotics. *Support Care Cancer* 1995;3:135-8.^A

880 *Fatigue*. In: National Cancer Institute CancerNet PDQ database, 2000. (http://cancernet.nci.nih.gov/pdq/, accessed 9 Dec 2000)

881 Homsi J, Walsh D, Nelson KA. Psychostimulants in supportive care. *Support Care Cancer* 2000;8:385-97.^A

882 Homsi J, et al. Methylphenidate for depression in advanced cancer (abstract). *J Pain Symptom Manage* 2000;20:S65

883 Masand PS, Pickett P, Murray GB. Hypomania precipitated by psychostimulant use in depressed medically ill patients. *Psychosomatics* 1995;36:145-7

884 Jenkins CA, Bruera E. Difficulties in diagnosing neuropsychiatric complications of corticosteroids in advanced cancer patients: two case reports. *J Pain Symptom Manage* 2000;19:309-17.^A

885 Foy A, et al. Confusion after admission to hospital in elderly patients using benzodiazepines. *Br Med J* 1986;293:1072

886 Barbato M, Rodriguez PJ. Thiamine deficiency in patients admitted to a palliative care unit. *Palliat Med* 1994;8:320-4.^A

887 Levine PM, Silberfarb PM, Lipowski ZJ. Mental disorders in cancer patients. A study of 100 psychiatric referrals. *Cancer* 1978;42:1385-91

888 Lee MA, Leng MEF, Tiernan EJJ. Risperidone: a useful adjunct for behavioural disturbance in primary cerebral tumours. *Palliat Med* 2001;15:255-56

889 Lodge P, Tanner M, McKeogh MM. Risperidone in the management of agitation in HIV dementia (letter). *Palliat Med* 1998;12:206-7

890 Kerr I, Taylor D. Acute disturbed or violent behaviour: principles of treatment. *J Psychopharmacol* 1997;11:271-77

891 Breitbart W, et al. A double-blind trial of haloperidol, chlorpromazine, and lorazepam in the treatment of delirium in hospitalized AIDS patients. *Am J Psychiatry* 1996;153:231-7.^A

892 Cook CCH, Thomson AD. B-complex vitamins in the prophylaxis and treatment of Wernicke-Korsakoff syndrome. *Br J Hosp Med* 1997;57:461-65

893 Jackson IK, Lipman AG. Delirium in palliative care patients. *J Pharm Care Pain Symptom Control* 1999;7:59-70.^A

894 *Delirium*. In: National Cancer Institute CancerNet PDQ database, 2000. (http://cancernet.nci.nih.gov/pdq/, accessed 9 Dec 2000)

895 Massie MJ, Holland J, Glass E. Delirium in terminally ill cancer patients. *Am J Psychiatry* 1983;140:1048-50

896 Caraceni A. Delirium in palliative medicine. *Eur J Palliat Care* 1995;2:62-7

897 Macleod AD. Clinical management. The management of delirium in hospice practice. *Eur J Palliat Care* 1997;4:116-20

898 Brown S, Degner LF. Delirium in the terminally-ill cancer patient: aetiology, symptoms and management. *Int J Palliat Nurs* 2001;7:266-72

899 Meagher DJ. Delirium: Optimising management. *Br Med J* 2001;322:144-49

900 Burke AL, et al. Terminal restlessness - its management and the role of midazolam. *Med J Aust* 1991;155:485-87

901 Stirling LC, Kurowska A, Tookman A. The use of phenobarbitone in the management of agitation and seizures at the end of life. *J Pain Symptom Manage* 1999;17:363-8.^A

902 Mercadante S, De Conno F, Ripamonti C. Propofol in terminal care. *J Pain Symptom Manage* 1995;10:639-42.^A

903 Moyle J. The use of propofol in palliative medicine. *J Pain Symptom Manage* 1995;10:643-6.^A

904 Burke AL. Palliative care: an update on "terminal restlessness". *Med J Aust* 1997;166:39-42.^A

905 Back IN. Terminal restlessness in patients with advanced malignant disease. *Palliat Med* 1992;6:293-98.^A

906 Sales JP. Sedation and terminal care. *Eur J Pall Care* 2001;8:97-100

907 Scott RC, Besag FM, Neville BG. Buccal midazolam and rectal diazepam for treatment of prolonged seizures in childhood and adolescence: a randomised trial. *Lancet* 1999;353:623-6.^A

908 Ellis SJ, Baddely L. Buccal midazolam and rectal diazepam for epilepsy (letter).

Lancet 1999;353:1796-7

909 Gambertoglio JG. Corticosteroids and anticonvulsants. *Drug Interactions Newsletter* 1983;3:55-58

910 Wong DD, et al. Phenytoin - dexamethasone: a possible drug-drug interaction. *JAMA* 1985;254:2062-63

911 Thompson AJ. Drug therapy in multiple sclerosis. *Prescribers Journal* 1999;39:72-80

912 The management of spasticity. *Drug Ther Bull* 2000;38:44-6.[A]

913 Lear J, Daniels RG. Muscle cramps related to corticosteroids (letter). *Br Med J* 1993;306:1169

914 Daniell HW. Simple cure for nocturnal leg cramps (letter). *New Engl J Med* 1979;301:216

915 Man-Song-Hing M, Wells G. Quinine for nocturnal leg cramps. A meta-analysis including unpublished data. *J Gen Intern Med* 1998;13:600-06

916 Young JB, Connolly MJ. Naftidrofuryl treatment for rest cramp. *Postgrad Med J* 1993;69:624-26

917 Roca AO, et al. Dialysis leg cramps. Efficacy of quinine versus vitamin E. *ASAIO J* 1992;38:481-85

918 Connolly PS, et al. Treatment of nocturnal leg cramps. A cross over trial of quinine versus vitamin E. *Arch Intern Med* 1992;152:1877-80

919 Poynard T, Valterio C. Meta-analysis of hydroxyethylrutosides in the treatment of chronic venous insufficiency. *Vasa* 1994;23:244-50.[A]

920 MacLennan WJ, et al. Hydroxyethylrutosides in elderly patients with chronic venous insufficiency: its efficacy and tolerability. *Gerontol* 1994;40:45-52.[A]

921 Merren MD. Gabapentin for treatment of pain and tremor: a large case series. *South Med J* 1998;91:739-44.[A]

922 Hallett M, et al. Controlled trial of isoniazid therapy for severe postural cerebellar tremor in multiple sclerosis. *Neurology* 1985;35:1374-77

923 Walters AS. Toward a better definition of the restless legs syndrome. The International Restless Legs Syndrome Study Group. *Mov Disord* 1995;10:634-42

924 Williams DC. Periodic limb movements of sleep and the restless legs syndrome. *Va Med Q* 1996;123:260-5.[A]

925 Lugaresi E, et al. Nocturnal myoclonus and restless legs syndrome. *Adv Neurol* 1986;43:295-307.[A]

926 Brodeur C, et al. Treatment of restless legs syndrome and periodic movements during sleep with L-dopa: a double-blind, controlled study. *Neurology* 1988;38:1845-8.[A]

927 O'Keeffe ST, Gavin K, Lavan JN. Iron status and restless legs syndrome in the elderly. *Age Ageing* 1994;23:200-3.[A]

928 O'Keeffe ST, Noel J, Lavan JN. Restless legs syndrome in the elderly. *Postgrad Med J* 1993;69:701-3.[A]

929 Bakshi R. Fluoxetine and restless legs syndrome. *J Neurol Sci* 1996;142:151-2

930 Hargrave R, Beckley DJ. Restless leg syndrome exacerbated by sertraline (letter). *Psychosomatics* 1998;39:177-8

931 Paik IH, et al. Mianserin-induced restless legs syndrome. *Br J Psychiatry* 1989;155:415-7.[A]

932 Sandyk R, et al. L-dopa in uremic patients with the restless legs syndrome. *Int J Neurosci* 1987;35:233-5.[A]

933 Scheele von. Levodopa in restless legs. *Lancet* 1986;2:426-7.[A]

934 Trenkwalder C, et al. L-dopa therapy of uremic and idiopathic restless legs syndrome: a double-blind, crossover trial. *Sleep* 1995;18:681-8.[A]

935 Allen RP, Earley CJ. Augmentation of the restless legs syndrome with carbidopa/levodopa. *Sleep* 1996;19:205-13.[A]

936 McQuillan R, Singh R. Restless legs syndrome (letter; comment). *Palliat Med* 1995;9:168-9

937 Marien P, Cole R. Restless legs syndrome (letter). *Palliat Med* 1994;8:256.[A]

938 Walters AS, et al. Successful treatment of the idiopathic restless legs syndrome in a randomized double-blind trial of oxycodone versus placebo. *Sleep* 1993;16:327-32.[A]

939 Montplaisir J, Lorrain D, Godbout R. Restless legs syndrome and periodic leg movements in sleep: the primary role of dopaminergic mechanism. *Eur Neurol* 1991;31:41-3.[A]

940 Montplaisir J, et al. The treatment of the restless leg syndrome with or without periodic leg movements in sleep. *Sleep* 1992;15:391-5.[A]

941 Winkelmann J, et al. Treatment of restless leg syndrome with pergolide--an open clinical trial. *Mov Disord* 1998;13:566-9.[A]

942 Staedt J, et al. Pergolide: treatment of choice in Restless Legs Syndrome (RLS) and Nocturnal Myoclonus Syndrome (NMS). Longterm follow up on pergolide. Short communication. *J Neural Transm* 1998;105:265-8.^

943 Noel S, Korri H, Vanderheyden JE. Low dosage of pergolide in the treatment of restless legs syndrome (letter). *Acta Neurol Belg* 1998;98:52-3

944 Mellick GA, Mellick LB. Management of restless legs syndrome with gabapentin (Neurontin) (letter). *Sleep* 1996;19:224-6

945 Peled R, Lavie P. Double-blind evaluation of clonazepam on periodic leg movements in sleep. *J Neurol Neurosurg Psychiatry* 1987;50:1679-81.^

946 Sandyk R, Kwo-on-Yuen PF, Bamford CR. The effects of baclofen in the restless legs syndrome: evidence for endogenous opioid involvement (letter). *J Clin Psychopharmacol* 1988;8:440-1

947 Sandyk R, Iacono RP, Bamford CR. Spinal cord mechanisms in amitriptyline responsive restless legs syndrome in Parkinson's disease. *Int J Neurosci* 1988;38:121-4.^

948 Ginsberg HN. Propranolol in the treatment of restless legs syndrome induced by imipramine withdrawal (letter). *Am J Psychiatry* 1986;143:938

949 Scharf MB, Brown L, Hirschowitz J. Possible efficacy of alprazolam in restless leg syndrome. *Hillside J Clin Psychiatry* 1986;8:214-23.^

950 Wagner ML, et al. Randomized, double-blind, placebo-controlled study of clonidine in restless legs syndrome. *Sleep* 1996;19:52-8.^

951 Bastani B, Westervelt FB. Effectiveness of clonidine in alleviating the symptoms of "restless legs" (letter). *Am J Kidney Dis* 1987;10:326

952 Bamford CR, Sandyk R. Failure of clonidine to ameliorate the symptoms of restless legs syndrome (letter). *Sleep* 1987;10:398-9

953 Clough C. Restless legs syndrome (editorial). *Br Med J (Clin Res Ed)* 1987;294:262-3

954 Bristow MF, Kohen D. How malignant is the neuroleptic malignant syndrome? *Br Med J* 1993;307:1223-24

955 Brook I, Frazier EH. Aerobic and anaerobic infection associated with malignancy. *Support Care Cancer* 1998;6:125-31.^

956 Vitetta L, Kenner D, Sali A. Bacterial infections in terminally Ill hospice patients. *J Pain Symptom Manage* 2000;20:326-34.^

957 Chocarro Martinez A, et al. Risk factors for esophageal candidiasis. *Eur J Clin Microbiol Infect Dis* 2000;19:96-100.^

958 Sheft DJ, Shrago G. Esophageal moniliasis: the spectrum of the disease. *JAMA* 1970;213:1859-62

959 Oravcova E, et al. Funguria in cancer patients: analysis of risk factors, clinical presentation and outcome in 50 patients. *Infection* 1996;24:319-23.^

960 Bowsher D. The effects of pre-emptive treatment of postherpetic neuralgia with amitriptyline: a randomized, double-blind, placebo-controlled trial. *J Pain Symptom Manage* 1997;13:327-31.^

961 Cunningham AL, Dworkin RH. The management of post-herpetic neuralgia. *Br Med J* 2000;321:778-9

962 Montes LF, Muchinik G, Fox CL. Response of varicella zoster virus and herpes zoster to silver sulfadiazine. *Cutis* 1986;38:363-5.^

963 Liu J, et al. The intracellular mechanism of insulin resistance in pancreatic cancer patients. *J Clin Endocrinol Metab* 2000;85:1232-8.^

964 Gullo L. Diabetes and the risk of pancreatic cancer. *Ann Oncol* 1999;10(S4):79-81.^

965 Boyd K. Diabetes mellitus in hospice patients: some guidelines. *Palliat Med* 1993;7:163-4

966 Poulson J. The management of diabetes in patients with advanced cancer. *J Pain Symptom Manage* 1997;13:339-46.^

967 Chye R, Lickiss N. Palliative Care rounds: The use of Corticosteroids in the management of bilateral malignant ureteric obstruction. *J Pain Symptom Manage* 1994;9:537-40

968 Bell D, Glynne-Jones R, Vernon CC. Cerebral metastases and dexamethasone: psychiatric aspects. *Palliat Med* 1987;1:132-35

969 Glynne-Jones R, Vernon CC, Bell G. Is steroid psychosis preventable by divided doses? (letter). *Lancet* 1986;ii:1404

970 MacDonald SM, Hagen N, Bruera E. Proximal muscle weakness in a patient with hepatocellular carcinoma. *J Pain Symptom Manage* 1994;9:346-50.^

971 Dropcho EJ, Soong S. Steroid-induced weakness in patients with primary brain tumours. *Neurology* 1991;41:1235-39

972 Eidelberg D. Neurological effects of steroid treatment. In: Rottenberg DA, ed.

Neurological complications of cancer treatment. Boston: Butterworth-Heinemann, 1991:173-91.

973   Braunstein PW, de Girolami U. Experimental corticosteroid myopathy. *Acta Neuropathologica* 1981;55:167-72

974   Falude G, Gotlieb J, Meyers J. Factors influencing the development of steroid-induced myopathies. *Ann N Y Acad Sci* 1966;138:61-72

975   Eastell R, et al. A UK Consensus Group on management of glucocorticoid-induced osteoporosis: an update. *J Intern Med* 1998;244:271-92.[A]

976   Adachi JD, et al. Intermittent etidronate therapy to prevent corticosteroid-induced osteoporosis. *N Engl J Med* 1997;337:382-7.[A]

977   Sebaldt RJ, et al. 36 month intermittent cyclical etidronate treatment in patients with established corticosteroid induced osteoporosis. *J Rheumatol* 1999;26:1545-9.[A]

978   Ringe JD, Welzel D. Salmon calcitonin in the therapy of corticoid-induced osteoporosis. *Eur J Clin Pharmacol* 1987;33:35-9.[A]

979   Sweeney C, Bruera E. New roles for old drugs: corticosteroids. *Prog Palliat Care* 2001;9:53-4

980   Hardy J. Clinical management. Corticosteroids in palliative care. *Eur J Palliat Care* 1998;5:46-50

981   Vecht CJ, et al. Dose-effect relationship of dexamethasone on Karnofsky performance in metastatic brain tumors: a randomized study of doses of 4, 8, and 16 mg per day. *Neurology* 1994;44:675-80.[A]

982   Tchekmedyian NS, et al. Megestrol acetate in cancer anorexia and weight loss. *Cancer* 1992;69:1268-74

983   Bruera E, et al. A controlled trial of megestrol acetate on appetite, caloric intake, nutritional status, and other symptoms in patients with advanced cancer. *Cancer* 1990;66:1279-83

984   Loprinzi CL, et al. Controlled trial of megestrol acetate for the treatment of cancer anorexia and cachexia. *J Natl Cancer Inst* 1990;82:1127-32

985   Loprinzi CL, et al. Randomized comparison of megestrol acetate versus dexamethasone versus fluoxymesterone for the treatment of cancer anorexia/cachexia. *J Clin Oncol* 1999;17:3299-306

986   Heckmayr M, Gatzemeier U. Treatment of cancer weight loss in patients with advanced lung cancer. *Oncology* 1992;49(S2):32-4.[A]

987   Tchekmedyian NS, Hickman M, Siau J. Treatment of cancer anorexia with megestrol acetate: impact on quality of life. *Oncology* 1990;4:185-92

988   Splinter TA. Cachexia and cancer: a clinician's view. *Ann Oncol* 1992;3(S3):25-7.[A]

989   Loprinzi CL, et al. Phase III evaluation of four doses of megestrol acetate as therapy for patients with cancer anorexia and/or cachexia. *J Clin Oncol* 1993;11:762-7.[A]

990   Vadell C, et al. Anticachectic efficacy of megestrol acetate at different doses and versus placebo in patients with neoplastic cachexia. *Am J Clin Oncol* 1998;21:347-51.[A]

991   Naing KK, et al. Megestrol acetate therapy and secondary adrenal suppression. *Cancer* 1999;86:1044-9.[A]

992   Loprinzi CL, et al. Effect of megestrol acetate on the human pituitary-adrenal axis. *Mayo Clin Proc* 1992;67:1160-2.[A]

993   Leinung MC, Liporace R, Miller CH. Induction of adrenal suppression by megestrol acetate in patients with AIDS. *Ann Intern Med* 1995;122:843-5.[A]

994   Subramanian S, et al. Clinical adrenal insufficiency in patients receiving megestrol therapy. *Arch Intern Med* 1997;157:1008-11.[A]

995   Castiel M. Management of menopausal symptoms in the cancer patient. *Oncology* 1999;13:1363-72; discussion 72, 77-83.[A]

996   Burger CW, et al. Hormone replacement therapy in women treated for gynaecological malignancy. *Maturitas* 1999;32:69-76.[A]

997   Jatoi I, Gore ME. Sex, pregnancy, hormones and melanoma. *Br Med J* 1993;307:2-3

998   Adsay NV, et al. Mixed epithelial and stromal tumor of the kidney. *Am J Surg Pathol* 2000;24:958-70.[A]

999   Hoibraaten E, Abdelnoor M, Sandset PM. Hormone replacement therapy with estradiol and risk of venous thromboembolism--a population-based case-control study. *Thromb Haemost* 1999;82:1218-21.[A]

1000   Grady D, et al. Postmenopausal hormone therapy increases risk for venous thromboembolic disease. The Heart and Estrogen/progestin Replacement Study. *Ann Intern Med* 2000;132:689-96.[A]

1001   Van Dijk JM. Hypercalcemia in prostatic carcinoma. Case report and review of the literature. *Am J Clin Oncol* 1993;16:329-31.[A]

1002 Sekine M, Takami H. Combination of calcitonin and pamidronate for emergency treatment of malignant hypercalcemia. *Oncol Rep* 1998;5:197-9.[A]

1003 Ralston SH, et al. Treatment of cancer associated hypercalcaemia with combined aminohydroxypropylidene diphosphonate and calcitonin. *Br Med J* 1986;292:1549-50

1004 Body JJ, Louviaux I, Dumon JC. Decreased efficacy of bisphosphonates for recurrences of tumor-induced hypercalcemia. *Support Care Cancer* 2000;8:398-404.[A]

1005 Pecherstorfer M, Thiebaud D. Treatment of resistant tumor-induced hypercalcaemia with escalating doses of pamidronate (APD). *Ann Oncol* 1992;3:661-63

1006 Major P, et al. Zoledronic acid is superior to pamidronate in the treatment of hypercalcaemia of malignancy: a pooled analysis of two randomized, controlled clinical trials. *J Clin Oncol* 2001;19:558-67

1007 Harrison M, et al. Somatostatin analogue treatment for malignant hypercalcaemia. *Br Med J* 1990;300:1313-14

1008 Wynick D, et al. Treatment of a malignant pancreatic endocrine tumour secreting parathyroid hormone related protein. *Br Med J* 1990;300:1314-15

1009 Dodwell D, et al. Treatment of a pancreatic tumour secreting parathyroid hormone related protein (letter). *Br Med J* 1990;300:1653

1010 Warrell RPJ, et al. Gallium nitrate for acute treatment of cancer-related hypercalcemia. A randomized, double-blind comparison to calcitonin. *Ann Intern Med* 1988;108:669-74.[A]

1011 Warrell RP, Jr. Gallium nitrate for the treatment of bone metastases. *Cancer* 1997;80:1680-5.[A]

1012 Hughes TE, Hansen LA. Gallium nitrate. *Ann Pharmacother* 1992;26:354-62.[A]

1013 Ostenstad B, Andersen OK. Disodium pamidronate versus mithramycin in the management of tumour-associated hypercalcaemia. *Acta Oncol* 1992;31:861-4.[A]

1014 Ralston SH, et al. Comparison of aminohydroxypropylidene diphosphonate, mithramycin, and corticosteroids / calcitonin in treatment of cancer-associated hypercalcaemia. *Lancet* 1985;ii:907-10

1015 Thiébaud D, et al. Effectiveness of salmon calcitonin administered as suppositories in tumor-induced hypercalcemia. *Am J Med* 1987;82:745-50.[A]

1016 Thiébaud D, Jacquet AF, Burckhardt P. Fast and effective treatment of malignant hypercalcemia. Combination of suppositories of calcitonin and a single infusion of 3-amino 1-hydroxypropylidene-1-bisphosphonate. *Arch Intern Med* 1990;150:2125-8.[A]

1017 Brautbar N, Luboshitzky R. Combined calcitonin and oral phosphate treatment for hypercalcemia in multiple myeloma. *Arch Intern Med* 1977;137:914-6.[A]

1018 *Hypercalcaemia.* In: National Cancer Institute CancerNet PDQ database, 2000. (http://cancernet.nci.nih.gov/pdq/, accessed 9 Dec 2000)

1019 Bilezikian JP. Management of hypercalcaemia. *J Clin Endocrinol Metab* 1993;77:1445-49

1020 Chisholm MA, Mulloy AL, Taylor AT. Acute management of cancer-related hypercalcemia. *Ann Pharmacother* 1996;30:507-13.[A]

1021 Kovacs CS, et al. Hypercalcemia of malignancy in the palliative care patient: a treatment strategy. *J Pain Symptom Manage* 1995;10:224-32.[A]

1022 Brogan G, et al. The importance of low magnesium in palliative care: two case reports. *Palliat Med* 2000;14:59-61

1023 Beckwith MC, Botros LR. Clinical implications of hypomagnesemia. *J Pharm Care Pain Symptom Control* 1998;6:65-77.[A]

1024 Crosby V, et al. The importance of low magnesium in palliative care. *Palliat Med* 2000;14:544

1025 Zylicz Z. Importance of magnesium in palliative medicine. *Prog Palliat Care* 2000;8:69-70

1026 Berghmans T, Paesmans M, Body JJ. A prospective study on hyponatraemia in medical cancer patients: epidemiology, aetiology and differential diagnosis. *Support Care Cancer* 2000;8:192-7.[A]

1027 Woo MH, Smythe MA. Association of SIADH with selective serotonin reuptake inhibitors. *Ann Pharmacother* 1997;31:108-10.[A]

1028 Asklin B, Cassuto J. Intravesical lidocaine in severe interstitial cystitis. Case report. *Scandinavian Journal of Urology and Nephrology* 1989;23:311-2.[A]

1029 Higson RH, Smith JC, Hills W. Intravesical lignocaine and detrusor instability. *Br J Urol* 1979;51:500-3.[A]

1030 Birch BR, Miller RA. Absorption characteristics of lignocaine following intravesical instillation. *Scandinavian Journal of Urology and Nephrology* 1994;28:359-64.[A]

1031   Labrecque M, et al. Efficacy of nonsteroidal anti-inflammatory drugs in the treatment of acute renal colic. A meta-analysis. *Arch Intern Med* 1994;154:1381-87.[A]

1032   Park JM, et al. Ketorolac suppresses postoperative bladder spasms after pediatric ureteral reimplantation. *Anesth Analg* 2000;91:11-5.[A]

1033   McInerney PD, et al. The effect of intravesical Marcain instillation on hyperreflexic detrusor contractions. *Paraplegia* 1992;30:127-30.[A]

1034   Vaidyananthan S, et al. Effect of intermittent urethral catheterization and oxybutynin bladder instillation on urinary continence status and quality of life in a selected group of spinal cord injury patients with neuropathic bladder dysfunction. *Spinal Cord* 1998;36:409-14.[A]

1035   Weese DL, et al. Intravesical oxybutynin chloride: experience with 42 patients. *Urology* 1993;41:527-30

1036   O'Flynn KJ, Thomas DG. Intravesical instillation of oxybutynin hydrochloride for detrusor hyper-reflexia. *Br J Urol* 1993;72:566-70

1037   Fowler CJ, et al. Intravesical capsaicin for treatment of detrusor hyperreflexia. *J Neurol Neurosurg Psychiatry* 1994;57:169-73

1038   Petersen T, Nielsen JB, Schroder HD. Intravesical capsaicin in patients with detrusor hyper-reflexia--a placebo-controlled cross-over study. *Scandinavian Journal of Urology and Nephrology* 1999;33:104-10.[A]

1039   Hilton J. Rest and pain. In: Jacobson WHA, ed. London: George Bell & Sons, 1907:273-75.

1040   Srinivasan V, Brown CH, Turner AG. A comparison of two radiotherapy regimens for the treatment of symptoms from advanced bladder cancer. *Clin Oncol* 1994;6:11-3.[A]

1041   Jenkins CN, McIvor J. Survival after embolization of the internal iliac arteries in ten patients with severe haematuria due to recurrent pelvic carcinoma. *Clin Radiol* 1996;51:865-8.[A]

1042   Anand AK, et al. Selective embolization of internal iliac artery for massive haemorrhage from bladder secondary to carcinoma. *Clinical Oncology (Royal College Of Radiologists)* 1991;3:348-50.[A]

1043   McIvor J, Williams G, Southcott RD. Control of severe vesical haemorrhage by therapeutic embolisation. *Clin Radiol* 1982;33:561-7.[A]

1044   Goswami AK, et al. How safe is 1% alum irrigation in controlling intractable vesical hemorrhage? *J Urol* 1993;149:264-7.[A]

1045   Praveen BV, Sankaranarayanan A, Vaidyanathan S. A comparative study of intravesical instillation of 15(s) 15 Me alpha and alum in the management of persistent hematuria of vesical origin. *Int J Clin Pharmacol Ther Toxicol* 1992;30:7-12.[A]

1046   Bullock N, Whitaker RH. Massive bladder haemorrhage. *Br Med J* 1985;291:1522-23

1047   Phelps KR, et al. Encephalopathy after bladder irrigation with alum: case report and literature review. *Am J Med Sci* 1999;318:181-5.[A]

1048   Shoskes DA, et al. Aluminum toxicity and death following intravesical alum irrigation in a patient with renal impairment. *J Urol* 1992;147:697-9.[A]

1049   Hampson SJ, Woodhouse CR. Sodium pentosanpolysulphate in the management of haemorrhagic cystitis: experience with 14 patients. *European Urology* 1994;25:40-2.[A]

1050   Parsons CL. Successful management of radiation cystitis with sodium pentosanpolysulfate. *J Urol (Baltimore)* 1986;136:813-14

1051   Pomer S, Karcher G, Simon W. Cutaneous ureterostomy as last resort treatment of intractable haemorrhagic cystitis following radiation. *Br J Urol* 1983;55:392-4.[A]

1052   Godec CJ, Gleich P. Intractable hematuria and formalin. *J Urol* 1983;130:688-91.[A]

1053   Dewan AK, Mohan GM, Ravi R. Intravesical formalin for hemorrhagic cystitis following irradiation of cancer of the cervix. *Int J Gynecol Obst* 1993;42:131-5.[A]

1054   Braam PF, Delaere KP, Debruyne FM. Fatal outcome of intravesical formalin instillation, with changes mimicking renal tuberculosis. *Urologia Internationalis* 1986;41:451-4.[A]

1055   Behnam K, Patil UB, Mariano E. Intravesical instillation of Formalin for hemorrhagic cystitis secondary to radiation for gynecologic malignancies. *Gynecol Oncol* 1983;16:31-3.[A]

1056   Ferrie BG, et al. Intravesical formalin in intractable haematuria. *Journal D Urologie* 1985;91:33-5.[A]

1057   Donahue LA, Frank IN. Intravesical formalin for hemorrhagic cystitis: analysis of therapy. *J Urol* 1989;141:809-12.[A]

1058 Giannakopoulos X, et al. Massive haemorrhage of inoperable bladder carcinomas: treatment by intravesical formalin solution. *Int Urol Nephrol* 1997;29:33-8.[A]

1059 Schultz M, van der Lelie H. Microscopic haematuria as a relative contraindication for tranexamic acid. *Br J Haematol* 1995;89:663-4.[A]

1060 Charytan C, Purtilo D. Glomerular capillary thrombosis and acute renal failure after epsilon-amino caproic acid therapy. *N Engl J Med* 1969;280:1102-4

1061 Itterbeek Hv, Vermylen J, Verstraete M. High obstruction of urine flow as a complication of the treatment with fibrinolysis inhibitors of haematuria in haemophiliacs. *Acta Haematologica* 1968;39:237-42

1062 Lindgardh G, Andersson L. Clot retention in the kidneys as a probable cause of anuria during treatment of haematuria with epsilon-aminocaproic acid. *Acta Medica Scandinavica* 1966;180:469-73

1063 Coggins JT, Allen TD. Insoluble fibrin clots within the urinary tract as a consequence of epsilon aminocaproioc acid therapy. *J Urol* 1972;107:647-9

1064 Ostroff EB, Chenault OW. Alum irrigation of the control of massive bladder haemorrhage. *J Urol* 1982;128:929-30

1065 Kennedy C, Snell ME, Witherow RO. Use of alum to control intractable vesical haemorrhage. *Br J Urol* 1984;56:673-75

1066 Arrizabalaga M, et al. Treatment of massive haematuria with aluminous salts. *Br J Urol* 1987;60:223-6.[A]

1067 Liu YK, et al. Treatment of radiation or cyclophosphamide induced hemorrhagic cystitis using conjugated estrogen. *J Urol* 1990;144:41-3.[A]

1068 Matthiesen TB, et al. A dose titration, and an open 6-week efficacy and safety study of desmopressin tablets in the management of nocturnal enuresis. *J Urol* 1994;151:460-3.[A]

1069 Major PP, et al. Oral bisphosphonates: A review of clinical use in patients with bone metastases. *Cancer* 2000;88:6-14.[A]

1070 Roemer-Becuwe C, et al. Safety of subcutaneous clodronate and efficacy in hypercalcemia of malignancy: a novel route of administration (abstract). *J Pain Symptom Manage* 2000;20:S54

1071 Walker P, et al. Subcutaneous clodronate: a study evaluating efficacy in hypercalcemia of malignancy and local toxicity. *Ann Oncol* 1997;8:915-6.[A]

1072 McIntyre E, Bruera E. Symptomatic hypocalcemia after intravenous pamidronate. *J Palliat Care* 1996;12:46-7.[A]

1073 Johnson MJ, Fallon MT. Symptomatic hypocalcemia with oral clodronate. *J Pain Symptom Manage* 1998;15:140-2.[A]

1074 Adami S, Zamberlan N. Adverse effects of bisphosphonates. A comparative review. *Drug Saf* 1996;14:158-70.[A]

1075 Bloomfield D, et al. *Use of bisphosphonates in patients with bone metastases from breast cancer.* In: Cancer Care Ontario Practice Guidelines Initiative, 1998. (http://hiru.mcmaster.ca/ccopgi, accessed 19 Sep 2000)

1076 Hillner BE, et al. American Society of Clinical Oncology guideline on the role of bisphosphonates in breast cancer. American Society of Clinical Oncology Bisphosphonates Expert Panel. *J Clin Oncol* 2000;18:1378-91.[A]

1077 Blamey RW. The British Association of Surgical Oncology Guidelines for surgeons in the management of symptomatic breast disease in the UK (1998 revision). BASO Breast Specialty Group. *Eur J Surg Oncol* 1998;24:464-76

1078 Pereira J, Mancini I, Walker P. The role of bisphosphonates in malignant bone pain: a review. *J Palliat Care* 1998;14:25-36

1079 Walker P. Clinical management. The use of bisphosphonates in palliative care. *Eur J Palliat Care* 2000;7:46-9

1080 Berenson JR. Skeletal metastases/Hypercalcemia. *Classic Papers and Current Comments* 1999;4:387-93

1081 Heatley S. Metastatic bone disease and tumour-induced hypercalcaemia: the role of bisphosphonates. *Int J Palliat Nurs* 2001;7:301-07

1082 Bloomfield DJ. Should bisphosphonates be part of the standard therapy of patients with multiple myeloma or bone metastases from other cancers? An evidence- based review. *J Clin Oncol* 1998;16:1218-25.[A]

1083 Body JJ. et al. Current use of bisphosphonates in oncology. International Bone and Cancer Study Group. *J Clin Oncol* 1998;16:3890-9.[A]

1084 Crandall C. Risedronate: a clinical review. *Arch Intern Med* 2001;161:353-60.[A]

1085 Diel IJ. Antitumour effects of bisphosphonates: first evidence and possible mechanisms. *Drugs* 2000;59:391-9.[A]

1086 Diel IJ, Mundy GR. Bisphosphonates in the adjuvant treatment of cancer: experimental evidence and first clinical results. International Bone and Cancer

Study Group (IBCG). *Br J Cancer* 2000;82:1381-6.[A]

1087 Bona RD, Hickey AD, Wallace DM. Efficacy and safety of oral anticoagulation in patients with cancer. *Thromb Haemost* 1997;78:137-40.[A]

1088 Johnson MJ. An audit of hospice inpatients taking warfarin (abstract). *Palliat Med* 1997;11:72-73

1089 Johnson MJ. Problems of anticoagulation within a palliative care setting: an audit of hospice patients taking warfarin. *Palliat Med* 1997;11:306-12.[A]

1090 Johnson MJ. Bleeding, clotting and cancer. *Clin Oncol* 1997;9:294-301

1091 Krauth D, et al. Safety and efficacy of long-term oral anticoagulation in cancer patients. *Cancer* 1987;59:983-5.[A]

1092 Guidelines on oral anticoagulation: third edition. *Br J Haematol* 1998;101:374-87

1093 Cowling MG. Filters inserted into the vena cava may be useful for some indications (letter). *Br Med J* 1998;316:1830

1094 Johnson MJ. Cancer patients with venous thromboembolism - A palliative care perspective. *CME Bulletin Palliat Med* 2000;2:45-48.[A]

1095 Lee AY, Levine MN. Management of venous thromboembolism in cancer patients. *Oncology* 2000;14:409-17, 21; discussion 22, 25-6.[A]

1096 Johnson M. Venous thromboembolism in advanced malignancy. *Palliat Care Today* 1999;8:6-7

1097 Bates SM, Hirsh J. Treatment of venous thromboembolism. *Thromb Haemost* 1999;82:870-7

1098 Wakefield TW. Treatment options for venous thrombosis. *Journal of Vascular Surgery* 2000;31:613-20

1099 Fennerty A, Campbell IA, Routledge PA. Anticoagulants in venous thromboembolism. *Br Med J* 1988;297:1285-8

1100 Lassauniere JM, et al. Platelet transfusions in advanced hematological malignancies: a position paper. *J Palliat Care* 1996;12:38-41.[A]

1101 Gardner FH, Helmer REd. Aminocaproic acid. Use in control of hemorrhage in patients with amegakaryocytic thrombocytopenia. *JAMA* 1980;243:35-7.[A]

1102 Gallardo RL, Gardner FH. Aminocaproic acid for bleeding in thrombocytopenic patients. *Texas Medicine* 1985;81:30-2

1103 Avvisati G, et al. Tranexamic acid for control of haemorrhage in acute promyelocytic leukaemia. *Lancet* 1989;2:122-4.[A]

1104 Bartholomew JR, Salgia R, Bell WR. Control of bleeding in patients with immune and nonimmune thrombocytopenia with aminocaproic acid. *Arch Intern Med* 1989;149:1959-61.[A]

1105 Ben-Bassat I, Douer D, Ramot B. Tranexamic acid therapy in acute myeloid leukemia: possible reduction of platelet transfusions. *Eur J Haematol* 1990;45:86-9.[A]

1106 Garewal HS, Durie BG. Anti-fibrinolytic therapy with aminocaproic acid for the control of bleeding in thrombocytopenic patients. *Scand J Haematol* 1985;35:497-500.[A]

1107 Shpilberg O, et al. A controlled trial of tranexamic acid therapy for the reduction of bleeding during treatment of acute myeloid leukemia. *Leukemia & Lymphoma* 1995;19:141-4.[A]

1108 Seto AH, Dunlap DS. Tranexamic acid in oncology. *Ann Pharmacother* 1996;30:868-70.[A]

1109 Benson K, et al. The platelet-refractory bone marrow transplant patient: prophylaxis and treatment of bleeding. *Semin Oncol* 1993;20:102-9.[A]

1110 Mezzano D, et al. Tranexamic acid inhibits fibrinolysis, shortens the bleeding time and improves platelet function in patients with chronic renal failure. *Thromb Haemost* 1999;82:1250-4.[A]

1111 Mannucci PM. Hemostatic drugs. *New Engl J Med* 1998;339:245-53

1112 Fain O, Mathieu E, Thomas M. Scurvy in patients with cancer. *Br Med J* 1998;316:1661-2

1113 Sindet-Pedersen S, Stenbjerg S, Ingerslev J. Control of gingival hemorrhage in hemophilic patients by inhibition of fibrinolysis with tranexamic acid. *J Periodontal Res* 1988;23:72-4

1114 Sindet-Pedersen S, et al. Management of oral bleeding in haemophilic patients (letter). *Lancet* 1988;2:566

1115 Borea G, et al. Tranexamic acid as a mouthwash in anticoagulant-treated patients undergoing oral surgery. An alternative method to discontinuing anticoagulant therapy. *Oral Surg Oral Med Oral Pathol* 1993;75:29-31.[A]

1116 Ramstrom G, et al. Prevention of postsurgical bleeding in oral surgery using tranexamic acid without dose modification of oral anticoagulants. *Journal of Oral & Maxillofacial Surgery* 1993;51:1211-6.[A]

1117 Kobrinsky NL, Israels ED, Bickis MG. Synergistic shortening of the bleeding time by desmopressin and ethamsylate in patients with various constitutional bleeding disorders. *Am J Pediatr Hematol Oncol* 1991;13:437-41.^

1118 Jamjian MC, Lipman AG. Bleeding problems in palliative care patients. *J Pharm Care Pain Symptom Control* 1999;7:37-46.^

1119 Marsland T, et al. Control of intraperitoneal haemorrhage with antifibrinolytic therapy in a patient with ovarian carcinoma (letter). *Thromb Haemost* 1981;46:566

1120 De Boer WA, et al. Tranexamic acid treatment of haemothorax in two patients with malignant mesothelioma. *Chest* 1991;100:847-48

1121 Cooke I, Lethaby A, Farquhar C. Antifibrinolytics for heavy menstrual bleeding. *Cochrane Database Syst Rev* 2000:CD000249.^

1122 Bonnar J, Sheppard BL. Treatment of menorrhagia during menstruation: randomised controlled trial of ethamsylate, mefenamic acid, and tranexamic acid. *Br Med J* 1996;313:579-82.^

1123 Hutton RA, et al. Studies on the action of ethamsylate (Dicynene) on haemostasis. *Thromb Haemost* 1986;56:6-8.^

1124 Harrison RF, Cambell S. A double-blind trial of ethamsylate in the treatment of primary and intrauterine-device menorrhagia. *Lancet* 1976;2:283-5.^

1125 Hutton RA, Hales M, Kernoff PB. A study of the effect of ethamsylate (Dicynene) on the bleeding time, von Willebrand factor level and fibrinolysis in patients with von Willebrand's disease. *Thromb Haemost* 1988;60:506-7.^

1126 Symes DM, et al. The effect of dicynene on blood loss during and after transurethral resection of the prostate. *Br J Urol* 1975;47:203-7.^

1127 Arora YR, Manford ML. Operative blood loss and the frequency of haemorrhage associated with adenotonsillectomy in children: a double-blind trial of ethamsylate. *Br J Anaesth* 1979;51:557-61.^

1128 Lyth DR, Booth CM. Does ethamsylate reduce haemorrhage in transurethral prostatectomy? *Br J Urol* 1990;66:631-4.^

1129 Kovacs L, Annus J. Effectiveness of etamsylate in intrauterine-device menorrhagia. *Gynecol Invest* 1978;9:161-5.^

1130 Daneshmend TK, et al. Failure of ethamsylate to reduce aspirin-induced gastric mucosal bleeding in humans. *Br J Clin Pharmacol* 1989;28:109-12.^

1131 Keith I. Ethamsylate and blood loss in total hip replacement. *Anaesthesia* 1979;34:666-70.^

1132 Vinazzer H. Clinical and experimental studies on the action of ethamsylate on haemostasis and on platelet functions. *Thromb Res* 1980;19:783-91

1133 Kasonde JM, Bonnar J. Effect of ethamsylate and aminocaproic acid on menstrual blood loss in women using intrauterine devices. *Br Med J* 1975;4:21-2

1134 Gray AJ, Noble WA. Ethamsylate and blood loss during dissection tonsillectomy. *Br J Anaesth* 1966;38:827-30

1135 Pilbrant A, Schannong M, Vessman J. Pharmacokinetics and bioavailability of tranexamic acid. *Eur J Clin Pharmacol* 1981;20:65-72.^

1136 Dunn CJ, Goa KL. Tranexamic acid: a review of its use in surgery and other indications. *Drugs* 1999;57:1005-32.^

1137 Monti M, et al. Use of red blood cell transfusions in terminally ill cancer patients admitted to a palliative care unit. *J Pain Symptom Manage* 1996;12:18-22.^

1138 Mercadante S, et al. Anaemia in cancer: pathophysiology and treatment. *Cancer Treat Rev* 2000;26:303-11.^

1139 Boyland L, Gleeson C. Clinical management. The management of anaemia. *Eur J Palliat Care* 1999;6:145-8

1140 Ludwig H, et al. Prediction of response to erythropoietin treatment in chronic anemia of cancer. *Blood* 1994;84:1056-63.^

1141 Quirt I, et al. Erythropoietin in the management of patients with nonhematologic cancer receiving chemotherapy. Systemic Treatment Program Committee. *Cancer Prev Control* 1997;1:241-8.^

1142 Khawaja HT, et al. Cost minimisation study of transdermal glyceryl trinitrate in reducing failures of peripheral intravenous infusion. *Br Med J* 1989;299:97

1143 Khawaja HT, Williams JD, Weaver PC. Transdermal glyceryl trinitrate to allow peripheral total parenteral nutrition: a double-blind placebo controlled feasibility study. *J R Soc Med* 1991;84:69-72.^

1144 O'Brien BJ, Buxton MJ, Khawaja HT. An economic evaluation of transdermal glyceryl trinitrate in the prevention of intravenous infusion failure. *J Clin Epidemiol* 1990;43:757-63.^

1145 Khawaja HT, Campbell MJ, Weaver PC. Effect of transdermal glyceryl trinitrate on the survival of peripheral intravenous infusions: a double-blind prospective clinical study. *Br J Surg* 1988;75:1212-5.^

1146 Wright A, Hecker JF, Lewis GB. Use of transdermal glyceryl trinitrate to reduce failure of intravenous infusion due to phlebitis and extravasation. *Lancet* 1985;2:1148-50.[A]

1147 Vrhovac B, et al. Pharmacokinetic changes in patients with oedema (Review). *Clin Pharmacokinet* 1995;28:405-18.[A]

1148 Beermann B, Midskov C. Reduced bioavailability and effect of furosemide given with food. *Eur J Clin Pharmacol* 1986;29:725-7.[A]

1149 Brater DC, et al. Bumetanide and furosemide. *Clin Pharmacol Ther* 1983;34:207-13.[A]

1150 Lawson DH, et al. Continuous infusion of frusemide in refractory oedema. *Br Med J* 1978;2:476

1151 Meyel VAN, et al. Continuous infusion of furosemide in the treatment of patients with congestive heart failure and diuretic resistance. *J Intern Med* 1994;235:329-34.[A]

1152 Lahav M, et al. Intermittent administration of furosemide vs continuous infusion preceded by a loading dose for congestive heart failure. *Chest* 1992;102:725-31.[A]

1153 Meyel VAN, et al. Diuretic efficiency of furosemide during continuous administration versus bolus injection in healthy volunteers. *Clin Pharmacol Ther* 1992;51:440-4.[A]

1154 Mapstone J, Houston B, Gogarty M. Role of spironolactone in heart failure should be emphasised. *Br Med J* 2000;321:706-7

1155 Reiffel JA. Selecting an antiarrhythmic agent for atrial fibrillation should be a patient-specific, data-driven decision. *Am J Cardiol* 1998;82:72N-81N.[A]

1156 Reiffel JA. Drug choices in the treatment of atrial fibrillation. *Am J Cardiol* 2000;85:12D-19D.[A]

1157 Taylor FC, Cohen H, Ebrahim S. Systematic review of long term anticoagulation or antiplatelet treatment in patients with non-rheumatic atrial fibrillation. *Br Med J* 2001;322:321-26.[A]

1158 Nademanee K, Kosar EM. Long-term antithrombotic treatment for atrial fibrillation. *Am J Cardiol* 1998;82:37N-42N.[A]

1159 Prasad AS. Clinical, endocrinological and biochemical effects of zinc deficiency. *Clinics in Endocrinology and Metabolism* 1985;14:567-89.[A]

1160 Prasad AS, et al. Zinc deficiency in elderly patients. *Nutrition* 1993;9:218-24.[A]

1161 Mahajan SK, et al. Zinc deficiency: a reversible complication of uremia. *Am J Clin Nutr* 1982;36:1177-83.[A]

1162 Lindsay AM, Piper BF. Anorexia, serum zinc, and immunologic response in small cell lung cancer patients receiving chemotherapy and prophylactic cranial radiotherapy. *Nutr Cancer* 1986;8:231-38

1163 Mossman KL. Taste acuity, plasma zinc, and weight loss during radiotherapy (letter). *Radiology* 1982;144:856

1164 Silverman JE, et al. Zinc supplementation and taste in head and neck cancer patients undergoing radiation therapy. *J Oral Med* 1983;38:14-6

1165 Pennypacker LC, et al. High prevalence of cobalamin deficiency in elderly outpatients. *Journal of the American Geriatrics Society* 1992;40:1197-204.[A]

1166 Healton EB, et al. Neurologic aspects of cobalamin deficiency. 1991;70:229-45.[A]

1167 Le Cacheux P, Gallet E, Charbonneau P. Prevention of nosocomial urinary tract infections in intensive care units. Evaluation of urinary acidification by ascorbic acid. *Medecine et Maladies Infectieuses* 1994;24:886-93.[A]

1168 Stahelin HB. Critical reappraisal of vitamins and trace minerals in nutritional support of cancer patients. *Support Care Cancer* 1993;1:295-7.[A]

1169 Fainsinger RL, et al. The use of hypodermoclysis for rehydration in terminally ill cancer patients. *J Pain Symptom Manage* 1994;9:298-302.[A]

1170 Dasgupta M, Binns MA, Rochon PA. Subcutaneous fluid infusion in a long-term care setting. *Journal of the American Geriatrics Society* 2000;48:795-9.[A]

1171 Schen R, Arieli S. Administration of potassium by subcutaneous infusion in elderly patients (letter). *Br Med J* 1982;285:1167

1172 Bruera E. Hypodermoclysis for the administration of fluids and narcotic analgesics in patients with advanced cancer. *J Pain Symptom Manage* 1990;5:218-20

1173 Constans T, Dutertre JP, Froge E. Hypodermoclysis in dehydrated elderly patients: local effects with and without hyaluronidase. *J Palliat Care* 1991;7:10-2.[A]

1174 Bruera Ede, et al. Comparison of two different concentrations of hyaluronidase in patients receiving one-hour infusions of hypodermoclysis. *J Pain Symptom Manage* 1995;10:505-9.[A]

1175 Bruera E, et al. Proctoclysis for hydration of terminally ill cancer patients. *J Pain Symptom Manage* 1998;15:216-9.[A]

1176 Ronayne C, Bray G, Robertson G. The use of aqueous cream to relieve pruritus in patients with liver disease. Br J Nurs 1993;2:527-8.^

1177 Thorns A, Edmonds P. Clinical management. The management of pruritus in palliative care patients. Eur J Palliat Care 2000;7:9-12

1178 Walt RP, et al. Effect of stanozolol on itching in primary biliary cirrhosis. Br Med J 1988;296:607

1179 Seymour CA, Summerton CB. Effect of stanozolol on itching in primary biliary cirrhosis (letter). Br Med J 1988;296:1066-7

1180 Price TJ, Patterson WK, Olver IN. Rifampicin as treatment for pruritus in malignant cholestasis. Support Care Cancer 1998;6:533-5.^

1181 Connolly CS, Kantor GR, Menduke H. Hepatobiliary pruritus: what are effective treatments? J Am Acad Dermatol 1995;33:801-5.^

1182 Dimitriou V, Voyagis GS. Opioid-induced pruritus: repeated vs single dose ondansetron administration in preventing pruritus after intrathecal morphine (letter). Br J Anaesth 1999;83:822-3

1183 Yeh HM, et al. Prophylactic intravenous ondansetron reduces the incidence of intrathecal morphine-induced pruritus in patients undergoing cesarean delivery. Anesth Analg 2000;91:172-5.^

1184 Borgeat A, Stirnemann HR. Ondansetron is effective to treat spinal or epidural morphine-induced pruritus. Anesthesiology 1999;90:432-6.^

1185 Larijani GE, Goldberg ME, Rogers KH. Treatment of opioid-induced pruritus with ondansetron: Report of four patients. Pharmacotherapy 1996;16:958-60.^

1186 Charuluxananan S, et al. Ondansetron for treatment of intrathecal morphine-induced pruritus after cesarean delivery. Reg Anesth Pain Med 2000;25:535-9.^

1187 Kyriakides K, Hussain SK, Hobbs GJ. Management of opioid-induced pruritus: A role for 5-HT3 antagonists? Br J Anaesth 1999;82:439-41.^

1188 Balaskas EV, et al. Histamine and serotonin in uremic pruritus: effect of ondansetron in CAPD-pruritic patients. Nephron 1998;78:395-402.^

1189 Jones EA, Bergasa NV. Evolving concepts of the pathogenesis and treatment of the pruritus of cholestasis. Can J Gastroenterol 2000;14:33-39.^

1190 Schworer H, Hartmann H, Ramadori G. Relief of cholestatic pruritus by a novel class of drugs: 5-hydroxytryptamine type 3 (5-HT3) receptor antagonists: effectiveness of ondansetron. Pain 1995;61:33-7.^

1191 Muller C, et al. Treatment of pruritus in chronic liver disease with the 5-hydroxytryptamine receptor type 3 antagonist ondansetron: a randomized, placebo-controlled, double-blind cross-over trial. Eur J Gastroenterol Hepatol 1998;10:865-70.^

1192 Quigley C, Plowman PN. 5HT3 receptor antagonists and pruritus due to cholestasis (letter). Palliat Med 1996;10:54

1193 Zylicz Z, Smits C, Krajnik M. Paroxetine for pruritus in advanced cancer. J Pain Symptom Manage 1998;16:121-4.^

1194 Drake LA, Millikan LE. The antipruritic effect of 5% doxepin cream in patients with eczematous dermatitis. Arch Dermatol 1995;131:1403-8.^

1195 Doxepin cream for eczema? Drug Ther Bull 2000;38:31-32.^

1196 Drake LA, et al. Pharmacokinetics of doxepin in subjects with pruritic atopic dermatitis. J Am Acad Dermatol 1999;41:209-14.^

1197 Nowak MA, et al. Generalized pruritus without primary lesions. Differential diagnosis and approach to treatment. Postgrad Med 2000;107:41-2, 45-6.^

1198 Fransway AF, Winkelmann RK. Treatment of pruritus. Semin Dermatol 1988;7:310-25

1199 Bymaster FP, et al. Radioreceptor binding profile of the atypical antipsychotic olanzapine. Neuropsychopharmacology 1996;14:87-96.^

1200 Blachley JD, et al. Uremic pruritus: skin divalent ion content and response to ultraviolet phototherapy. Am J Kidney Dis 1985;5:237-41.^

1201 Tan JK, Haberman HF, Coldman AJ. Identifying effective treatments for uremic pruritus. J Am Acad Dermatol 1991;25:811-8.^

1202 De Marchi S, et al. Relief of pruritus and decreases in plasma histamine concentrations during erythropoietin therapy in patients with uremia. N Engl J Med 1992;326:969-74.^

1203 Watson WC. Intravenous lignocaine for relief of intractable itch. Lancet 1973;1:211

1204 McCormick PA, et al. Thalidomide as therapy for primary biliary cirrhosis: a double-blind placebo controlled pilot study. J Hepatol 1994;21:496-9.^

1205 Silva SR, et al. Thalidomide for the treatment of uremic pruritus: a crossover randomized double-blind trial. Nephron 1994;67:270-3.^

1206 Wang JJ, Ho ST, Tzeng JI. Comparison of intravenous nalbuphine infusion versus naloxone in the prevention of epidural morphine-related side effects. Reg Anesth

Pain Med 1998;23:479-84.[A]

1207 Saiah M, et al. Epidural-morphine-induced pruritus: propofol versus naloxone. Anesth Analg 1994;78:1110-3.[A]

1208 Wolfhagen FH, et al. Oral naltrexone treatment for cholestatic pruritus: a double-blind, placebo-controlled study. Gastroenterology 1997;113:1264-9.[A]

1209 Peer G, et al. Randomised crossover trial of naltrexone in uraemic pruritus. Lancet 1996;348:1552-4.[A]

1210 Borgeat A, et al. Subhypnotic doses of propofol relieve pruritus induced by epidural and intrathecal morphine. Anesthesiology 1992;76:510-2.[A]

1211 Borgeat A, Wilder_Smith OH, Mentha G. Subhypnotic doses of propofol relieve pruritus associated with liver disease. Gastroenterology 1993;104:244-7.[A]

1212 Horta ML, Horta BL. Inhibition of epidural morphine-induced pruritus by intravenous droperidol. Regional Anesthesia 1993;18:118-20.[A]

1213 Pruritus. In: National Cancer Institute CancerNet PDQ database, 2000. (http://cancernet.nci.nih.gov/pdq/, accessed 9 Dec 2000)

1214 Krajnik M, Zylicz Z. Understanding puritus in systemic disease. J Pain Symptom Manage 2001;21:151-68.[A]

1215 Robertson KE, Mueller BA. Uremic pruritus. Am J Health Syst Pharm 1996;53:2159-70; quiz 215-6 15;53(20):523.[A]

1216 Smith EB, King CA, Baker MD. Crotamiton lotion in pruritus. Int J Dermatol 1984;23:684-5.[A]

1217 Moyle J. Clinical management. The management of malodour. Eur J Palliat Care 1998;5:148-51

1218 Goode HF, Burns E, Walker BE. Vitamin C depletion and pressure sores in elderly patients with femoral neck fracture. Br Med J 1992;305:925-27

1219 Taylor TV, et al. Ascorbic acid supplementation in the treatment of pressure-sores. Lancet 1974;2:544-6.[A]

1220 Wilkinson EA, Hawke CI. Oral zinc for arterial and venous leg ulcers. 2000:CD001273.[A]

1221 Wilkinson EA, Hawke CI. Does oral zinc aid the healing of chronic leg ulcers? A systematic literature review. Arch Dermatol 1998;134:1556-60.[A]

1222 Hallböök T, Lanner E. Serum-zinc and healing of venous leg ulcers. Lancet 1972;2:780-2

1223 Finlay IG, et al. The effect of topical 0.75% metronidazole gel on malodorous cutaneous ulcers. J Pain Symptom Manage 1996;11:158-62.[A]

1224 Hampson JP. The use of metronidazole in the treatment of malodorous wounds. J Wound Care 1996;5:421-5

1225 Newman V, Allwood M, Oakes RA. The use of metronidazole gel to control the smell of malodorous lesions. Palliat Med 1989;3:303-05

1226 Metronidazole gel for smelly tumours. Drug Ther Bull 1992;30:18-19

1227 Jepson BA. Relieving the pain of pressure sores (letter). Lancet 1992;503

1228 Farncombe M. Management of bleeding in a patient with colorectal cancer: a case study. Support Care Cancer 1993;1:159-60.[A]

1229 Grocott P. Clinical management. The management of malignant wounds. Eur J Palliat Care 2000;7:126-9

1230 Tamoxifen in breast cancer. Drug Ther Bull 1986;24:65-67

1231 Hanley H, Rodgers J. An outline of lymphoedema management. CME Bulletin Palliat Med 2000;2:21-26

1232 Arm oedema following breast cancer treatment. Drug Ther Bull 2000;38:41-3.[A]

1233 Ling J, et al. Lymphorrhoea in palliative care. Eur J Palliat Care 1997;4:50-2.[A]

1234 Casley-Smith JR, Morgan RG, Piller NB. Treatment of lymphedema of the arms and legs with 5,6-benzo-alpha-pyrone. N Engl J Med 1993;329:1158-63

1235 Loprinzi CL, et al. Lack of effect of coumarin in women with lymphedema after treatment for breast cancer. N Engl J Med 1999;340:346-50.[A]

1236 Klastersky J, et al. Fever of unexplained origin in patients with cancer. Eur J Cancer 1973;9:649-56

1237 Gobbi PG, et al. Night sweats in Hodgkin's disease. A manifestation of preceding minor febrile pulses. Cancer 1990;65:2074-7.[A]

1238 Loprinzi CL, et al. Megestrol Acetate for the prevention of hot flashes. N Engl J Med 1994;331:347-52

1239 Loprinzi CL, et al. Venlafaxine in management of hot flashes in survivors of breast cancer: a randomised controlled trial. Lancet 2000;356:2059-63.[A]

1240 Barlow DH. Venlafaxine for hot flushes. Lancet 2000;356:2025-6

1241 Stearns V, et al. A pilot trial assessing the efficacy of paroxetine hydrochloride (Paxil) in controlling hot flashes in breast cancer survivors. Ann Oncol 2000;11:17-22.[A]

1242 Roth AJ, Scher HI. Sertraline relieves hot flashes secondary to medical castration as treatment of advanced prostate cancer. *Psycho-oncology* 1998;7:129-32

1243 Chang JC, Gross HM. Neoplastic fever responds to the treatment of an adequate dose of naproxen. *J Clin Oncol* 1985;3:552-58.^

1244 Tsavaris N, et al. A randomised trial of the effect of three non-steroid anti-inflammatory agents in ameliorating cancer-induced fever. *J Int Med* 1990;228:451-55.^

1245 Economos K, et al. The effect of naproxen on fever in patients with advanced gynecologic malignancies. *Gynecol Oncol* 1995;56:250-4.^

1246 Klaber M, Catterall M. Treating hyperhidrosis. Anticholinergic drugs were not mentioned. *Br Med J* 2000;321:703

1247 Mercadante S. Hyoscine in opioid-induced sweating (letter). *J Pain Symptom Manage* 1998;15:214-5

1248 Canaday BR, Stanford RH. Propantheline bromide in the management of hyperhidrosis associated with spinal cord injury. *Ann Pharmacother* 1995;29:489-92.^

1249 Pandya KJ, et al. Oral clonidine in postmenopausal patients with breast cancer experiencing tamoxifen-induced hot flashes: a University of Rochester Cancer Center Community Clinical Oncology Program study. *Ann Intern Med* 2000;132:788-93.^

1250 Bressler LR, et al. Use of clonidine to treat hot flashes secondary to leuprolide or goserelin. *Ann Pharmacother* 1993;27:182-5.^

1251 Smith JA, Jr. Management of hot flushes due to endocrine therapy for prostate carcinoma. *Oncology (Hunting)* 1996;10:1319-22; discussion 24.^

1252 Eaton AC, McGuire N. Cyproterone acetate in treatment of post-orchidectomy hot flushes. Double-blind cross-over trial. *Lancet* 1983;2:1336-7.^

1253 Miller JI, Ahmann FR. Treatment of castration-induced menopausal symptoms with low dose diethylstilbestrol in men with advanced prostate cancer. *Urology* 1992;40:499-502.^

1254 Towlerton G, et al. Acupuncture in the control of vasomotor symptoms caused by tamoxifen (letter). *Palliat Med* 1999;13:445

1255 Calder K, Bruera E. Thalidomide for night sweats in patients with advanced cancer (letter). *Palliat Med* 2000;14:77-8

1256 Deaner P. Thalidomide for distressing night sweats in advanced malignant disease (letter). *Palliat Med* 1998;12:208-9

1257 Deaner PB. The use of thalidomide in the management of severe sweating in patients with advanced malignancy: Trial report. *Palliat Med* 2000;14:429-31

1258 Watkinson D. Hot flushes. *CME Bulletin Palliat Med* 1999;1:95-97

1259 Hami F, Trotman I. Clinical management. The treatment of sweating. *Eur J Palliat Care* 1999;6:184-7

1260 Cowap J, Hardy J. Thioridazine in the management of cancer-related sweating (letter). *J Pain Symptom Manage* 1998;15:266

1261 Regnard C. Use of low dose thioridazine to control sweating in advanced cancer (Research abstract). *Palliat Med* 1996;10:78-79

1262 Rudolph RL, Derivan AT. The safety and tolerability of venlafaxine hydrochloride: analysis of the clinical trials database. *J Clin Psychopharmacol* 1996;16:54S-59S; discussion 59S-61S.^

1263 Garber A, Gregory RJ. Benztropine in the treatment of venlafaxine-induced sweating (letter). *J Clin Psychiatry* 1997;58:176-7

1264 Pierre JM, Guze BH. Benztropine for venlafaxine-induced night sweats (letter). *J Clin Psychopharmacol* 2000;20:269

1265 Schwartz TL. Diaphoresis and pruritus with extended-release venlafaxine (letter). *Ann Pharmacother* 1999;33:1009

1266 Shaw JE, et al. A randomised controlled trial of topical glycopyrrolate, the first specific treatment for diabetic gustatory sweating. *Diabetologia* 1997;40:299-301

1267 Seukeran DC, Highet AS. The use of topical glycopyrrolate in the treatment of hyperhidrosis. *Clinical And Experimental Dermatology* 1998;23:204-5.^

1268 Urman JD, Bobrove AM. Diabetic gustatory sweating successfully treated with topical glycopyrrolate: report of a case and review of the literature. *Arch Intern Med* 1999;159:877-8.^

1269 Elrington G. The Lambert-Eaton myasthenic syndrome. *Palliat Med* 1992;6:9-17.^

1270 Stone P, Richards M, Hardy J. Fatigue in patients with cancer. *Eur J Cancer* 1998;34:1670-6.^

1271 Richardson A. Fatigue in cancer patients: a review of the literature. *Eur J Cancer Care* 1995;4:20-32.^

1272 Tyler LS, Lipman AG. Fatigue in palliative care patients. *J Pharm Care Pain*

Symptom Control 2000;8:129-41.[A]

1273 Krupp LB, et al. Fatigue therapy in multiple sclerosis: results of a double-blind, randomized, parallel trial of amantadine, pemoline, and placebo. *Neurology* 1995;45:1956-61.[A]

1274 A randomized controlled trial of amantadine in fatigue associated with multiple sclerosis. The Canadian MS Research group. *Can J Neurol Sci* 1987;14:273-8.[A]

1275 Cohen RA, Fisher M. Amantadine treatment of fatigue associated with multiple sclerosis. *Archives Of Neurology* 1989;46:676-80.[A]

1276 Stein DP, Dambrosia JM, Dalakas MC. A double-blind, placebo-controlled trial of amantadine for the treatment of fatigue in patients with the post-polio syndrome. *Ann N Y Acad Sci* 1995;753:296-302.[A]

1277 Davies AN, Mitchell M. Methotrimeprazine and UV light (letter). *Palliat Med* 1996;10:264

1278 Sykes NP, Oliver DJ. Isotonic methotrimeprazine by continuous infusion in terminal cancer care (letter). *Lancet* 1987;1:393-4

1279 Regnard C, Pashley S, Westrope F. Anti-emetic/diamorphine mixture compatibility in infusion pumps. *Br J Pharm Prac* 1986;August:218-20

1280 Allwood MC. Diamorphine mixed with anti-emetic drugs in plastic syringes. *Br J Pharm Pract* 1984;6:88-90

1281 Allwood MC. The stability of diamorphine alone and in combination with anti-emetics in plastic syringes. *Palliat Med* 1991;5:330-33

1282 Grassby PF, Hutchings L. Drug combinations in syringe drivers: the compatibility and stability of diamorphine with cyclizine and haloperidol. *Palliat Med* 1997;11:217-24.[A]

1283 Allwood MC, Brown PW, Lee M. Stability of injections containing diamorphine and midazolam in plastic syringes. *Int J Pharm Pract* 1994;3:57-59

1284 Back IN. Database of drug compatibility for syringe drivers: www.pallmed.net, 2001.

1285 McNamara P, Minton M, Twycross RG. Use of midazolam in palliative care. *Palliat Med* 1991;5:244-49

1286 Johnson I, Patterson S. Drugs used in combination in the syringe driver - a survey of hospice practice. *Palliat Med* 1992;6:125-30.[A]

1287 Oliver DJ. The use of the syringe driver in terminal care. *Br J Clin Pharmacol* 1985;20:515-16

1288 Fielding H, et al. The compatibility and stability of octreotide acetate in the presence of diamorphine hydrochloride in polypropylene syringes. *Palliat Med* 2000;14:205-07.[A]

1289 Mendenhall A, Hoyt DB. Incompatibility of ketorolac tromethamine with haloperidol lactate and thiethylperazine maleate. *Am J Hosp Pharm* 1994;51:2964

1290 Dover SB. Syringe driver in terminal care. *Br Med J* 1987;294:553-55

1291 Bradley K. Swap data on drug compatibilities. *Pharm Pract* 1996;6:69-72

1292 Nicholson H. The success of the syringe driver. *Nurs Times* 1986;82:49-51

1293 Dawkins L, et al. A randomized trial of winged Vialon cannulae and metal butterfly needles. *Int J Palliat Nurs* 2000;6:110-16

1294 Youssef MS, Atkinson RE. Comparison of Teflon cannulas and metal needles for subcutaneous infusion in terminal care: a pilot study. *Br Med J* 1990;300:847

1295 Shvartzman P, Bonneh D. Local skin irritation in the course of subcutaneous morphine infusion: a challenge. *J Palliat Care* 1994;10:44-5.[A]

1296 Hussey HJ, Tisdale MJ. Effect of a cachectic factor on carbohydrate metabolism and attenuation by eicosapentaenoic acid. *Br J Cancer* 1999;80:1231-5.[A]

1297 Burns CP, et al. Phase I clinical study of fish oil fatty acid capsules for patients with cancer cachexia: cancer and leukemia group B study 9473. *Clin Cancer Res* 1999;5:3942-7.[A]

1298 Ernst E, Cassileth BR. How useful are unconventional cancer treatments? *Eur J Cancer* 1999;35:1608-13.[A]

1299 Kaegi E. Unconventional therapies for cancer: 1. Essiac. *Can Med Assoc J* 1998;158:897-902

1300 Kaegi E. Unconventional therapies for cancer: 2. Green tea. *Can Med Assoc J* 1998;158:1033-35

1301 Kaegi E. Unconventional therapies for cancer: 3. Iscador. *Can Med Assoc J* 1998;158:1157-59

1302 Kaegi E. Unconventional therapies for cancer: 5. Vitamins A, C and E. *Can Med Assoc J* 1998;158:1483-88

1303 Miller DR, et al. Phase I/II trial of the safety and efficacy of shark cartilage in the treatment of advanced cancer. *J Clin Oncol* 1998;16:3649-55.[A]

1304 Chlebowski RT, et al. Hydrazine sulfate in cancer patients with weight loss. A placebo-controlled clinical experience. *Cancer* 1987;59:406-10.[A]

1305 Chlebowski RT, et al. Hydrazine sulfate influence on nutritional status and survival in non-small-cell lung cancer. *J Clin Oncol* 1990;8:9-15.[A]

1306 Filov VA, et al. Experience of the treatment with Sehydrin (Hydrazine Sulfate, HS) in the advanced cancer patients. *Investigational New Drugs* 1995;13:89-97.[A]

1307 Gold J. Hydrazine sulfate: a current perspective. *Nutrition & Cancer* 1987;9:59-66.[A]

1308 Kosty MP, et al. Cisplatin, vinblastine, and hydrazine sulfate in advanced, non-small-cell lung cancer: a randomized placebo-controlled, double-blind phase III study of the Cancer and Leukemia Group B. *J Clin Oncol* 1994;12:1113-20.[A]

1309 Loprinzi CL, et al. Randomized placebo-controlled evaluation of hydrazine sulfate in patients with advanced colorectal cancer. *J Clin Oncol* 1994;12:1121-5.[A]

1310 Tayek JA, Heber D, Chlebowski RT. Effect of hydrazine sulphate on whole-body protein breakdown measured by 14C-lysine metabolism in lung cancer patients. *Lancet* 1987;2:241-4.[A]

1311 Kaegi E. Unconventional therapies for cancer: 4. Hydrazine sulfate. *Can Med Assoc J* 1998;158:1327-30

1312 Findlay GFG. Adverse effects of the management of malignant spinal cord compression. *J Neurol Neurosurg Psychiatr* 1984;47:761-68

1313 Kim RY, et al. Extradural spinal cord compression: analysis of factors determining functional prognosis - prospective study. *Radiology* 1990;176:279-82.[A]

1314 Cowap J, Hardy JR, A'Hern R. Outcome of malignant spinal cord compression at a cancer center: implications for palliative care services. *J Pain Symptom Manage* 2000;19:257-64.[A]

1315 Kramer JA. Spinal cord compression in malignancy (review). *Palliat Med* 1992;6:202-11.[A]

1316 Hillier R, Wee B. Clinical management. Palliative management of spinal cord compression. *Eur J Palliat Care* 1997;4:189-92

1317 Abrahm JL. Management of pain and spinal cord compression in patients with advanced cancer. ACP-ASIM End-of-life Care Consensus Panel. American College of Physicians-American Society of Internal Medicine. *Ann Intern Med* 1999;131:37-46.[A]

1318 Bach F, et al. Metastatic spinal cord compression. Occurrence, symptoms, clinical presentations and prognosis in 398 patients with spinal cord compression. *Acta Neurochir (Wien)* 1990;107:37-43.[A]

1319 Loblaw DA, Laperriere NJ. Emergency treatment of malignant extradural spinal cord compression: an evidence-based guideline. *J Clin Oncol* 1998;16:1613-24.[A]

1320 Vecht CJ, et al. Initial bolus of conventional versus high-dose dexamethasone in metastatic spinal cord compression. *Neurology* 1989;39:1255-7.[A]

1321 Heimdal K, et al. High incidence of serious side effects of high-dose dexamethasone treatment in patients with epidural spinal cord compression. *J Neurooncol* 1992;12:141-4.[A]

1322 Ethical decision-making. CPR for people who are terminally ill. *Eur J Palliat Care* 1997;4:125

1323 Willard C. Cardiopulmonary resuscitation for palliative care patients: a discussion of ethical issues. *Palliat Med* 2000;14:308-12.[A]

1324 Ethical decision-making in palliative care. *Cardiopulmonary resuscitation (CPR) for people who are terminally ill:* National Council for Hospice and Specialist Palliative Care, 1997.

1325 Decisions relating to cardiopulmonary resuscitation. A joint statement from the British Medical Association, the Resuscitation Council (UK) and the Royal College of Nursing, 2001. (http://www.resus.org.uk, accessed Mar 2001)

1326 Dunphy K. Advance directives. *Palliat Care Today* 1998;7:24-25

1327 Stern K. Living wills in English law. *Palliat Med* 1993;7:283-8.[A]

1328 Voltz R, et al. End-of-life decisions and advance directives in palliative care: a cross-cultural survey of patients and health-care professionals. *J Pain Symptom Manage* 1998;16:153-62.[A]

1329 British Medical Association. *Advance Statements about Medical Treatment - Code of Practice*, 1995. (http://web.bma.org.uk, accessed Mar 2001)

1330 Referral criteria to Cancer Genetics Service. Cardiff: Medical Genetics Department, University of Wales Hospital, 2000.

1331 Atkinson RE. Medicolegal aspects of pain management. *Pain Reviews* 2000;7:25-36

1332 Makin M. Wish you were here? Advice for foreign travel. *Palliat Care Today* 1999;7:39-40

1333 Myers K. Travel. Flying home: helping patients to arrange international air travel.

Eur J Palliat Care 1999;6:158-61

1334 Bruera E, et al. The cognitive effects of the administration of narcotic analgesics in patients with cancer pain. *Pain* 1989;39:13-16

1335 Hanks GW, et al. The cognitive and psychomotor effects of opioid analgesics. II. A randomized controlled trial of single doses of morphine, lorazepam and placebo in healthy subjects. *Eur J Clin Pharmacol* 1995;48:455-60

1336 Chesher GB. The influence of analgesic drugs in road crashes. *Accid Anal Prev* 1985;17:303-9.[A]

1337 Vainio A, et al. Driving ability in cancer patients receiving long-term morphine analgesia. *Lancet* 1995;346:667-70.[A]

1338 Galski T, Williams JB, Ehle HT. Effects of opioids on driving ability. *J Pain Symptom Manage* 2000;19:200-8.[A]

1339 *At a glance guide to the current medical standards of fitness to drive.* Swansea: DVLA, 2001.

1340 Brydak LB, et al. Humoral immune response after vaccination against influenza in patients with breast cancer. *Support Care Cancer* 2001;9:65-68.[A]

1341 Major advances in the treatment of HIV-1 infection. *Drug Ther Bull* 1997;35:25-9.[A]

1342 Feder G, et al. Guidelines for the prevention of falls in people over 65. The Guidelines' Development Group. *Br Med J* 2000;321:1007-11

1343 Scott N, ed. *Procedures in practice.* 3rd ed. London: BMJ Publishing Group, 1994.

1344 Planas R, et al. Dextran-70 versus albumin as plasma expanders in cirrhotic patients with tense ascites treated with total paracentesis. *Gastroenterology* 1990;99:1736-44

1345 Blackwell N, Burrows M. A sticky tip (letter). *Palliat Med* 1994;8:256-7.[A]

1346 Grodzin CJ, Balk RA. Indwelling small pleural catheter needle thoracentesis in the management of large pleural effusions. *Chest* 1997;111:981-8.[A]

1347 Hussain SA, Burton GM, Yuce M. Symptomatic loculated malignant pleural effusion treatment with indwelling Tenckhoff catheter (letter). *Chest* 1990;97:766-7

1348 Twycross R. *Pain relief in advanced cancer.* Edinburgh: Churchill Livingstone, 1994.

1349 Anderson R, et al. Accuracy at equianalgesic dosing: conversion dilemmas. *J Pain Symptom Manage* 2001;21:397-406

1350 Gordon DB, et al. Opioid equianalgesic calculations. *J Palliat Med* 1999;2:209-18.[A]

1351 Cherny NI. Opioid analgesics: comparative features and prescribing guidelines. *Drugs* 1996;51:713-37.[A]

1352 Bernard SA, Bruera E. Drug interactions in palliative care. *J Clin Oncol* 2000;18:1780-99.[A]

1353 Harder S, Thurmann P. Clinically important drug interactions with anticoagulants. An update. *Clin Pharmacokinet* 1996;30:416-44.[A]

1354 Jackson T, Ditmanson L, Phibbs B. Torsade de pointes and low-dose oral haloperidol. *Arch Intern Med* 1997;157:2013-5.[A]

1355 Browne B, Linter S. Monoamine oxidase inhibitors and narcotic analgesics. A critical review of the implications for treatment. *Br J Psychiatry* 1987;151:210-2.[A]

1356 Yap YG, Camm J. Risk of torsades de pointes with non-cardiac drugs. Doctors need to be aware that many drugs can cause qt prolongation. *Br Med J* 2000;320:1158-9

1357 Brady M. Treatment of common symptoms in paediatric palliative care. *CME Bulletin Palliat Med* 1999;1:63-68

1358 Royal College of Paediatrics and Child Health. *Medicines in children.* London: RCPCH, 1999.

1359 IASP Task Force on Taxonomy. *Classification of chronic pain.* In: IASP, 1999. (http://www.halcyon.com/iasp/terms-p.html, accessed 20 Jan 2001)

1360 Emanuel EJ, Emanuel LL. The promise of a good death. *Lancet* 1998;351(SII):21-29

1361 American Psychiatric Association. *DSM-IV,* 1994.

1362 Endicott J. Measurement of depression in patients with cancer. *Cancer* 1984;53:2243-9.[A]

1363 Folstein MF, Folstein SE, McHugh PR. 'Mini-Mental State': a practical method for grading the cognitive state of patients for the clinician. *J Psychiatr Res* 1975;12:189-98

1364 Folstein MF, et al. Cognitive assessment of cancer patients. *Cancer* 1984;53(S):2250

1365 Lindop E, Read S. District nurses' needs: palliative care for people with learning disabilities. *Int J Palliat Nurs* 2000;6:117-22

366 Tuffrey-Wijne I. Social care. Bereavement in people with learning disabilities. *Eur*

J Palliat Care 1997;4:170-3

1367 Keenan P, McIntosh P. Learning disabilities and palliative care. *Palliat Care Today* 2000;9:11-13

1368 *Positive partnerships: palliative care for adults with severe mental health problems*: National Council for Hospice and Specialist Palliative Care, 2000.

INDEX